CULPEPER'S COMPLETE HERBAL

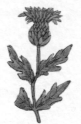

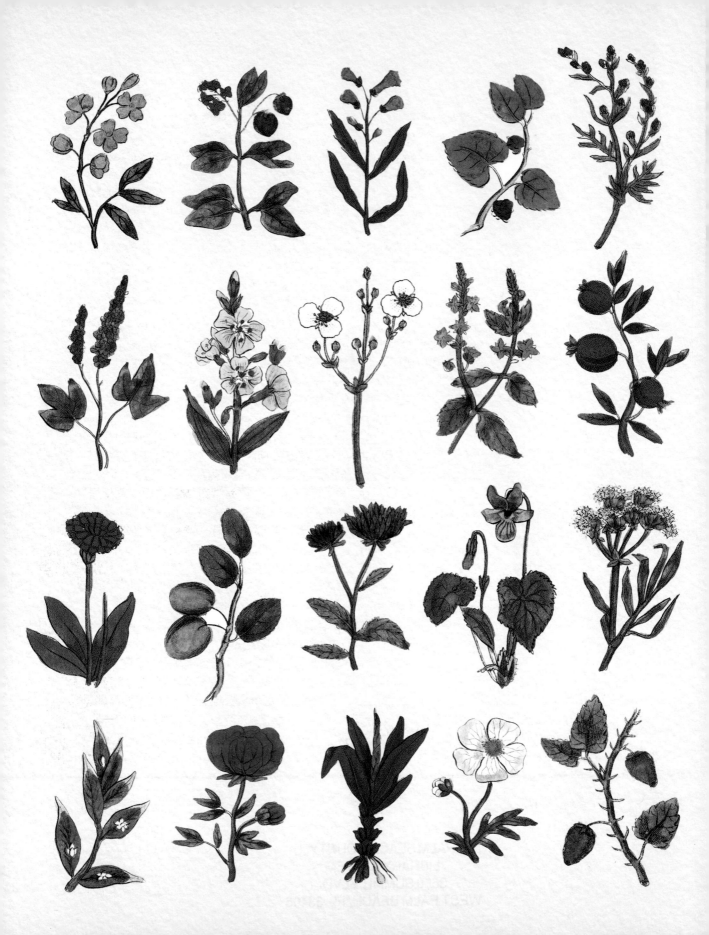

CULPEPER's
COMPLETE HERBAL

ILLUSTRATED & ANNOTATED EDITION

Nicholas Culpeper

EDITED BY STEVEN FOSTER

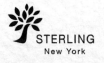

STERLING
New York

STERLING
New York

An Imprint of Sterling Publishing, Co., Inc.
1166 Avenue of the Americas
New York, NY 10016

ISBN 978-1-4549-3287-1

Distributed in Canada by Sterling Publishing Co., Inc.
c/o Canadian Manda Group, 664 Annette Street
Toronto, Ontario M6S 2C8, Canada
Distributed in the United Kingdom by GMC Distribution Services
Castle Place, 166 High Street, Lewes, East Sussex BN7 1XU, England
Distributed in Australia by NewSouth Books
University of New South Wales, Sydney, NSW 2052, Australia

For information about custom editions, special sales, and premium and corporate purchases, please
contact Sterling Special Sales at 800-805-5489 or specialsales@sterlingpublishing.com.

Manufactured in China

2 4 6 8 10 9 7 5 3 1

sterlingpublishing.com

Cover and interior design by Lorie Pagnozzi
Author photograph by Melanie Myhre Photography
Picture credits—see page 276

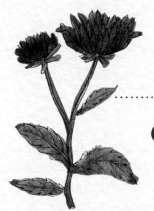

CONTENTS

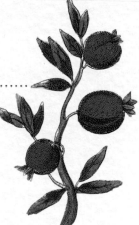

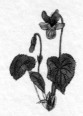

EDITOR'S NOTE
CONTEMPLATING CULPEPER

In 1518, the Royal College of Physicians in London was chartered by the edict of Henry VIII. Nearly a century later, at the beginning of the Reign of James I in 1617, the English monarch extended control of the medical profession(s) to the Royal College by forming the Worshipful Society of Apothecaries, who were given the exclusive right to compound drugs. A year later, the Royal College jointly published the first *Pharmacopoeia Londinensis* [now th British Pharmacopoeia, the official compendium of drugs that apothecaries used to dispense drugs on behalf of physicians. Published in Latin, its content was only available to the academic elite.

Two years earlier, on October 18, 1616, Nicholas Culpeper was born. Eventually Culpeper entered Cambridge; he left without completing his studies, but became adept in Latin. Later apprenticed to an apothecary, he abandoned that indenture and instead joined the rebellious cause of Oliver Cromwell and his Parliamentarians against the Cavaliers of King Charles I.

The life of Nicholas Culpeper and his works reflect the social, political, and religious upheaval of mid-seventeenth century England. He sparked a revolution in access to medical information for the common person amid the revolt known as the English Civil War (1642–51). In 1649, King Charles I was tried and executed. His son Charles II was exiled, and the victorious Parliamentarians led by Oliver Cromwell established the Commonwealth of England. The major publications for which Nicholas Culpeper is best remembered were published during the social turbulence between 1649–53, concurrent with the end of the first English Civil War, and the 1653 ascension of Oliver Cromwell as Lord Protector of the Commonwealth of England, Scotland, and Ireland. Nicholas Culpeper received a chest wound in battle in service to Cromwell's rebels, which probably contributed to his untimely death in his thirty-ninth year, on January 10, 1654, when he was consumed by pulmonary tuberculosis.

In 1649, Culpeper crossed a line that would change medical history. He translated the Latin *Pharmacopoeia Londinensis* into English, published as *A Physical Directory or a Translation of the London Dispensatory*. Proclaiming "THE LIBERTY OF THE SUBJECT" [in capital letters], Culpeper snarled, "The Liberty of our *Common-Wealth* . . . is most infringed by three sorts of men, *Priests, Physitians* [Physicians], *Lawyers*." The monopoly on medical authority by credentialed physicians had been stripped bare by Nicholas Culpeper, gent, astrologer, herbalist, author, and translator. But his most famous work would come three years later.

In 1652, Culpeper authored *The English Phystian or an Astrologo-physical Discourse of the Vulgar Herbs of this Nation*—famously known as "Culpeper's Herbal." The following year, a second expanded edition appeared. For more than 366 years, various editions of "Culpeper's Herbal" have been in print making it the best-selling herbal of all time.

Why is this archaic mix of astrology and domestic medicine the best-selling herbal of all time? Part of the answer lies in the price. Culpeper managed to condense the information on English herbs from the 1,755-page *Theatrum Botanicum* of John Parkinson down to a pocket-sized book of 324 pages and three pence, which was 150 times cheaper than Parkinson's massive herbal. As the title page of the 1652 edition proclaimed, the book intend to be "A compleat method of Physick whereby a man may preserve his Body in health; or cure himself, being sick, for three pence charge, with such things only as grow in England, they being most fit for English bodies."

Besides the affordable price, in part made possible because it contained no costly illustrations, another factor that contributed to the book's long success was the intended audience—the literate gentlewoman. Culpeper brought herbal medicine to the common people in the form of an affordable book intended for those who gathered herbs, kept household medicinal information, and dispensed herbs when needed—the female head of household. By the end of the 1600s, over twenty editions of *The English Physician* had been published. The first medical book published in North America was the 1708 Boston edition of Culpeper's work. Dozens of editions of his *English Physician* were published throughout the eighteenth, nineteenth, and twentieth centuries, and continue to be published into the twenty-first century.

The present volume is an annotated, edited edition with a lineage originating from the 1653 second edition at its foundation, then reprinted with additions and edits from an 1850 edition published by Thomas Kelly of London as *The Complete Herbal . . . or English Physician Enlarged*. That book included twenty colored plates with stylized botanical license, borrowed from other editions as early as 1814, some of which are reproduced here along with supplemental illustrations.

In this edition, we have added modern scientific names, since the 1653 *English Physician* predates by a century the 1753 work of Carl Linnaeus, *Species Plantarum*, the starting point of modern scientific names. Common names reflect current use. Culpeper, himself, used folk names in common use in Surrey County, England. We have heavily edited his descriptions and place of occurrence to reflect modern plant distribution and concepts. To capture the flavor and charm of the original, Culpeper's entries on "government and virtues" remain largely intact. Each of the plant entries includes a brief section on "modern uses" with "cautions" as appropriate.

Culpeper's *English Physician*, published at a time of populist uprising, led to the concept of "teaching every man and woman to be their own doctor"—an idea of lasting appeal that itself has contributed to and accentuated a five-hundred-year-long schism between herbalism and medicine that still exists today. This is Culpeper's overarching legacy.

—STEVEN FOSTER

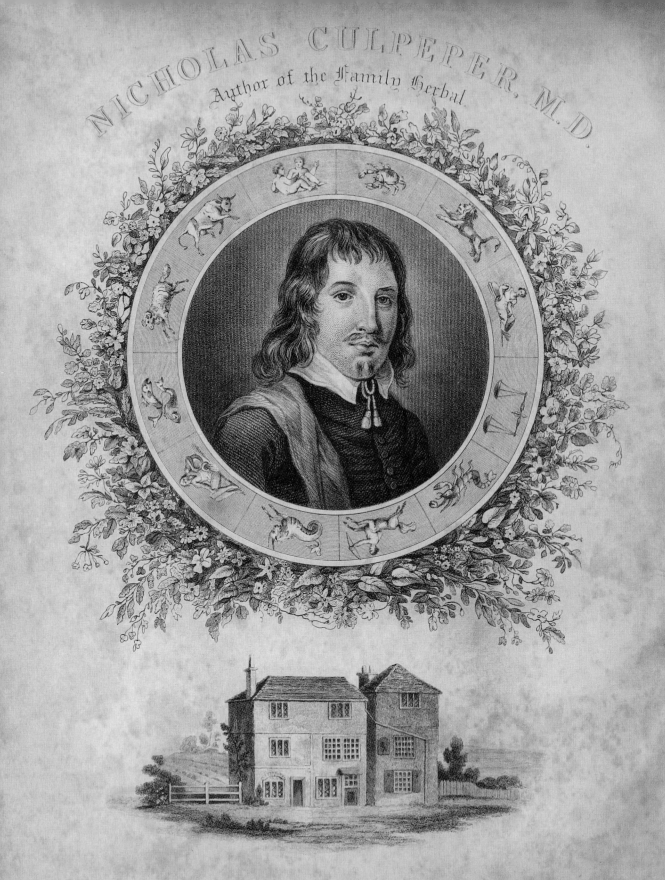

NICHOLAS CULPEPER, M.D.

Author of the Family Herbal.

RED LION HOUSE, SPITALFIELDS,
IN WHICH CULPEPER LIVED, STUDIED AND DIED.

CULPEPER's ORIGINAL
EPISTLE TO THE READER

All other Authors that have written of the nature of Herbs, give not a bit of reason why such an Herb was appropriated to such a part of the body, nor why it cured such a disease. Truly my own body being sickly, brought me easily into a capacity, to know that health was the greatest of all earthly blessings, and truly he was never sick that doth not believe it. Then I considered that all medicines were compounded of Herbs, Roots, Flowers, Seeds, &c., and this first set me to work in studying the nature of simples, most of which I knew by sight before; and indeed all the Authors I could read gave me but little satisfaction in this particular, or none at all. I cannot build my faith upon Authors' words, nor believe a thing because they say it, and could wish everybody were of my mind in this,—to labour to be able to give a reason for everything they say or do. They say Reason makes a man differ from a Beast; if that be true, pray what are they that, instead of reason for their judgment, quote old Authors? Perhaps their authors knew a reason for what they wrote, perhaps they did not; what is that to us? Do we know it? Truly in writing this work first, to satisfy myself, I drew out all the virtues of the vulgar or common Herbs, Plants, and Trees, &c., out of the best or most approved authors I had, or could get; and having done so, I set myself to study the reason of them. I knew well enough the whole world, and everything in it, was formed of a composition of contrary elements, and in such a harmony as must needs show the wisdom and power of a great God. I knew as well this Creation, though thus composed of contraries, was one united body, and man an epitome of it: I knew those various affections in man, in respect of sickness and health, were caused naturally (though God may have other ends best known to himself) by the various operations of the Microcosm; and I could not be ignorant, that as the cause is, so must the cure be; and therefore he that would know the reason of the operation of the Herbs, must look up as high as the

Stars, astrologically. I always found the disease vary according to the various motions of the Stars; and this is enough, one would think, to teach a man by the effect where the cause lies. Then to find out the reason of the operation of Herbs, Plants, &c., by the Stars went I; and herein I could find but few authors, but those as full of nonsense and contradiction as an egg is full of meat. This not being pleasing, and less profitable to me, I consulted with my two brothers, Dr. Reason and Dr. Experience, and took a voyage to visit my mother Nature, by whose advice, together with the help of Dr. Diligence, I at last obtained my desire; and, being warned by Mr. Honesty, a stranger in our days, to publish it to the world, I have done it.

But you will say, *what need I have written on this Subject, seeing so many famous and learned men have written so much of it in the English Tongue, much more than I have done?*

To this I answer, neither Gerard nor Parkinson, or any that ever wrote in the like nature, ever gave one wise reason for what they wrote, and so did nothing else but train up young novices in Physic in the School of tradition, and teach them just as a parrot is taught to speak; an Author says so, therefore it is true; and if all that Authors say be true, why do they contradict one another? But in mine, if you view it with the eye of reason, you shall see a reason for everything that is written, whereby you may find the very ground and foundation of Physic; you may know what you do, and wherefore you do it; and this shall call me Father, it being (that I know of) never done in the world before.

I have now but two things to write, and then I have done.

What the profit and benefit of this Work is.

Instructions in the use of it.

The profit and benefit arising from it, or that may occur to a wise man from it are many; so many that should I sum up all the particulars, my Epistle would be as big as my Book; I shall quote some few general heads.

First. The admirable Harmony of the Creation is herein seen, in the influence of Stars upon Herbs and the Body of Man, how one part of the Creation is subservient to another, and all for the use of Man, whereby the infinite power and wisdom of God in the creation appear; and if I do not admire at the simplicity of the Ranters, never trust me; who but viewing the Creation can hold such a sottish opinion, as that it was from eternity, when the mysteries of it are so clear to every eye? but that Scripture shall be verified to them, *Rom.* i. 20: "*The invisible things of him from the Creation of the World are clearly seen, being understood by the things that are made, even his Eternal Power and Godhead; so that they are without excuse.*"—And a Poet could teach them a better lesson;

"*Because out of thy thoughts God shall not pass,*

"*His image stamped is on every grass.*"

This indeed is true, God has stamped his image on every creature, and therefore the abuse of the creature is a great sin; but how much the more do the wisdom and excellency of God appear, if we consider the harmony of the Creation in the virtue and operation of every Herb!

Secondly, hereby you may know what infinite knowledge *Adam* had in his innocence, that by looking upon a creature, he was able to give it a name according to its nature; and by knowing that, thou mayest know how great thy fall was and be humbled for it even in this respect, because hereby thou art so ignorant.

Thirdly, here is the right way for thee to begin at the study of Physic, if thou art minded to begin at the right end, for here thou hast the reason of the whole art. I wrote before in certain Astrological Lectures, which I read, and printed, entitled, *Astrological Judgment of Diseases*, what planet caused (as a second cause) every disease, how it might be found out what planet caused it; here thou hast what planet cures it by *Sympathy* and *Antipathy*; and this brings me to my last promise, *viz.*

INSTRUCTIONS FOR THE RIGHT USE OF THE BOOK

And herein let me premise a word or two. The Herbs, Plants, &c. are now in the book appropriated to their proper planets. Therefore, First, consider what planet causeth the disease; that thou mayest find it in my aforesaid Judgment of Diseases.

Secondly, consider what part of the body is afflicted by the disease, and whether it lies in the flesh, or blood, or bones, or ventricles.

Thirdly, consider by what planet the afflicted part of the body is governed: that my Judgment of Diseases will inform you also.

Fourthly, you may oppose diseases by Herbs of the planet, opposite to the planet that causes them: as diseases of *Jupiter* by herbs of *Mercury*, and the contrary; diseases of the *Luminaries* by the herbs of *Saturn*, and the contrary; diseases of *Mars* by herbs of *Venus*, and the contrary.

Fifthly, there is a way to cure diseases sometimes by *Sympathy*, and so every planet cures his own disease; as the *Sun* and *Moon* by their Herbs cure the Eyes, *Saturn* the Spleen, *Jupiter* the liver, *Mars* the Gall and diseases of choler [bile], and *Venus* diseases in the instruments of Generation.

NICH. CULPEPER.
From my House in Spitalfields,
next door to the Red Lion,
September 5, 1653.

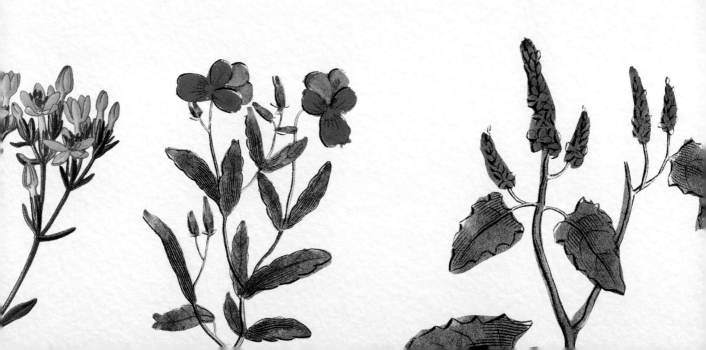

A–Z COMPENDIUM *of* HERBS

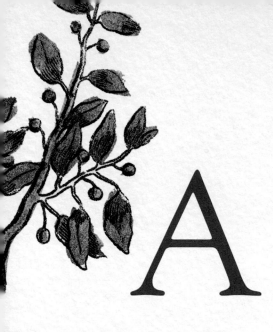

A

ADDER'S TONGUE

(OPHIOGLOSSUM VULGATUM)

Serpent's Tongue

DESCRIPTION: This herb has but one leaf [actually, it is a small fern with a single broad leaf], which grows with the stalk a finger's length above the ground, being flat, like the tongue of an adder serpent (only this is as useful as they are formidable).

PLACE: It grows in moist meadows, and such like places. [Widespread in the Northern Hemisphere, including Europe, Asia, and southeastern North America.]

GOVERNMENT AND VIRTUES: It is an herb under the dominion of the Moon and Cancer, and therefore if the weakness of the retentive faculty be caused by an evil influence of Saturn in any part of the body governed by the Moon, or under the dominion of Cancer, this herb cures it by sympathy: It cures these diseases after specified, in any part of the body under the influence of Saturn, by antipathy.

It is temperate in respect of heat, but dry in the second degree. The juice of the leaves, drank with the distilled water of Horsetail, is a singular remedy for all manner of wounds in the breast, bowels, or other parts of the body, and is given with good success to those that are troubled with casting, vomiting, or bleeding at the mouth or nose, or otherwise downwards. The said juice given in the distilled water of Oaken-buds, is very good for women who have their usual courses, or the whites flowing down too abundantly. It helps sore eyes. Of the leaves infused or boiled in oil, omphacine [oil of unripe olives] or unripe olives, set in the sun four certain days, or the green leaves sufficiently boiled in the said oil, is made an excellent green balsam, not only for green and fresh wounds, but also for old and inveterate ulcers, especially if a little fine clear turpentine be dissolved therein. It also stays and refreshes all inflammations that arise upon pains by hurts and wounds.

MODERN USES: Preparations of adder's tongue in olive oil are historically known in English folk medicine as "green oil of charity." Topical ointments made from frond extracts have been experimentally confirmed as of use for burns and wounds. Recent research confirms traditional use for wound healing and anti-inflammatory, antioxidant, and antiviral activity.

....

AGRIMONY
(AGRIMONIA EUPATORIA)

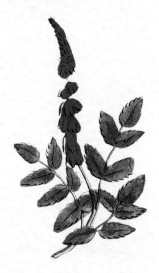

DESCRIPTION: This has diverse long leaves, among which arises up one hairy stalk, two or three feet high [with] many small yellow flowers in long spikes.

PLACE: [Native to grassy banks and fields throughout Great Britain and Europe; a scattered weed in North America.]

GOVERNMENT AND VIRTUES: It is an herb under Jupiter, and the sign Cancer; and strengthens those parts under the planet and sign, and removes diseases in them by sympathy, and those under Saturn, Mars and Mercury by antipathy, if they happen in any part of the body governed by Jupiter, or under the signs Cancer, Sagittarius, or Pisces, and therefore must needs be good for the gout, either used outwardly in oil or ointment, or inwardly in an electuary, or syrup, or concerted juice.

It is of a cleansing and cutting faculty, without any manifest heat, moderately drying and binding. It opens and cleanses the liver, helps the jaundice, and is very beneficial to the bowels, healing all inward wounds, bruises, hurts, and other distempers. The decoction of the herb made with wine, and drank, is good against the biting and stinging of serpents, and helps them that make foul, troubled or bloody water [urine]. This herb also helps the cholic, cleanses the breast, and rids away the cough. A draught of the decoction taken warm before the fit, first removes, and in time rids away the tertian or quartan agues [malaria]. The leaves and seeds taken in wine, stays the bloody flux [dysentery]; outwardly applied, being stamped with old swine's grease, it helps old sores, cancers, and inveterate ulcers, and draws forth thorns and splinters of wood, nails, or any other such things gotten in the flesh. It helps to strengthen the members that be out of joint: and being bruised and applied, or the juice dropped in it, helps foul and imposthumed [abscessed] ears.

It is a most admirable remedy for such whose livers are annoyed either by heat or cold. The liver is the former of blood, and blood the nourisher of the body, and Agrimony a strengthener of the liver. I cannot stand to give you a reason in every herb why it cures such diseases; but if you please to pursue my judgment in the herb Wormwood, you shall find them there, and it will be well worth your while to consider it in every herb, you shall find them true throughout the book.

MODERN USES: A clinical study from 2013 found lipid-lowering and antioxidant effects for a water extract of agrimony in patients with elevated liver enzymes. Anti-inflammatory, antioxidant, antimicrobial, mild astringent, and analgesic effects are also described for water extracts. Agrimony is traditionally used in tea for the symptomatic relief of mild diarrhea and mild inflammation of the mouth and throat; applied externally for minor, superficial wounds.

....

ALDER
(ALNUS GLUTINOSA)

The Common Alder–Tree

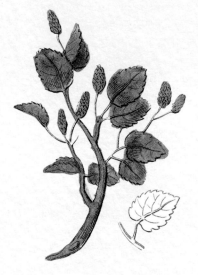

DESCRIPTION: It is so generally known to country people, that I conceive it needless to tell that which is no news.

PLACE: It delights to grow in moist woods, and watery places. [Alder grows plentifully near brooks, damp woods, and rivers throughout Europe and North Africa; introduced in north-central North America, Chile, and New Zealand.]

GOVERNMENT AND VIRTUES: It is a tree under the dominion of Venus, and of some watery sign or others, I suppose Pisces; and therefore the decoction, or distilled water of the leaves, is excellent against burnings and inflammations, either with wounds or without, to bathe the place grieved with, and especially for that inflammation in the breast, which the vulgar call an ague [fever]. If you cannot get the leaves (as in Winter, it is impossible) make use of the bark in the same manner.

The leaves and bark of the Alder-tree are cooling, drying, and binding. The fresh leaves, laid upon swellings, dissolve them, and stay the inflammation. The leaves put under the bare feet galled with travelling, are a great refreshing to them. The said leaves, gathered while the morning dew is on them, and brought into a chamber troubled with fleas, will gather them thereunto, and will rid the chamber of those troublesome bed-fellows.

MODERN USES: The habit and leaves of alder buckthorn and alder (see below) are similar, so the bark of alder has sometimes appeared as a contaminant or adulterant to alder buckthorn. Leaf and bark tea was used externally in European folk medicine to reduce swelling and inflammation. Alder and its preparations are seldom used today. Wound-healing, anti-inflammatory, and antioxidant activity are suggested by the presence of the bioactive compound shikimic acid.

．．．．．．．．．．．．．．．．．

ALDER BUCKTHORN

(*FRANGULA ALNUS*; SYN. *RHAMNUS FRANGULA*)

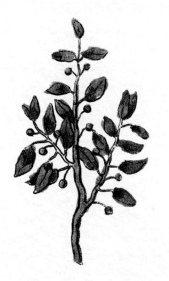

DESCRIPTION: This tree seldom grows to any great bigness; the inner bark is yellow, which being chewed, will turn the spittle near into a saffron colour.

PLACE: This tree or shrub may be found [plentifully in moist woods and streamsides throughout Europe. It is a serious invasive alien in eastern North America].

GOVERNMENT AND VIRTUES: It is a tree of Venus, and perhaps under the celestial sign Cancer. The inner yellow bark hereof purges downwards both choler [bile] and phlegm, and the watery humours of such that have the dropsy, and strengthens the inward parts again by binding. It purges and strengthens the liver and spleen, cleansing them from such evil humours and hardness as they are afflicted with. It is to be understood that these things are performed by the dried bark; for the fresh green bark taken inwardly provokes strong vomiting, pains in the stomach, and griping in the belly; yet if the decoction may stand and settle two or three days, until the yellow colour be changed black, it will not work so strongly as before, but will strengthen the stomach, and procure an appetite to meat. The outward bark contrariwise doth bind the body, and is helpful for all lasks [diarrhea] and fluxes thereof, but this also must be dried first, whereby it will work the better. The inner bark thereof boiled in vinegar is an approved remedy to kill lice, to cure the itch, and take away scabs, by drying them up in a short time. It is singularly good to wash the teeth, to take away the pains, to fasten those that are loose, to cleanse them, and to keep them sound. The leaves are good fodder for kine [cows], to make them give more milk.

If in the Spring-time you use the herbs before mentioned, and will take but a handful of each of them, and to them add an handful of alder buds, and having bruised them all, boil them in a gallon of ordinary beer, when it is new; and having boiled them half an hour, add to this three gallons more, and let them work together, and drink a draught of it every morning, half a pint or thereabouts; it is an excellent purge for the Spring, to consume the phlegmatic quality the Winter hath left behind it, and withal to keep your body in health, and consume those evil humours which the heat of Summer will readily stir up. Esteem it as a jewel.

MODERN USES: The dried aged inner bark of alder buckthorn is used as a stimulant laxative, due to the stimulant purgative effects of anthraquinone glycoside constituents. The dosage for occasional constipation for adults is 0.5–2.5 grams of the dried bark. Often used in standardized product forms to restrict dosage. Long-term use and abuse of stimulant laxatives should be avoided and may cause diarrhea, in addition to fluid and electrolyte loss. After one to two weeks seek medical supervision.

....

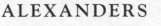

ALEXANDERS

(*SMYRNIUM OLUSATRUM*)

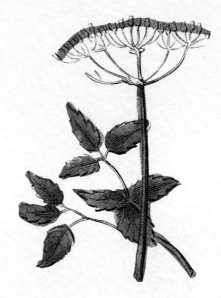

It is called Alisander, Horse-parsley, and Wild-parsley, [Wild-celery], and the Black Pot-herb; the seed of it is that which is usually sold in apothecaries' shops for Macedonian Parsley-seed.

DESCRIPTION AND PLACE: [Native to Mediterranean Europe and grown in gardens in Europe and North Africa. Found along roads, ditches, and wastelands, often by the sea.]

GOVERNMENT AND VIRTUES: It is an herb of Jupiter, and therefore friendly to nature, for it warms a cold stomach, and opens a stoppage of the liver and spleen; it is good to move women's courses, to expel the afterbirth, to break wind, to provoke urine, and helps the strangury [painful, frequent urination]; and these things the seeds will likewise. If either of them be boiled in wine, or being bruised and taken in wine, is also effectual against the biting of serpents. And you know what Alexander pottage is good for, that you may no longer eat it out of ignorance but out of knowledge.

MODERN USES: Alexanders was used as a celery-like food into the Middle Ages; the roots were boiled and used in soups. Of research interest for its anti-protozoal activity against African trypanosomiasis (sleeping sickness). Seldom used today.

....

ALKANET

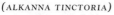

(*ALKANNA TINCTORIA*)

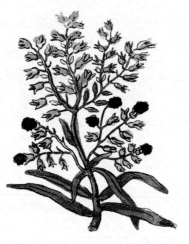

Besides the common name, it is called Orchanet, and Spanish Bugloss, and by apothecaries, Enchusa.

DESCRIPTION: It hath a great and thick root, of a reddish colour, long, narrow, hairy leaves; the stalks rise up compassed round about, thick with leaves; the flowers are small and reddish.

PLACE: [A perennial herb of high rocky meadows in southern Europe. Cultivated in gardens.]

GOVERNMENT AND VIRTUES: It is an herb under the dominion of Venus, and indeed one of her darlings, though somewhat hard to come by. It helps old ulcers, hot inflammations, burnings by common fire, and St. Anthony's fire, by antipathy to Mars; for these uses, your best way is to make it into an ointment; also, if you make a vinegar of it, as you make vinegar of roses, it helps the morphew [skin blemishes] and leprosy. It helps the yellow jaundice, spleen, and gravel in the kidneys. Dioscorides saith it helps such as are bitten by a venomous beast, whether it be taken inwardly, or applied to the wound; nay, he saith further, if any one that hath newly eaten it, do but spit into the mouth of a serpent, the serpent instantly dies [don't try this at home]. It stays the flux of the belly, kills worms, helps the fits of the mother. Its decoction made in wine, and drank, strengthens the back, and eases the pains thereof: It helps bruises and falls, and is as gallant a remedy to drive out the small pox and measles as any is; an ointment made of it, is excellent for green wounds, pricks or thrusts.

MODERN USES: Alkanna red, a dye formerly extracted from alkanet root, was used as a coloring agent for fish products. Components of the root and leaves (alkannin derivatives) are considered to be wound-healing, antimicrobial, and antiphlogistic. Used in Greece, Turkey, and Iran in topical products for wound healing, leg ulcers, and burns. Clinical study shows that an ointment of alkanet may accelerate wound healing. **CAUTION:** May contain liver-toxic pyrrolizidine alkaloids, common in the borage family (Boraginaceae).

....

AMARANTH

(AMARANTHUS CAUDATUS)

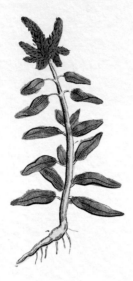

Besides its common name, by which it is best known by the florists of our days, it is called Flower Gentle, Flower Velure Floramor, and Velvet Flower [also Love-lies-bleeding, Tasselflower, Purple Amaranth].

DESCRIPTION: It [is] a garden flower, and well known to everyone that keeps it.

PLACE: [From South America, cultivated in gardens and escaped from cultivation.]

GOVERNMENT AND VIRTUES: It is under the dominion of Saturn, and is an excellent qualifier of the unruly actions and passions of Venus, though Mars also should join with her. The flowers dried and beaten into powder, stop the terms in women, and so do almost all other red things. And by the icon, or image of every herb, the ancients at first found out their virtues. Modern writers laugh at them for it; but I wonder in my heart, how the virtues of herbs came at first to be known, if not by their signatures; the moderns have them from the writings of the ancients; the ancients had no writings to have them from, but to proceed. The flowers stop all fluxes of blood; whether in man or woman, bleeding either at the nose or wound. There is also a sort of Amaranthus that bears a white flower, which stops the whites [vaginal discharges] in women, and is a most gallant antivenereal, and a singular remedy for the French pox [syphilis].

MODERN USES: An ancient Andean food crop, amaranth was brought to Europe from Peru in the sixteenth century. It is now regarded as a protein-rich health food, high in dietary fiber and antioxidants. The leaves and flowering tops of this and related amaranth species are used in tea as a mild astringent for diarrhea and dysentery and to stop bleeding.

....

ANGELICA

(ANGELICA ARCHANGELICA)

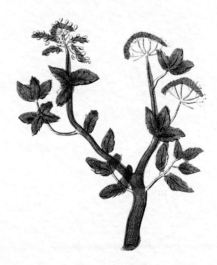

In time of Heathenism, when men had found out any excellent herb, they dedicated it to their gods; as the bay-tree to Apollo, the Oak to Jupiter, the Vine to Bacchus, the Poplar to Hercules. Our physicians must imitate like apes (though they cannot come off half so cleverly) for they blasphemously call Phansies [Pansies] or Heartsease, *an herb of the Trinity*, because it is of three colours; and a certain ointment, *an ointment of the Apostles*, because it consists of twelve ingredients. Certainly they have read so much in old rusty authors, that they have lost all their divinity. The Heathens and infidels were bad, and ours worse; the idolaters give idolatrous names to herbs for their virtues sake, not for their fair looks; and therefore some called this an herb of the *Holy Ghost*; others, more moderate, called it Angelica, because of its angelical virtues, and that name it retains still, and all nations follow it so near as their dialect will permit.

PLACE: [Angelica grows in damp soils near riverbanks and ditches. Frequently cultivated in herb gardens. Native to the northern European continent. Naturalized in Great Britain and northeastern North America.]

GOVERNMENT AND VIRTUES: It is an herb of the Sun in Leo; let it be gathered when he is there, the Moon applying to his good aspect; let it be gathered either in his hour, or in the hour of Jupiter, let Sol be angular; observe the like in gathering the herbs of other planets, and you may happen to do wonders. In all epidemical diseases caused by Saturn, that is as good a preservative as grows: It resists poison, by defending and comforting the heart, blood, and spirits; it doth the like against the plague and all epidemical diseases, if the root be taken in powder to the weight of half a dram at a time, with some good treacle in Carduus water, and the party thereupon laid to sweat in his bed; if treacle be not to be had taken it alone in Carduus or Angelica-water. The stalks or roots can-

died and eaten fasting, are good preservatives in time of infection; and at other times to warm and comfort a cold stomach. The root also steeped in vinegar, and a little of that vinegar taken sometimes fasting, and the root smelled unto, is good for the same purpose. A water distilled from the root simply, as steeped in wine, and distilled in a glass, is much more effectual than the water of the leaves; and this water, drank two or three spoonfuls at a time, easeth all pains and torments coming of cold and wind, so that the body be not bound; and taken with some of the root in powder at the beginning, helpeth the pleurisy, as also all other diseases of the lungs and breast, as coughs, phthisic [tuberculosis], and shortness of breath; and a syrup of the stalks do the like. It helps pains of the cholic, the strangury and stoppage of the urine, procureth women's courses, and expelleth the after-birth, openeth the stoppings of the liver and spleen, and briefly easeth and discusseth all windiness and inward swellings. The decoction drank before the fit of an ague, that they may sweat (if possible) before the fit comes, will, in two or three times taking, rid it quite away; it helps digestion and is a remedy for a surfeit. The juice or the water, being dropped into the eyes or ears, helps dimness of sight and deafness; the juice put into the hollow teeth, easeth their pains. The root in powder, made up into a plaster with a little pitch, and laid on the biting of mad dogs, or any other venomous creature, doth wonderfully help. The juice or the waters dropped, or tent wet therein, and put into filthy dead ulcers, or the powder of the root (in want of either) doth cleanse and cause them to heal quickly, by covering the naked bones with flesh; the distilled water applied to places pained with the gout, or sciatica, doth give a great deal of ease.

The wild Angelica is not so effectual as the garden; although it may be safely used to all the purposes aforesaid.

MODERN USES: A tea of the roots, seeds, and leaves of angelica has traditionally been used as an appetite stimulant and to treat dyspepsia with gas and mild gastrointestinal cramps. **CAUTION**: When ingested, angelica may cause photosensitivity due to its content of furanocoumarins, a group of compounds that causes mild to serious inflammatory skin reactions when the skin is exposed to direct sunlight (photodermatitis).

....

ARTICHOKES

(CYNARA CARDUNCULUS VAR. SCOLYMUS; SYN. CYNARA SCOLYMUS)

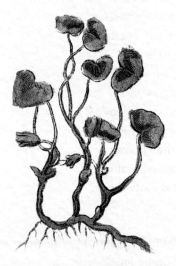

The Latins call them Cinera, only our college calls them Artichocus.

PLACE: [Native to the Mediterranean region. Introduced to gardens in England and elsewhere; sometimes naturalized or persisting in cultivation.]

GOVERNMENT AND VIRTUES: They are under the dominion of Venus, and therefore it is no marvel if they provoke lust, as indeed they do, being somewhat windy meat; and yet they stay the involuntary course of natural seed in man, which is commonly called nocturnal pollutions. And here I care not

greatly if I quote a little of Galen's nonsense in his treatise of the faculties of nourishment. He saith, they contain plenty of choleric juice, (which notwithstanding I can scarcely believe,) of which he saith is engendered melancholy juice, and of that melancholy juice thin choleric blood. But, to proceed; this is certain, that the decoction of the root boiled in wine, or the root bruised and distilled in wine in an alembic, and being drank, purges by urine exceedingly.

MODERN USES: Artichokes are best known as a food; the bracts of flowerbuds are eaten. The leaves are used in the form of tea or extracts for dyspepsia, particularly to increase bile flow and secretions from the liver (to detoxify and protect it), as well as to normalize liver and gallbladder function. It has also been shown to lower cholesterol.

....

ASARABACCA

(ASARUM EUROPAEUM)

DESCRIPTION: Asarabacca appears like an evergreen. The roots are small and whitish, spreading diverse ways in the ground. They are somewhat sweet in smell, but more when they are dry than green; and of a sharp and not unpleasant taste.

PLACE: [It grows frequently in shaded gardens in much of Europe, England, and Scotland.]

GOVERNMENT AND VIRTUES: It is a plant under the dominion of Mars, and therefore inimical to nature. This herb being drank, not only provokes vomiting, but purges downwards, and by urine also, purges both choler [bile] and phlegm: If you add to it some spikenard, with the whey of goat's milk, or honeyed water, it is made more strong, but it purges phlegm more manifestly than choler, and therefore does much help pains in the hips, and other parts; being boiled in whey, it wonderfully helps the obstructions of the liver and spleen, and therefore profitable for the dropsy and jaundice; being steeped in wine and drank, it helps those continual agues that come by the plenty of stubborn humours; an oil made thereof by setting in the sun, with some laudanum [tincture of opium] added to it, provokes sweating (the ridge of the back being anointed therewith), and thereby drives away the shaking fits of the ague. It will not abide any long boiling, for it lost its chief strength thereby; nor much beating, for the finer powder provokes vomits and urine, and the coarser purgeth downwards.

The common use hereof is, to take the juice of five or seven leaves in a little drink to cause vomiting; the roots have also the same virtue, though they do not operate so forcibly; they are very effectual against the biting of serpents. The leaves and roots being boiled in lye, and the head often washed therewith while it is warm, comforts the head and brain that is ill affected by taking cold, and helps the memory.

I shall desire ignorant people to forbear the use of the leaves; the roots purge more gently, and may prove beneficial to such as have cancers, or old putrefied ulcers, or fistulas upon their bodies, to take a dram of them in powder in a quarter of a pint of white wine in the morning. The truth is, I fancy purging and vomiting medicines as little as any man breathing doth, for they weaken nature, nor shall ever advise them to be used, unless upon urgent necessity. If a physician be nature's servant, it is his duty to strengthen his mistress as much as he can, and weaken her as little as may be.

MODERN USES: No longer in use. As Culpeper himself states, asarabacca induces vomiting and purging, clues pointing to its toxicity. It contains a chemical compound called beta-asarone, which induces nausea followed by vomiting. **CAUTION:** Avoid during pregnancy and lactation. In fact, just avoid ingesting it.

....

ASH TREE
(FRAXINUS EXCELSIOR)

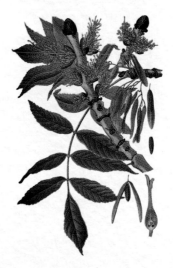

This is so well known, that time would be misspent in writing a description of it; therefore I shall only insist upon the virtues of it.

PLACE: [One of Great Britain's most common tree species, found in damp woods and now in serious decline. Ash species in both Europe and North America are threatened with extinction by an Asian beetle called the emerald ash borer.]

GOVERNMENT AND VIRTUES: It is governed by the Sun: and the young tender tops, with the leaves, taken inwardly, and some of them outwardly applied, are singularly good against the bitings of viper, adder, or any other venomous beasts; and the water distilled therefrom being taken, a small quantity every morning fasting, is a singular medicine for those that are subject to dropsy, or to abate the greatness of those that are too gross or fat. The decoction of the leaves in white wine helps to break the stone, and expel it, and cures the jaundice. The ashes of the bark of the Ash made into lye, and those heads bathed therewith which are leprous, scabby, or scald, they are thereby cured. The kernels within the husks, commonly called Ashen Keys, prevail against stitches and pains in the sides, proceeding of wind, and voideth away the stone by provoking urine.

I can justly except against none of all this, save only the first, *viz.* that Ash-tree tops and leaves are good against the bitings of serpents and vipers. I suppose this had its rise from Gerard or Pliny, both which hold that there is such an antipathy between an adder and an Ash-tree, that if an adder be encompassed round with Ash-tree leaves, she will sooner run through the fire than through the leaves: The contrary to which is the truth, as both my eyes are witnesses. The rest are virtues something likely, only if it be in Winter when you cannot get the leaves, you may safely use the bark instead of them. The keys [winged fruits] you may easily keep all the year, gathering them when they are ripe.

MODERN USES: Both the bark of young ash branches and the leaves have been used traditionally in herbal medicine. Bark preparations were used for fevers. Ash leaf tea was used for arthritis, gout, and as a diuretic for bladder complaints. Experiments have shown fresh ash bark to have anti-inflammatory and pain-relieving qualities. Modern research stimulated by the words of Culpeper suggests that preparations made from the fruits may benefit obese individuals with impaired glucose tolerance, insulin resistance, and inflammation.

....

ASPARAGUS

(*ASPARAGUS OFFICINALIS*)

Sparagus, or Sperage

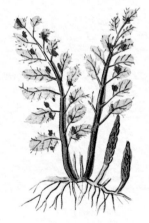

DESCRIPTION: Asparagus rises up with green scaly heads, very brittle or easy to break while they are young.

PLACE: [Native to the European continent and grown as a vegetable for many centuries. Naturalized in sandy soils and near gardens in Great Britain and throughout the continental United States.]

GOVERNMENT AND VIRTUES: It is under the dominion of Jupiter. The young buds or branches boiled in ordinary broth, make the belly soluble and open, and boiled in white wine, provoke urine, being stopped, and is good against the strangury or difficulty of making water; it expelleth the gravel and stone out of the kidneys, and helpeth pains in the lower back. And boiled in white wine or vinegar, it is prevalent for them that have their arteries loosened, or are troubled with the hip-gout or sciatica. The decoction of the roots boiled in wine and taken, is good to clear the sight, and being held in the mouth easeth the toothache. The decoction of the root in white wine, and the back and belly bathed therewith, or kneeling or lying down in the same, or sitting therein as a bath, has been found effectual against pains of the kidneys and bladder, pains of the mother and cholic, and generally against all pains that happen to the lower parts of the body, and no less effectual against stiff and benumbed sinews, or those that are shrunk by cramps and convulsions, and helps the sciatica.

MODERN USES: Aptly described by Culpeper, the spring shoots are what we know as asparagus. Asparagus root preparations are traditionally used as a diuretic and laxative, for inflammatory disease of the urinary tract, and to prevent kidney stones. The dried, cut rhizome is used in infusions or tinctures. **CAUTION:** Rare allergic skin reactions have been reported.

. . . .

AVENS, WOOD AVENS

(GEUM URBANUM)

Colewort, and Herb Bonet

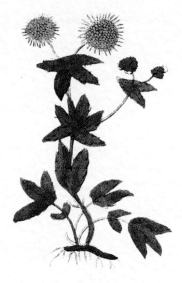

DESCRIPTION: On the tops of the branches stand small, pale, yellow flowers, like the flowers of Cinquefoil, but larger.

PLACE: They grow wild in many places under hedge's sides, and by the path-ways in fields; yet they rather delight to grow in shadowy than sunny places. [A common plant throughout Europe.]

GOVERNMENT AND VIRTUES: It is governed by Jupiter, and that gives hopes of a wholesome healthful herb. It is good for the diseases of the chest or breast, for pains, and sti[t]ches in the side, and to expel crude and raw humours from the belly and stomach, by the sweet savour and warming quality. It dissolves the inward congealed blood happening by falls or bruises, and the spitting of blood, if the roots, either green or dry, be boiled in wine and drank; as also all manner of inward wounds or outward, if washed or bathed therewith. The decoction also being drank, comforts the heart, and strengthens the stomach and a cold brain, and therefore is good in the spring times to open obstructions of the liver, and helps the wind cholic; it also helps those that have fluxes, or are bursten, or have a rupture; it takes away spots or marks in the face, being washed therewith. The juice of the fresh root, or powder of the dried root, has the same effect with the decoction. The root in the Springtime steeped in wine, gives it a delicate savour and taste, and being drank fasting every morning, comforts the heart, and is a good preservative against the plague, or any other poison. It helps indigestion, and warms a cold stomach, and opens obstructions of the liver and spleen.

MODERN USES: The essential oil of the fresh avens root contains eugenol, the same compound that gives cloves their characteristic flavor and fragrance. As a folk medicine, especially in Eastern Europe, the root or the dried herb has been used to treat diarrhea, fevers, and bleeding. It is also used to treat ulcerative colitis and dyspepsia. Recent research focuses on antimicrobial and antioxidant potential from the root's tannins. Avoid excess use.

....

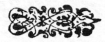

B

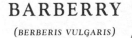

BARBERRY
(BERBERIS VULGARIS)

The shrub is so well known by every boy or girl that has but attained to the age of seven years, that it needs no description.

PLACE: [Found in hedges and field edges throughout Eurasia; a widely naturalized weedy shrub in North America; a noxious weed in Connecticut, Michigan, and New Hampshire.]

GOVERNMENT AND VIRTUES: Mars owns the shrub, and presents it to the use of my countrymen to purge their bodies of choler [bile]. The inner rind [bark] of the Barberry-tree boiled in white wine, and a quarter of a pint drank each morning, is an excellent remedy to cleanse the body of scabs, itch, tetters, ringworms, yellow jaundice, boils, etc. It is excellent for hot agues, burnings, scaldings, heat of the blood, heat of the liver, bloody-flux [dysentery]; for the berries are as good as the bark, and more pleasing: they get a man a good stomach to his victuals, by strengthening the attractive faculty which is under Mars. The hair washed with the lye made of the tree and water, will make it turn yellow, *viz.* of Mars' own colour. The fruit and rind of the shrub, the flowers of broom and of heath, cleanse the body of choler by sympathy, as the flowers, leaves, and bark of the peach-tree do by antipathy, because these are under Mars, that under Venus.

MODERN USES: In Iran, the edible red barberry fruit is cooked with rice. The fruits are high in antioxidants, vitamin C, and vitamin K and are used to treat acne, high blood pressure, and type 2 diabetes. The inner bark, colored bright yellow by its alkaloid, berberine, is used traditionally to treat fever, cough, depression, liver diseases, bleeding, high cholesterol, and high blood sugar. **CAUTION:** May cause gastrointestinal upset and interact with prescription drugs. Avoid use during pregnancy and lactation.

....

BARLEY

(HORDEUM VULGARE)

The continual usefulness hereof hath made all in general so acquainted herewith that it is altogether needless to describe it. The virtues thereof take as follow.

PLACE: [Barley is an ancient cultivated grain that, as known in the modern sense, originates in the Middle East to the Caucasus between the Red Sea and the Caspian Sea. It is widely distributed as a cultivated crop throughout the world.]

GOVERNMENT AND VIRTUES: It is a notable plant of Saturn: if you view diligently its effects by sympathy and antipathy, you may easily perceive a reason of them, as also why barley bread is so unwholesome for melancholy people. Barley in all the parts and compositions thereof (except malt) is more cooling than wheat, and a little cleansing. And all the preparations thereof, as barley-water and other things made thereof, give great nourishment to persons troubled with fevers and heats in the stomach: A poultice made of barley meal or flour boiled in vinegar and honey, and a few dry figs put into them, dissolves all imposthumes [abscesses], and assuages inflammations, being thereto applied. The meal of barley boiled with vinegar and quince eases the pains of the gout; barley-flour, white salt, honey, and vinegar mingled together, takes away the itch speedily and certainly. The water distilled from the green barley in the end of May, is very good for those that have defluctions of humours fallen into their eyes, and eases the pain, being dropped into them; or white bread steeped therein, and bound on the eyes, does the same.

MODERN USES: Better known as a food than an herb, or the stuff of which beer is brewed, barley has been valued for its anti-inflammatory and antioxidant benefits. Barley grain infused in water has been used as a nutritive food for convalescing patients. It is considered soothing to irritated mucous membranes. **CAUTION:** May affect glucose regulation; diabetics should use with caution. Some individuals are allergic to barley.

....

BASIL

(OCIMUM BASILICUM)

Garden Bazil, or Sweet Bazil

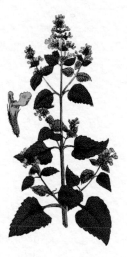

DESCRIPTION: [A tender annual widely grown as a culinary herb.]

PLACE: It grows in gardens. It must be sowed late, and flowers in the heart of Summer, being a very tender plant. [Basil may have originated in India and Southeast Asia. It reached Mediterranean shores in ancient times and is cultivated for flavor, fragrance, and medicine. Today, it is widespread in southern Asia, tropical Africa, Central America, South America, and northeastern Australia.]

GOVERNMENT AND VIRTUES: This is the herb which all authors are together by the ears about, and rail at one another (like lawyers). Galen and Dioscorides hold it not fit to be taken inwardly; Pliny, and the Arabian physicians defend it. For my own part, I presently found that speech true: *Non nostrium inter nos tantas componere lites* ["There is great debate among us"]. And away to Dr. Reason went I, who told me it was an herb of Mars, and under the Scorpion, and perhaps therefore called

Basilicon; and it is no marvel if it carry a kind of virulent quality with it. Being applied to the place bitten by venomous beasts, or stung by a wasp or hornet, it speedily draws the poison to it; *Every like draws his like.* Something is the matter; this herb and rue will not grow together, no, nor near one another: and we know rue is as great an enemy to poison as any that grows.

MODERN USES: Better known today as the culinary base of pesto rather than a treatment for scorpion bites, basil is considered antibacterial, antioxidant, and antiviral, among other effects. A weak basil tea is used to treat flatulence; externally, the leaves are poulticed for insect stings. **CAUTION:** Some individuals may be allergic to basil.

BAY

(LAURUS NOBILIS)

The Bay Tree

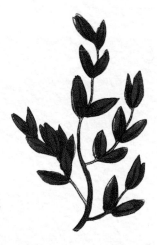

This is so well known that it needs no description: I shall therefore only write the virtues thereof, which are many.

PLACE: [Native to dry, gravelly soils in countries bordering the Mediterranean; planted elsewhere in Europe since ancient times.]

GOVERNMENT AND VIRTUES: I shall but only add a word or two to what my friend has written, *viz.*, that it is a tree of the sun, and under the celestial sign Leo, and resists witchcraft very potently, as also all the evils old Saturn can do to the body of man, and they are not a few; for it is the speech of one, and I am mistaken if it were not Mizaldus, that neither witch nor devil, thunder nor lightning, will hurt a man in the place where a Bay-tree is. Galen said, that the leaves or bark do dry and heal very much, and the berries more than the leaves; the bark of the root is less sharp and hot, but more bitter, and hath some astriction [astringency] withal whereby it is effectual to break the stone, and good to open obstructions of the liver, spleen, and other inward parts, which bring the jaundice, dropsy, etc. The berries are very effectual against all poison of venomous creatures, and the sting of wasps and bees; as also against the pestilence, or other infectious diseases, and therefore put into sundry treacles for that purpose; they likewise procure women's courses, and seven of them given to woman in sore travail of child-birth, do cause a speedy delivery, and expel the after-birth, and therefore not to be taken by such as have not gone out their time, lest they procure abortion, or cause labour too soon. They wonderfully help all cold and rheumatic distillations from the brain to the eyes, lungs or other parts; and being made into an electuary with honey, do help the consumption, old coughs, shortness of breath, and thin rheums; as also the megrim [spirits]. They mightily expel the wind, and provoke urine; help the mother, and kill the worms. The leaves also work the like effect. A bath of the decoction of leaves and berries is singularly good for women to sit in, that are troubled with the mother, or the diseases thereof, or the stoppings of their courses, or for the diseases of the bladder, pains in the bowels by wind and stoppage of the urine. The oil made of the berries is very comfortable in all cold griefs of the joints, nerves, arteries, stomach, belly, or womb, and helps palsies, convulsions, cramp, aches, tremblings, and numbness in any part, weariness also, and pains that come by sore travelling. All griefs and pains proceeding from wind, either in the head, stomach, back, belly, or womb, by anointing the parts affected therewith. And pains in the ears are also cured by dropping in some of the oil, or by receiving into the ears the fume of the decoction of the berries through a funnel. The oil takes away the marks of the skin and flesh by bruises, falls, &c. and dissolves the congealed blood in them. It helps also the itch, scabs, and weals in the skin.

MODERN USES: Primarily used for flavoring food, bay leaves have antimicrobial and antioxidant benefits. In the Middle East, the leaves are used in herbal preparations to treat nervous conditions. **CAUTION:** May cause contact dermatitis.

....

BEANS
(VICIA FABA)

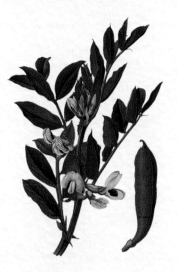

Both the garden and field beans are so well known, that it saves me the labour of writing any description of them. The virtues follow.

PLACE: [Cultivated for many centuries; origin uncertain. Widely cultivated worldwide and casually naturalized near cultivated fields.]

GOVERNMENT AND VIRTUES: They are plants of Venus, and the distilled water of the flower of garden beans is good to clean the face and skin from spots and wrinkles, and the meal or flour of them, or the small beans doth the same. The water distilled from the green husk is held to be very effectual against the stone, and to provoke urine. Bean flour is used in poultices to assuage inflammations arising from wounds, and the swelling of women's breasts caused by the curdling of their milk, and represses their milk. Flour of beans and Fenugreek mixed with honey, and applied to felons, boils, bruises, or blue marks by blows, or the imposthumes [abscesses] in the kernels of the ears, helps them all. If a bean be parted in two, the skin being taken away, and laid on the place where the leech hath been set that bleeds too much, stays the bleeding. Bean flour boiled to a poultice with wine and vinegar, and some oil put thereto, eases both pains and swelling of the privities [private parts]. The husk boiled in water to the consumption of a third part thereof, stays a lask [diarrhea]; and the ashes of the husks, made up with old hog's grease, helps the old pains, contusions, and wounds of the sinews, the sciatica and gout. The field beans have all the aforementioned virtues as the garden beans.

Beans eaten are extremely windy meat; but if after the they are half boiled you husk them and then stew them, they are wholesome food.

MODERN USES: Beans are a significant source of vegetable protein. As an obscure folk medicine, they are used as a diuretic and expectorant. **CAUTION:** Safe use assumes beans are cooked.

....

BEANS, FRENCH
(PHASEOLUS VULGARIS)

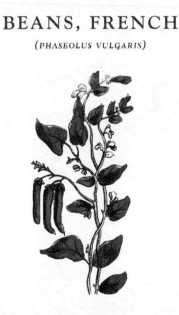

DESCRIPTION: French or kidney Bean arises at first but with one stalk, sustained with sticks or poles.

Flowers are like pea blossoms, of the same colour; after which come long and slender flat pods, some crooked, some straight.

PLACE: [An ancient crop native to Mexico and Central America, beans are now cultivated worldwide and casually grow wild near cultivated fields in South America, Africa, and much of Asia.]

GOVERNMENT AND VIRTUES: These also belong to Dame Venus, and being dried and beat to powder, are as great strengtheners of the kidneys as any are; neither is there a better remedy than it; a dram at a time taken in white wine to prevent the stone, or to cleanse the kidneys of gravel or stoppage. The ordinary French Beans are of an easy digestion; they move the belly, provoke urine, enlarge the breast that is straightened with shortness of breath, engender sperm, and incite to venery. And the scarlet coloured Beans, in regard of the glorious beauty of their colour, being set near a quickset hedge, will much adorn the same, by climbing up thereon, so that they may be discerned a great way, not without admiration of the beholders at a distance. But they will go near to kill the quicksets by clothing them in scarlet.

MODERN USES: French beans are used as a source of vegetable protein. **CAUTION:** Safe use assumes beans are cooked.

....

BEAR'S-BREECHES

(ACANTHUS MOLLIS)

Brank Ursine

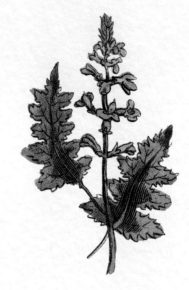

Besides the common name Brank-Ursine, it is also called Bear's-breach, and Acanthus, though I think our English names to be more proper; for the Greek word *Acanthus*, signifies any thistle whatsoever.

DESCRIPTION: This thistle shoots forth very many large, thick, sad green smooth leaves, with a very thick and juicy middle rib; the leaves are parted with sundry deep gashes on the edges. The flowers are hooded and gaping, being white in colour.

PLACE: [Native to the central Mediterranean region; grown as a garden plant and escaped cultivation.]

GOVERNMENT AND VIRTUES: It is an excellent plant under the dominion of the Moon; I could wish such as are studious would labour to keep it in their gardens. The leaves being boiled and used in clysters [enemas], is excellent good to mollify the belly, and make the passage slippery. The decoction drank inwardly, is excellent and good for the bloody-flux [dysentery]; the leaves being bruised, or rather boiled and applied like a poultice are excellent good to unite broken bones and strengthen joints that have been put out. The decoction of either leaves or roots being drank, and the decoction of leaves applied to the place, is excellent good for the king's evil [unusual swelling of lymph nodes or scrofula] that is broken and runs; for by the influence of the moon, it revives the ends of the veins which are relaxed. There is scarce a better remedy to be applied to such places as are burnt with fire than this is, for it fetches out the fire, and heals it without a scar. This is an excellent remedy for such as are bursten, being either taken inwardly, or applied to the place. In like manner used, it helps the cramp and the gout. It is excellently good in hectic fevers, and restores radical moisture to such as are in consumptions.

MODERN USES: Bear's-breeches is a European folk medicine for inflamed mucous membranes of the respiratory and digestive tract; it is also used externally for wound healing. The herb contains active chemical compounds such as mucilage, phenols, and flavonoids, which contribute anti-inflammatory, antioxidant, and antifungal properties, suggesting a scientific basis for some of Culpeper's claimed benefits.

. . . .

BEECH TREE
(FAGUS SYLVATICA)

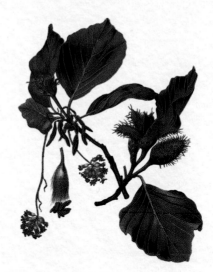

I suppose it is needless to discribe it, being already well known to my countrymen.

PLACE: It grows in woods amongst oaks and other trees, and in parks, forests, and chases, to feed deer; and in other places to fatten swine.

GOVERNMENT AND VIRTUES: It is a plant of Saturn, and therefore performs his qualities in these operations. The leaves of the Beech tree are cooling and binding, and therefore good to be applied to hot swellings to discuss them; the nuts do much nourish such beasts as feed thereon. The water that is found in the hollow places of decaying Beeches will cure both man and beast of any scurf, or running tetters, if they be washed therewith; you may boil the leaves into a poultice, or make an ointment of them when time of year serves.

MODERN USES: Seldom used today, beech leaves, bark, and nuts were used in European folk traditions. The leaves and bark were claimed to be useful astringent and antiseptic agents for diarrhea, indigestion, and fevers. A medicinal creosote historically distilled from the wood was used as an expectorant for bronchitis. Bitter, astringent, and largely unpalatable green beechnuts were consumed as a worm expellant. **CAUTION:** Once roasted, beechnuts are considered edible, but may cause allergic reactions in some individuals.

....

BEETS

(BETA VULGARIS)

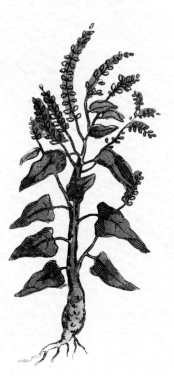

Of Beets there are two sorts, which are best known generally, and whereof I shall principally treat at this time, *viz.* the white and red Beets and their virtues.

DESCRIPTION: The common white beet has many great leaves next the ground, somewhat large and of a whitish green colour. The common red Beet leaves and roots are somewhat red.

PLACE: [Cultivated for hundreds of years. Wild relatives of the familiar common beet are native to fields in much of northern Europe, northern Africa, and east to India. Widely naturalized elsewhere as a relic from cultivation.]

GOVERNMENT AND VIRTUES: The government of these two sorts of Beets are far different; the red Beet being under Saturn and the white under Jupiter; therefore take the virtues of them apart, each by itself. The white Beet much loosens the belly, and is of a cleansing, digesting quality, and provokes urine. The juice of it opens obstructions both of the liver and spleen, and is good for the head-ache and swimmings therein, and turnings of the brain; and is effectual also against all venomous creatures; and applied to the temples, stays inflammations of the eyes; it helps burnings, being used with oil, and with a little alum put to it, is good for St. Anthony's fire. It is good for all wheals, pushes, blisters, and blains in the skin: the herb boiled, and laid upon chilblains or kibes, helps them. The decoction thereof in water and some vinegar, heals the itch, if bathed therewith; and cleanses the head of dandruff, scurf, and dry scabs, and does much good for fretting and running sores, ulcers, and cankers in the head, legs, or other parts, and is much commended against baldness and shedding the hair.

The red Beet is good to stay the bloody-flux [dysentery], women's courses, and the whites [vaginal discharges], and to help the yellow jaundice; the juice of the root put into the nostrils, purges the head, helps the noise in the ears, and the tooth-ache; the juice snuffed up the nose, helps a stinking breath, if the cause lie in the nose, as many times it does, if any bruise has been there: as also want of smell coming that way.

MODERN USES: Beets are primarily used as a food, though beet juice (often combined with other vegetable juices) is believed to be diuretic and a folk cancer remedy. About 14 percent of individuals who consume red beets may experience *beeturia*—red urine after eating beets—due to increased intestinal absorption of the red-colored anti-oxidant, betalaine.

....

BETONY

(*BETONICA OFFICINALIS; SYN. STACHYS OFFICINALIS*)

Wood Betony

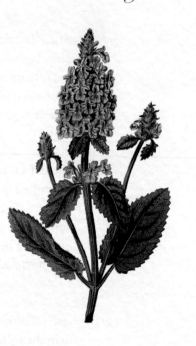

DESCRIPTION: Common or Wood Betony has many leaves rising from the root, leaves thereon to a piece at the joints, smaller than the lower, whereon are set several spiked heads of flowers like Lavender.

PLACE: It grows frequently in woods, and delights in shady places [in much of Europe. Elsewhere it's grown as a garden ornamental].

GOVERNMENT AND VIRTUES: The herb is appropriated to the planet Jupiter, and the sign Aries. Antonius Musa, physician to the Emperor Augustus Cæsar, wrote a peculiar book of the virtues of this herb; and among other virtues saith of it, that it preserves the liver and bodies of men from the danger of epidemical diseases, and from witchcraft also; it helps those that loath and cannot digest their meat, those that have weak stomachs and sour belchings, or continual rising in their stomachs, using it familiarly either green or dry; either the herb, or root, or the flowers, in broth, drink, or meat, or made into conserve, syrup, water, electuary, or powder, as everyone may best frame themselves unto, or as the time and season requires; taken any of the aforesaid ways, it helps the jaundice, falling sickness, the palsy, convulsions, or shrinking of the sinews, the gout and those that are inclined to dropsy, those that have continual pains in their heads, although it turn to phrensy. The powder mixed with pure honey is no less available for all sorts of coughs or colds, wheezing, or shortness of breath, distillations of thin rheum [watery discharge] upon the lungs, which causes consumptions. It helps also to break and expel the stone, either in the bladder or kidneys. The decoction with wine gargled in the mouth, eases the tooth-ache. It is commended against the stinging and biting of venomous serpents, or mad dogs, being used inwardly and applied outwardly to the place. A dram of the powder of Betony taken with a little honey in some vinegar, does wonderfully refresh those that are over-wearied by travelling. It stays bleeding at the mouth or nose, and helps those that void or spit blood, and those that are bursten or have a rupture, and is good for such as are bruised by any fall or otherwise. The green herb bruised, or the juice applied to any inward hurt, or outward green wound in the head or body, will quickly heal and close it up; as also any vein or sinews that are cut, and will draw forth any broken bone or splinter, thorn or other things got into the flesh. It is no less profitable for old sores or filthy ulcers, yea, tho' they be fistulous and hollow. The root of Betony is displeasing both to the taste and stomach, whereas the leaves and flowers, by their sweet and spicy taste, are comfortable both to meat and medicine.

These are some of the many virtues Anthony Muse, an expert physician (for it was not the practice of Octavius Cæsar to keep fools about him), appropriates to Betony; it is a very precious herb, that is certain, and most fitting to be kept in a man's house, both in syrup, conserve, oil, ointment and plaster. The flowers are usually conserved.

MODERN USES: Betony, an herb that Culpeper describes as so eminently useful, has fallen into disuse despite potential antioxidant and anti-inflammatory activity. Today, it's a folk remedy for cuts and wounds. In Eastern Europe, betony tea is used as a bitter tonic to aid digestion, alleviate headaches, and improve neuralgia.

....

BILBERRIES
(VACCINIUM MYRTILLUS)

Whorts, Whortle–Berries

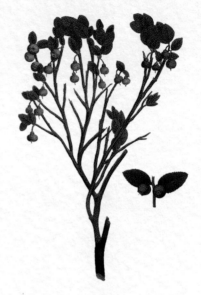

DESCRIPTION: Of these I shall only speak of two sorts which are common in England, *viz.* The black [*Vaccinium myrtillus*] and red [*Vaccinium vitis-idaea*] berries. And first of the black.

The small bush creeps along upon the ground, scarcely rising half a yard high, with diverse small green leaves set in the green branches and small round berries of the size and colour of juniper berries, but of a purple, sweetish sharp taste. This loses its leaves in Winter.

The Red Bilberry, or Whortle-Bush, rises up like the former, having sundry hard leaves, like the Box-tree leaves, at the top, come forth diverse round, reddish, sappy berries, when they are ripe, of a sharp taste. [The leaves are evergreen.]

PLACE: The first grows in forests [and hillsides throughout Europe]. The red grows in the north parts of [the Northern Hemisphere].

GOVERNMENT AND VIRTUES: They are under the dominion of Jupiter. It is a pity they are used no more in physic than they are. The black Bilberries are good in hot agues and to cool the heat of the liver and stomach; they do somewhat bind the belly, and stay vomiting and loathings; the juice of the berries made in a syrup, or the pulp made into a conserve with sugar, is good for the purposes aforesaid, as also for an old cough, or an ulcer in the lungs, or other diseases therein. The Red Worts are more binding, and stops women's courses, spitting of blood, or any other flux of blood or humours, being used as well outwardly as inwardly.

MODERN USES: Pity no more, Culpeper! Today the bilberry is widely used in herbal medicine. For over fifty years, European researchers have studied its benefits for vision. During the Second World War, British pilots reported better night vision after eating bilberry jam. Antioxidant components in the fruits strengthen blood capillaries and help to build healthy cellular connective tissue. It's claimed that bilberry products aid in the management of varicose veins and hemorrhoids while reducing capillary fragility and a tendency to bruising. Culpeper's "red bilberry" is best known today as lingonberry, which is also high in antioxidant compounds.

....

BIRCH
(BETULA PENDULA AND BETULA PUBESCENS)
The Birch Tree

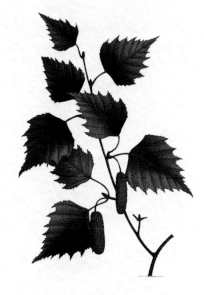

DESCRIPTION: This grows a goodly tall straight tree. The leaves at the first breaking out are crumpled, and afterwards like the beech leaves, but smaller and greener.

PLACE: It usually grows in woods.

GOVERNMENT AND VIRTUES: It is a tree of Venus; the juice of the leaves, while they are young, or the distilled water of them, or the water that comes from the tree being bored with an auger, and distilled afterwards; any of these being drank for some days together, is available to break the stone in the kidneys and bladder, and is good also to wash sore mouths.

MODERN USES: Birch leaf tea and extracts are widely used as a diuretic for the treatment of urinary tract problems like bacterial infections and inflammation such as cystitis and urethritis. Birch is also traditionally used for gout and rheumatism and as a springtime "blood purifier" (to remove toxic compounds from the blood and facilitate blood flow after a long winter with no fresh vegetables). European folk use has led to scientific studies on its potential anticancer, anti-inflammatory, antioxidant, antidiabetic, and antiarthritic activity, among other effects.

....

BISHOP'S-WEED

(*AMMI MAJUS*)

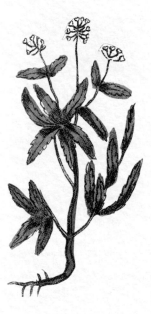

Besides the common name Bishop's-weed, it is usually known by the Greek name *Ammi* and *Ammois*; some call it Ethiopian Cumin-seed, and others Cumin-royal, as also Herb William, and Bull-wort.

DESCRIPTION: Common Bishop's-weed rises up three or four feet high, having at the top small umbels of white flowers, which turn into small round seeds little bigger than Parsley seeds, of a quick hot scent and taste.

PLACE: [Native to southern Europe and Mediterranean North Africa; cultivated and escaped elsewhere in wastelands and fields.]

GOVERNMENT AND VIRTUES: It is hot and dry in the third degree, of a bitter taste, and somewhat sharp withal; it provokes lust to purpose; I suppose Venus owns it. It digests humours, provokes urine and women's courses, dissolves wind, and being taken in wine it eases pains and griping in the bowels, and is good against the biting of serpents; it is used to good effect in those medicines which are given to hinder the poisonous operation of Cantharides, upon the passage of the urine: being mixed with honey and applied to black and blue marks, coming of blows or bruises, it takes them away; and being drank or outwardly applied, it abates a high colour, and makes it pale; and the fumes thereof taken with rosin or raisins, cleanses the mother.

MODERN USES: Bishop's-weed is used in traditional medicine in the Middle East and elsewhere for the treatment of skin disorders including vitiligo and psoriasis. A compound in the seeds, xanthotoxin, is used in controlled clinical settings for the treatment of these disorders in conjunction with the controlled administration of UV radiation. In essence, a photodermatitis reaction is induced, causing irritation and inflammation, which, after about two weeks, results in a deep brown pigmentation of the skin that persists for several months. **CAUTION:** Use only under medical supervision.

....

BISTORT

(*BISTORTA OFFICINALIS*; SYN. *PERSICARIA BISTORA, POLYGONUM BISTORT*)

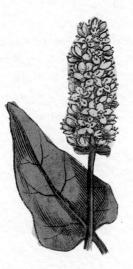

It is called Snakeweed, English Serpentary, Dragon-wort, Osterick, and Passions.

DESCRIPTION: This has a thick short knobbed root, blackish without, and somewhat reddish within, of a hard astringent taste, two feet high, bearing a spiky bush of pale-coloured flowers.

PLACE: [Found in grassy areas. Native to Europe, Morocco, and temperate regions of Asia. Escaped from gardens elsewhere.]

GOVERNMENT AND VIRTUES: It belongs to Saturn, and is in operation cold and dry; both the leaves and roots have a powerful faculty to resist all poison. The root, in powder, taken in drink expels the venom of the plague, the small-pox, measles, purples, or any other infectious disease, driving it out by sweating. The root in powder, the decoction thereof in wine being drank, stays all manner of inward bleeding, or spitting of blood, and any fluxes in the body of either man or woman, or vomiting. It is also very available against ruptures, or burstings, or all bruises from falls, dissolving the congealed blood, and easing the pains that happen thereupon; it also helps the jaundice.

The water, distilled from both leaves and roots, is a singular remedy to wash any place bitten or stung by any venomous creature; as also for any of the purposes before spoken of, and is very good to wash any running sores or ulcers. The leaves, seed, or roots are all very good in decoction, drinks, or lotions, for inward or outward wounds, or other sores. And the powder, strewed upon any cut or wound in a vein, stays the immoderate bleeding thereof. The distilled water is very effectual to wash sores or cankers in the nose, or any other part; if the powder of the root be applied thereunto afterwards. It is good also to fasten the gums, and to take away the heat and inflammations that happen in the jaws, almonds of the throat, or mouth, if the decoction of the leaves, roots, or seeds bruised, or the juice of them, be applied; but the roots are most effectual to the purposes aforesaid.

MODERN USES: Bistort is considered astringent (due to the presence of tannins), anti-inflammatory, and antidiarrheal. An infusion of the herb is used to treat diarrhea, dysentery, and discharges associated with upper respiratory tract inflammation. Only for short-term use due to concerns about the long-term toxicity of tannins. In traditional Chinese medicine, the root in decoction is used for dysentery, diarrhea with gastroenteritis, and acute respiratory infections; used externally for hemorrhoids.

....

BITTERSWEET

(SOLANUM DULCAMARA)

Woody Nightshade, Amara Dulcis

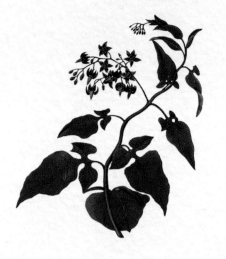

Considering diverse shires in this nation give diverse names to [this] herb, and that the common name which it bears in one county, is not known in another; I shall take the pains to set down all the names that I know of each herb: pardon me for setting that name first, which is most common to myself. Besides Amara Dulcis, some call it Mortal, others Bitter-sweet; some Woody Night-shade, and others Felon-wort.

DESCRIPTION: It grows up with woody stalks even to a man's height, and sometimes higher. The flowers are of a purple colour, or of a perfect blue, like to violets. The berries are very red.

PLACE: [Common along fence rows, hedges, ditches, and walls. Native to Europe, a common naturalized weed in North America.]

GOVERNMENT AND VIRTUES: It is under the planet Mercury, and a notable herb of his also, if it be rightly gathered under his influence. It is excellently good to remove witchcraft both in men and beasts, as also all sudden diseases whatsoever. Being tied round about the neck, is one of the most admirable remedies for the vertigo or dizziness in the head; and that is the reason the people in Germany commonly hang it about their cattle's necks, when they fear any such evil hath betided them: Country people commonly take the berries of it, and having bruised them, apply them to felons, and thereby soon rid their fingers of such troublesome guests.

MODERN USES: The bittersweet stem, which contains steroidal alkaloids and saponins, is used. Topical preparations of bittersweet are traditional in European phytomedicine for the supportive symptomatic relief of mild recurrent eczema. The action is astringent, antimicrobial, anticholinergic, and antiphlogistic. **CAUTION:** Irritating to mucous membranes. Solanine glycoalkaloids can cause gastrointestinal irritation. Preparations may cause contact dermatitis. Not recommended for children under eighteen years of age.

....

BLACKBERRY

(RUBUS FRUTICOSUS)

Bramble, Black–Berry Bush

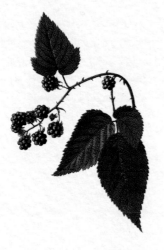

It is so well known that it needs no description. [Originated in Europe; cultivated elsewhere.] The virtues thereof are as follows:—

GOVERNMENT AND VIRTUES: It is a plant of Venus in Aries. If any ask the reason why Venus is so prickly? Tell them it is because she is in the house of Mars. The buds, leaves, and branches, while they are green, are of a good use in the ulcers and putrid sores of the mouth and throat, and of the quinsy, and likewise to heal other fresh wounds and sores; but the flowers and fruit unripe are very binding, and so profitable for the bloody flux [dysentery], lasks [diarrhea], and are a fit remedy for spitting of blood. Either the decoction of the powder or of the root taken, is good to break or drive forth gravel and the stone in the kidneys. The leaves and brambles, as well green as dry, are exceeding good lotions for sores in the mouth, or secret parts. The decoction of them, and of the dried branches, do much bind the belly and are good for too much flowing of women's courses. The berries are a powerful remedy against the poison of the most venomous serpents; as well drank as outwardly applied, helps the sores of the fundament and the piles; the juice of the berries mixed with the juice of mulberries, do bind more effectally, and helps all fretting and eating sores and ulcers wheresoever. The distilled water of the branches, leaves, and flowers, or of the fruit, is very pleasant in taste, and very effectual in fevers and hot distempers of the body, head, eyes, and other parts, and for the purposes aforesaid. The leaves boiled in lye, and the head washed there-with, heals the itch and running sores thereof, and makes the hair black. The powder of the leaves strewed on cankers and running ulcers, wonderfully helps to heal them. Some use to con-densate the juice of the leaves, and some the juice of the berries, to keep for their use all the year, for the purposes aforesaid.

MODERN USES: Most blackberry varieties are used similarly. Both the root and leaves are valued as toning astringents. They are used in tea for mild diarrhea and as a gargle for mouth and throat inflammation. This is a highly variable plant group with hundreds of described varieties.

....

BLACK HELLEBORE

(HELLEBORUS NIGER)

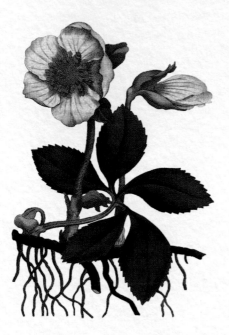

It is also called Setter-wort, Setter-grass, Bear's-foot, Christmas-herb, and Christmas-flowers.

DESCRIPTION: It hath sundry fair green leaves rising from the root, each of them standing about a handful high from the earth; each leaf is divided into seven, eight, or nine parts, green all the Winter; about Christmas-time, the flowers appear consisting of five large, round, white, sometimes purple [petals] towards the edges.

PLACE: [It] is maintained in gardens. [Originated in western Asia; widely cultivated as an ornamental plant and escaped from gardens.]

GOVERNMENT AND VIRTUES: It is an herb of Saturn, and therefore no marvel if it has some sullen conditions with it, and would be far safer, being purified by the art of the alchemist than given raw. If any have taken any harm by taking it, the common cure is to take goat's milk: If you cannot get goat's milk, you must make a shift with such as you can get. The roots are very effectual against all melancholy diseases, especially such as are of long standing, as quartan agues [malaria recurring every four days] and madness; it helps the falling sickness, the leprosy, both the yellow and black jaundice, the gout, sciatica, and convulsions; and this was found out by experience, that the root of that which grows wild in our country, works not so churlishly as those do which are brought from beyond sea, as being maintained by a more temperate air. The root used as a pessary, provokes the terms exceedingly; also being beaten into powder, and strewed upon foul ulcers, it consumes the dead flesh, and instantly heals them; nay, it will help gangrenes in the beginning. Twenty grains taken inwardly is a sufficient dose for one time, and let that be corrected with half so much cinnamon; country people used to rowel their cattle with it. If a beast be troubled with a cough, or have taken any poison, they bore a hole through the ear, and put a piece of the root in it, this will help him in 24 hours' time. Many other uses farriers put it to which I shall forbear.

MODERN USES: Black hellebore is not used today. It contains various irritant saponins and the toxin protoanemonin (typical of the buttercup family, Ranunculaceae) and may also contain heart-toxic compounds. **CAUTION:** Poisonous plant. Do not ingest.

....

BLESSED THISTLE

(CNICUS BENEDICTUS; SYN. CENTAUREA BENEDICTA)

Carduus Benedictus

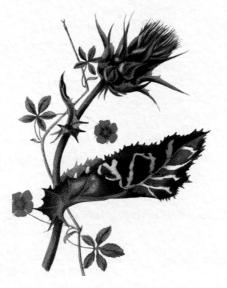

It is called Carduus Benedictus, or Blessed Thistle, or Holy Thistle. I suppose the name was put upon it by some that had little holiness themselves.

I shall spare a labour in writing a description of this as almost everyone that can but write at all, may describe them from his own knowledge.

PLACE: [Common annual weed found in fields and disturbed ground throughout Europe and elsewhere. Seed spread by birds.]

GOVERNMENT AND VIRTUES: It is an herb of Mars, and under the sign of Aries. Now, in handling this herb, I shall give you a rational pattern of all the rest; and if you please to view them throughout the book, you shall, to your content, find it true. It helps swimming and giddiness of the head, or the disease called vertigo, because Aries is in the house of Mars. It is an excellent remedy against the yellow jaundice and other infirmities of the gall, because Mars governs choler [bile]. It strengthens the attractive faculty in man, and clarifies the blood, because the one is ruled by Mars. The continual drinking the decoction of it, helps red faces, tetters, and ringworms, because Mars causes them. It helps the plague, sores, boils, and itch, the bitings of mad dogs and venomous beasts, all which infirmities are under Mars; thus you see what it doth by sympathy.

By antipathy to other planets it cures the French pox [syphilis]. By antipathy to Venus, who governs it, it strengthens the memory, and cures deafness by antipathy to Saturn, who has his fall in Aries, which rules the head. It cures quartan agues [malaria recurring every four days], and other diseases of melancholy, and adust choler, by sympathy to Saturn, Mars being exalted in Capricorn. Also provokes urine, the stopping of which is usually caused by Mars or the Moon.

MODERN USES: As a dried herb, blessed thistle is used in modern herbal medicine in the supportive treatment of gastrointestinal conditions. The primary indications are to treat anorexia, loss of appetite, and dyspepsia. In tea or tincture it's used as a simple bitter, digestive tonic, and digestive stimulant. Its extremely bitter principle, cnicin, is largely responsible for the production of saliva and gastric secretions, hence its value in stimulating appetite. Blessed thistle has also been used traditionally to help promote milk flow.

....

BORAGE

(*BORAGO OFFICINALIS*)

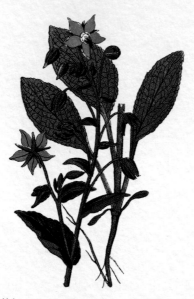

[It] so well known to the inhabitants in every garden that I hold it needless to describe [it].

PLACE: [Native to the Mediterranean region in southern Europe and North Africa; elsewhere widely grown as a garden plant. It has also escaped and grows on wastelands.]

GOVERNMENT AND VIRTUES: [It is an herb of] Jupiter and under Leo, a great cordial, and great strengthener of nature. The leaves and roots are to very good purpose used in putrid and pestilential fevers, to defend the heart, and help to resist and expel the poison, or the venom of other creatures. The seed is of the like effect; and the seed and leaves are good to increase milk in women's breasts. The leaves, flowers, and seed, all or any of them, are good to expel pensiveness and melancholy; it helps to clarify the blood, and mitigate heat in fevers. The flowers candied or made into a conserve, are helpful in the former cases, but are chiefly used as a cordial, and are good for those that are weak in long sickness, and to comfort the heart and spirits of those that are in a consumption, or troubled with often swoonings, or passions of the heart. The distilled water is no less effectual to all the purposes aforesaid, and helps the redness and inflammations of the eyes, being washed therewith; the herb dried is never used, but the green; yet the ashes thereof boiled in mead, or honied water, is available against the inflammations and ulcers in the mouth or throat, to gargle it therewith.

MODERN USES: Borage flowers are eaten in salads or candied. Traditionally, the herb is believed to be useful to treat coughs (as an expectorant), reduce sweating, promote milk flow, and treat depression. It's also claimed to be a diuretic, antiinflammatory, and pain-relieving agent. As a source of gamma-linolenic acid, borage seed oil is sold as a substitute for evening primrose oil.

CAUTION: Borage herb, flowers, and seeds (but apparently not the seed oil) may contain livertoxic pyrrolizidine alkaloids, which cause venoocclusive liver disease. The risks outweigh the benefits.

....

BROOKLIME

(VERONICA BECCABUNGA)

Water–Pimpernel

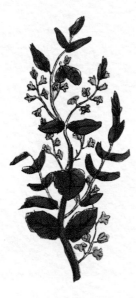

DESCRIPTION: [It has] a creeping root, diverse and sundry green stalks, [with] somewhat broad, round, deep green, and thick leaves, with sundry small blue flowers on them.

PLACE: They grow in small standing waters, and usually near Water-Cresses.

GOVERNMENT AND VIRTUES: It is a hot and biting martial plant. Brooklime and Watercress are generally used together in diet-drink, with other things serving to purge the blood and body from all ill humours that would destroy health, and are helpful to the scurvy. They do all provoke urine, and help to break the stone, and pass it away; they procure women's courses. Being fried with butter and vinegar, and applied warm, it helps all manner of tumours, swellings, and inflammations.

MODERN USES: Brooklime is used in traditional medicine as a diuretic and blood purifier, and to treat water retention, fevers, and dyspepsia. The young shoots are eaten to treat scurvy. One of the most important antiscorbutic plants before Culpeper.

BRYONY

(BRYONIA ALBA; SYN. BRYONIA DIOICA)

Briony, Wild Vine

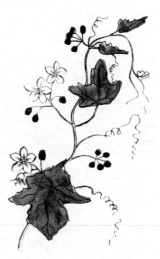

It is called Wild, and Wood Vine, Tamus, or Ladies' Seal. The white is called White Vine by some; and the black, Black Vine.

DESCRIPTION: The common White Bryony grows upon hedges, sending forth many long, rough, very tender branches, with many very rough, and broad leaves cut into five partitions. At the several joints comes forth a long stalk bearing many whitish flowers. [The small fruits, very red when they are ripe, are] of no good scent, but of a most loathsome taste [that] provokes vomit.

PLACE: It grows on banks, or under hedges, through this land; the roots lie very deep. [Found throughout much of Europe; scattered in North America.]

GOVERNMENT AND VIRTUES: They are furious martial plants. The root of Briony purges the belly with great violence, troubling the stomach and burning the liver, and therefore not rashly to be taken; but being corrected, is very profitable for the diseases of the head, as falling sickness, giddiness, and swimmings, by drawing away much phlegm and rheumatic humours that oppress the head, as also the joints and sinews; and is therefore good for palsies, convulsions, cramps, stitches in the sides, and the dropsy, and for provoking urine. The leaves, fruit, and root do cleanse old and filthy sores, are good against fretting and running cankers, gangrenes, and tetters and therefore the berries are by some people called tetter-berries. The root cleanses the skin from all black and blue spots, freckles, morphew [blemishes], leprosy, foul scars, or other deformity whatsoever; also all running scabs and manginess are healed by the powder of the dried root, or the juice thereof, but especially by the fine white hardened juice. The distilled water of the root works the same effects, but more weakly; the root bruised and applied of itself to any place where the bones are broken, helps to draw them forth, as also splinters and thorns in the flesh; and being applied with a little wine mixed therewith, it breaks boils, and helps whitlows on the joints. For all these latter, beginning at sores, cancers, etc., apply it outwardly, mixing it with a little hog's grease, or other convenient ointment. As for the former diseases where it must be taken inwardly, it purges very violently, and needs an abler hand to correct it than most country people have.

MODERN USES AND CAUTION: As you might guess from Culpeper's described "virtues," bryony is more likely to be found in a book on poisonous plants rather than an herbal. It contains toxic bitter terpenoids called cucurbitacins, which act as a strong laxative and induce vomiting. **CAUTION:** Avoid use.

....

BUCK'S-HORN PLANTAIN

(PLANTAGO CORONOPUS)

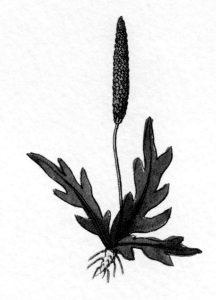

DESCRIPTION: [It has] long, narrow, hairy, dark green leaves like grass, but those that follow are gashed in on both sides and pointed at the ends, resembling a buck's horn (whereof it took its name), and bearing a small, long spiky head, like to those of the common Plantain.

PLACE: They grow in sandy grounds. [Native to Africa, temperate Asia, Europe, and Pakistan.]

GOVERNMENT AND VIRTUES: It is under the dominion of Saturn, and is of a gallant, drying, and binding quality. This boiled in wine and drank, and some of the leaves put to the hurt place, is an excellent remedy for the biting of the viper or adder. The same being also drank, helps those that are troubled with the stone in the kidneys, by cooling the heat of the part afflicted, and strengthens them; also weak stomachs that cannot retain, but cast up their meat. It stays all bleeding both at mouth or nose; bloody urine or the bloody-flux [dysentery], and stops the lask [diarrhea] of the belly and bowels. The leaves hereof bruised and laid to their sides that have an ague, suddenly ease the fits; and the leaves and roots applied to the wrists, works the same effect. The herb boiled in ale and wine, and given for some mornings and evenings together, stays the distillation of hot and sharp rheums falling into the eyes from the head, and helps all sorts of sore eyes.

MODERN USES: A lost vegetable of European gardens, buck's-horn plantain—also known as "star-of-the-earth"—has slipped into obscurity. During the early modern era from the 1500s to the 1800s, it was grown as a garden vegetable in England and France. It was still seen in seed lists in the early eighteenth century, but disappeared from gardens by the early nineteenth century. John Gerarde in his *Herball* (1633) suggests that to treat fevers nine whole buck's-horn plantain plants ("roots and all") can be hung around the neck of a man, and seven plants around the necks of women or children.

. . . .

BUGLE
(*AJUGA REPTANS*)

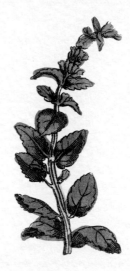

DESCRIPTION: The square stalk rises up to be half a yard high sometimes, with the leaves set by couples, the flowers of a blueish colour.

PLACE: They grow in woods, copses, and fields, generally throughout England. [Introduced to flower gardens centuries ago, bugle is widely naturalized in eastern North America and native throughout Europe, temperate Asia, and East Africa.]

GOVERNMENT AND VIRTUES: This herb belongs to Dame Venus: If the virtues of it makes you fall in love with it (as they will if you be wise) keep a syrup of it to take inwardly, an ointment and plaster of it to use outwardly, always by you.

The decoction of the leaves and flowers made in wine, and taken, dissolves the congealed blood in those that are bruised inwardly by a fall, or otherwise is very effectual for any inward wounds, thrusts, or stabs in the body or bowels; and it is an especial help in all wound-drinks, and for those that are liver-grown (as they call it.) It is wonderful in curing all manner of ulcers and sores, whether new and fresh, or old and inveterate; yea, gangrenes and fistulas also, if the leaves bruised and applied, or their juice be used to wash and bathe the place; and the same made into a lotion, and some honey and alum, cures all sores in the mouth and gums, be they ever so foul, or of long continuance; and works no less powerfully and effectually for such ulcers and sores as happen in the secret parts of men and women. Being also taken inwardly, or outwardly applied, it helps those that have broken any bone, or have any member out of joint.

The truth is, I have known this herb cure some diseases of Saturn, of which I thought good to quote one. Many times such as give themselves much to drinking are troubled with strange fancies, strange sights in the night time, and some with voices, as also with the disease Ephialtes, or the Mare. I take the reason of this to be (according to Fernelius) a melancholy vapour made thin by excessive drinking strong liquor, and, so flies up and disturbs the fancy, and breeds imaginations like itself, *viz.* fearful and troublesome. Those I have known cured by taking only two spoonfuls, of the syrup of this herb after supper two hours, when you go to bed. But whether this does it by sympathy, or antipathy, is some doubt in astrology. I know there is great antipathy between Saturn and Venus in matter of procreation; yea, such a one, that the barrenness of Saturn can be removed by none but Venus! Nor the lust of Venus be repelled by none but Saturn; but I am not of opinion this is done this way, and my reason is, because these vapours though in quality melancholy, yet by their flying upward, seem to be something aerial; therefore I rather think it is done by antipathy; Saturn being exalted in Libra, in the house of Venus.

MODERN USES: A small, attractive member of the mint family, bugle is used in tea to slow internal and external bleeding. Considered to be astringent, mildly laxative, and wound healing. Various compounds in bugle suggest a rational, scientific basis for the wound-healing claims of old, including antioxidant and anti-inflammatory activity.

....

BURDOCK

(ARCTIUM LAPPA)

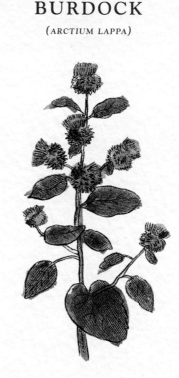

It is so well known, even by the little boys, who pull off the burs to throw and stick upon each other, that I shall spare to write any description of it.

PLACE: They grow plentifully by ditches and watersides, and by the highways almost everywhere through this land. [Found in fields, wasteland, and roadsides; native throughout Europe and Asia and naturalized in North America.]

GOVERNMENT AND VIRTUES: Venus challenges this herb for her own, and by its leaf or seed you may draw

the womb which way you please, either upwards by applying it to the crown of the head, in case it falls out; or downwards in fits of the mother, by applying it to the soles of the feet; or if you would stay it in its place, apply it to the navel, and that is one good way to stay the child in it. The Burdock leaves are cooling, moderately dry-ing, and discussing withal, whereby it is good for old ulcers and sores. The juice of the leaves, or rather the roots themselves, given to drink with old wine, doth wonderfully help the biting of any serpents. The juice of the leaves being drank with honey, provokes urine, and remedies the pain of the bladder. The seed being drank in wine forty days together, doth wonderfully help the sciatica. The leaves bruised with the white of an egg, and applied to any place burnt with fire, takes out the fire, gives sudden ease, and heals it up afterwards. The roots may be preserved with sugar, and taken fasting, or at other times, for the same purposes, and for consumptions, the stone, and the lask [diarrhea]. The seed is much commended to break the stone, and cause it to be expelled by urine, and is often used with other seeds and things to that purpose.

MODERN USES: Dried burdock roots are used in Western herbal traditions for gastrointestinal ailments, gout, arthritis, and as a "blood purifier" to help clear skin conditions. Burdock is consid-ered diuretic, antidiabetic, anti-inflammatory, antioxidant, and antimicrobial. It is commonly grown in Japanese and Korean vegetable gardens for the edible roots. The leaves are used similarly to the root, and, when young, are used in salads. In traditional Chinese medicine, the seeds are used to relieve sore throat and reduce swelling, among other uses.

....

BUR MARIGOLD

(BIDENS TRIPARTITA)

Water Agrimony

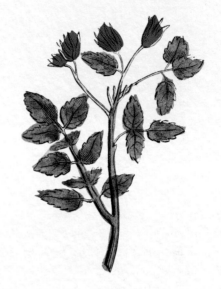

DESCRIPTION: The stalk grows up about two feet high, sometimes higher. They are of a dark purple colour. The leaves are fringed. The flowers at the top [are] of a brown yellow colour, spotted with black spots. If you rub them between your fingers, they smell like rosin or cedar when it is burnt.

PLACE: [A worldwide annual weed found in wet soils near ponds, ditches, and marshy fields.]

GOVERNMENT AND VIRTUES: It is a plant of Jupiter, as well as the other Agrimony, only this belongs to the celestial sign Cancer. It heals and dries, cuts and cleanses thick and tough humours of the breast, and for this I hold it inferior to but few herbs that grow. It helps the cachexia or evil disposition of the body, the dropsy and yellow-jaundice. It opens obstructions of the liver, molli-fies the hardness of the spleen, being applied out-wardly. It breaks imposthumes [abscesses] away inwardly. It is an excellent remedy for the third

day ague [malarial fever]. It provokes urine and the terms; it kills worms, and cleanses the body of sharp humours, which are the cause of itch and scabs; the herb being burnt, the smoke thereof drives away flies, wasps, etc. It strengthens the lungs exceedingly. Country people give it to their cattle when they are troubled with the cough, or broken-winded.

MODERN USES: Recent studies confirm the anti-oxidant, antimicrobial, antifungal, and antidiabetic activity of water extracts of bur marigold. Traditionally, an infusion of the aboveground dried herb has been used for acute respiratory infections, gout, colitis, and allergies. Also used for urinary tract infections, fevers, and ulcerative colitis. In developing countries, it is used in modern herbal practice for dysentery and acute enteritis; also applied as an ointment for psoriasis.

....

BURNET

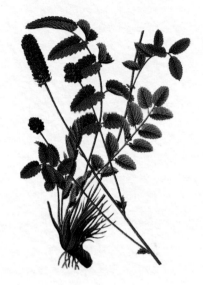

The common garden Burnet is so well known, that it needs no description. There is another sort which is wild [*Poterium sanguisorba*; syn. *Sanguisorba minor*].

PLACE: It first grows frequently in gardens. The wild kind grows in diverse counties of this land. [Garden Burnet (*Sanguisorba officinalis*) is widespread in wet soils and along streams in Europe, Asia, and western North America.]

GOVERNMENT AND VIRTUES: This is an herb the Sun challenges dominion over, and is a most precious herb, little inferior to Betony; the continual use of it preserves the body in health, and the spirits in vigour. They are accounted to be both of one property, but the lesser is more effectual because quicker and more aromatic. It is a friend to the heart, liver, and other principal parts of a man's body. Two or three of the stalks, with leaves put into a cup of wine, especially claret, are known to quicken the spirits, refresh and cheer the heart,

and drive away melancholy. It is a special help to defend the heart from noisome vapours, and from infection of the pestilence, the juice thereof being taken in some drink, and the party laid to sweat thereupon. They have also a drying and an astringent quality, whereby they are available in all manner of fluxes of blood or humours, to staunch bleedings inward or outward, lasks [diarrhea], scourings, the bloody-flux [dysentery], women's too abundant flux of courses, the whites, and the choleric belchings and castings of the stomach, and is a singular wound-herb for all sorts of wounds, both of the head and body, either inward or outward, for all old ulcers, running cankers, and most sores, to be used either by the juice or decoction of the herb, or by the powder of the herb or root, or the water of the distilled herb, or ointment by itself, or with other things to be kept. The seed is also no less effectual both to stop fluxes, and dry up moist sores, being taken in powder inwardly in wine, or steeled water, that is, wherein hot rods of steel have been quenched; or the powder, or the seed mixed with the ointments.

MODERN USES: Herb use often has a cultural context. Chinese medicinal preparations of burnet root are used in conjunction with patients receiving chemotherapy or radiation. It is believed that saponins in the root induce the production of mature blood cells from the bone marrow, which may be suppressed during conventional cancer treatment. This combination of Western medicine and traditional Chinese medicine is practiced mostly in China or other Asian countries where herb use is a normal part of medical practice. The root and leaves staunch bleeding and lessen diarrhea. Pharmacological studies suggest anti-inflammatory, antioxidant, astringent, styptic, wound-healing, and neuroprotective properties. Science is just beginning to unlock this herb's potential.

....

BURNET SAXIFRAGE

(*PIMPINELLA SAXIFRAGA, PIMPINELLA MAJOR*)

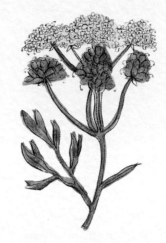

DESCRIPTION: The greater sort of our English Burnet Saxifrage grows up with diverse long stalks of winged leaves, set directly opposite one to another on both sides. At the top of the stalks stand umbels of white flowers. Our lesser Burnet Saxifrage hath much finer leaves than the former, and very small. The umbels of the flowers are white, and the seed very small.

PLACE: These grow in moist meadows. [Burnet saxifrage is found throughout much of Europe.]

GOVERNMENT AND VIRTUES: They are both of them herbs of the Moon. The Saxifrages are hot as pepper. They have the same properties the parsleys have, but in provoking urine, and causing the pains thereof, and of the wind and colic, are much more effectual, the roots or seed being used either in powder, or in decoctions, or any other way; and likewise helps the windy pains of the mother, and to procure their courses, and to break and void the stone in the kidneys, to digest cold, viscous, and tough phlegm in the stomach, and is an especial remedy against all kind of venom. Some do use to make the seeds into comfits (as

they do caraway seeds) which is effectual to all the purposes aforesaid. The juice of the herb dropped into the most grievous wounds of the head, dries up their moisture, and heals them quickly. Some women use the distilled water to take away freckles or spots in the skin or face; and to drink the same sweetened with sugar for all the purposes aforesaid.

MODERN USES: The roots and leaves of both the burnet saxifrage (*Pimpinella saxifraga*) and the greater burnet saxifrage (*Pimpinella major*) are used as folk medicines for their mild expectorant and antitussive effects in the treatment of upper respiratory tract infections and catarrhs. The tea was also gargled for sore throat. The leaves were formerly used for stimulating digestion and as a wash for varicose veins. Not commonly in use except as ingredients in polyherbal formulations.

....

BUTCHER'S-BROOM

(*RUSCUS ACULEATUS*)

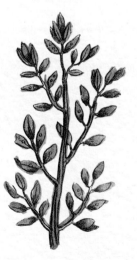

It is called Ruscus, and Bruscus, Kneeholm, Knee-holly, Kneehulver, and Pettigree.

DESCRIPTION: The first shoots that sprout from the root of Butcher's Broom are thick, whitish, and short, somewhat like those of Asparagus, but are spread into diverse [green] branches, whereon are set somewhat broad and almost round hard leaves and prickly. It has small whitish green flowers, consisting of four small round pointed [petals].

PLACE: It grows in copses, and upon heaths and wastelands. [Common throughout Europe and North Africa; naturalized in Mexico.]

GOVERNMENT AND VIRTUES: It is a plant of Mars, being of a gallant cleansing and opening quality. The decoction of the root made with wine opens obstructions, provokes urine, helps to expel gravel and the stone, the strangury and women's courses, also the yellow jaundice and the head-ache; and with same honey or sugar put thereunto, cleanses the breast of phlegm, and the chest of such clammy humours gathered therein. The decoction of the root drank, and a poultice made of the berries and leaves applied, are effectual in knitting and consolidating broken bones or parts out of joint. The common way of using it, is to boil the root of it, and Parsley, and Fennel, and Smallage in white wine, and drink the decoction, adding the like quantity of Grass-root to them: The more of the root you boil, the stronger will the decoction be; I hope you have wit enough to give the strongest decoction to the strongest bodies.

MODERN USES: Butcher's-broom is used traditionally as a diuretic and mild laxative. Extracts are considered anti-inflammatory and used to treat symptoms of varicose veins and chronic venous insufficiency, helping to relieve cramps, itching, swelling, and minor pain. Topical preparations are used for hemorrhoids. **CAUTION:** May cause contact dermatitis or irritation.

....

BUTTERBUR

(PETASITES HYBRIDUS)

Petasites

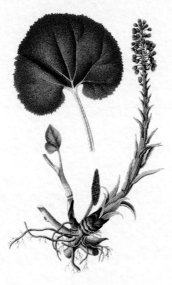

DESCRIPTION: This rises up in February, with a thick stalk about a foot high, and at the top a long spiked head; flowers of a blue or deep red colour, according to the soil where it grows, and before the stalk with the flowers have abiden a month above ground, it will be withered and gone, and blow away with the wind, and the leaves will begin to spring, which being full grown, are very large and broad.

PLACE AND TIME: They grow in low and wet grounds by rivers and water sides. Their flower (as is said) rising and decaying in [spring], before their leaves. [Butterbur is common in moist ground throughout Europe.]

GOVERNMENT AND VIRTUES: It is under the dominion of the Sun, and therefore is a great strengthener of the heart, and clearer of the vital spirit. The roots thereof are by long experience found to be very available against the plague and pestilential fevers by provoking sweat; if the powder thereof be taken in wine, it also resists the force of any other poison. The decoction of the root in wine, is singularly good for those that wheeze much, or are short-winded. It provokes urine also, and women's courses, and kills the flat and broad worms in the belly. The powder of the root doth wonderfully help to dry up the moisture of the sores that are hard to be cured, and takes away all spots and blemishes of the skin. It were well if gentlewomen would keep this root preserved, to help their poor neighbors. *It is fit the rich should help the poor, for the poor cannot help themselves.*

MODERN USES: Herbs were once called "simples," but modern understanding of butterbur root and leaf extracts is anything but simple. Different chemotypes or chemical types may have different effects. The plant also contains liver-toxic pyrrolizidine alkaloids; therefore, producers of modern butterbur herbal extracts must remove the toxic components. Modern use includes treatment of acute spastic pain of the urinary tract (such as in cases of urinary stones) as well as gastrointestinal spasms. Proprietary products are also formulated to reduce spasms for chronic headaches and migraines. Still other products are formulated for use in treating allergic rhinitis and asthma. **CAUTION:** Only properly prepared extracts (with toxic alkaloids removed) should be used. See product labels.

....

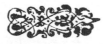

BUTTERCUP

(RANUNCULUS ACRIS)

Crowfoot

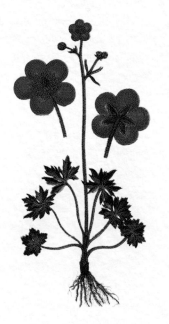

Many are the names this furious biting herb has obtained, almost enough to make up a Welshman's pedigree, if he fetch no farther than John of Gaunt, or William the Conqueror; for it is called Frog's-foot, from the Greek name Barrakion: Crowfoot, Gold Knobs, Gold Cups, King's Knob, Baffiners, Troilflowers, Polts, Locket Gouions, and Butterflowers.

Abundance are the sorts of this herb, that to describe them all would tire the patience of Socrates himself, but because I have not yet attained to the spirit of Socrates, I shall but describe the most usual.

DESCRIPTION: The most common Buttercup has many thin great leaves, cut into diverse parts, in taste biting and sharp, biting and blistering the tongue: It bears many flowers, and those of a bright, resplendent, yellow colour. I do not remember, that I ever saw anything yellower. Virgins, in ancient time, used to make powder of them to furrow bride beds.

PLACE: They grow very common everywhere; unless you turn your head into a hedge you cannot but see them as you walk.

GOVERNMENT AND VIRTUES: This fiery and hot-spirited herb of Mars is no way fit to be given inwardly, but an ointment of the leaves or flowers will draw a blister, and may be so fitly applied to the nape of the neck to draw back rheum [watery discharge] from the eyes. The herb being bruised and mixed with a little mustard, draws a blister as well, and as perfectly as Cantharides, and with far less danger to the vessels of urine, which Cantharides naturally delight to wrong. I knew the herb once applied to a pestilential rising that was fallen down, and it saved life even beyond hope; it were good to keep an ointment and plaster of it, if it were but for that.

MODERN USES: Culpepper aptly describes the visual features and appropriate dangers of handling or ingesting the common buttercup. The fresh plant of this and other *Ranunculus* species contain the highly irritating (and blistering) toxic protoanemonin, which causes intense pain, inflammation, and ulceration, both internally and externally. Culpepper foreshadows recent science when he observes, "I do not remember that I ever saw anything yellower." Physicists have revealed that buttercups' brilliant yellow flowers have mirror-like glossy cells that produce iridescent flashes—a color adaptation seen in animals but rarely in plants.

....

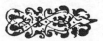

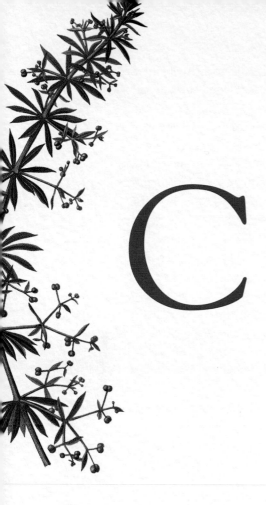

C

CALENDULA
(CALENDULA OFFICINALIS)

Marigolds, Pot Marigold

These being so plentiful in every garden, and so well known that they need no description. [Native to south-central Europe and North Africa. Widely cultivated in herb gardens since ancient times.]

GOVERNMENT AND VIRTUES: It is an herb of the Sun, and under Leo. They strengthen the heart exceedingly, and are very expulsive, and a little less effectual in the small-pox and measles than saffron. The juice of Calendula leaves mixed with vinegar, and any hot swelling bathed with it, instantly gives ease, and assuages it. The flowers, either green or dried, are much used in possets, broths, and drink, as a comforter of the heart and spirits, and to expel any malignant or pestilential quality which might annoy them. A plaster made with the dry flowers in powder, hog's-grease, turpentine, and rosin, applied to the breast, strengthens and succors the heart infinitely in fevers, whether pestilential or not.

MODERN USES: In both traditional and modern use, calendula—as a lotion, tincture, ointment, or a wash of the cooled tea—is applied externally to speed the healing of sprains, bruises, cuts, minor infections, sores, slow-to-heal wounds, and burns. It is also used as a gargle to reduce the inflammation of a sore throat or the oral mucosa. Effects include helping to rebuild cellular tissue at the site of a wound, reducing swelling and discharges, and lessening scarring from burns, abscesses, or abrasions. Calendula and its preparations have anti-inflmmatory and immunostimulant activity.

....

CARAWAY

(CARUM CARVI)

Carraway

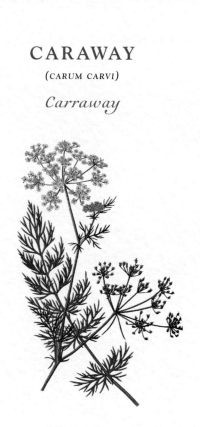

It is on account of the seeds principally that the Caraway is cultivated.

DESCRIPTION: It bears diverse stalks of fine cut leaves, and at the top small umbels of white flowers, which turn into small blackish seed, smaller than the Aniseed, and of a quicker and hotter taste.

PLACE: It is usually sown with us in gardens. [It is cultivated and found in fields and wastelands throughout Europe and Asia; naturalized in cool, temperate regions of North America.]

GOVERNMENT AND VIRTUES: This is also a Mercurial plant. Caraway seed has a moderate sharp quality, whereby it breaks wind and provokes urine, which also the herb doth. The root is better food than the parsnip; it is pleasant and comfortable to the stomach, and helps digestion. The seed is conducing to all cold griefs of the head and stomach, bowels, or mother, as also the wind in them, and helps to sharpen the eye-sight. The powder of the seed put into a poultice, takes away black and blue spots of blows and bruises. The herb itself, or with some of the seed bruised and fried, laid hot in a bag or double cloth, to the lower parts of the belly, eases the pains of the wind cholic.

The roots of Caraway eaten as men do parsnips, strengthen the stomach of ancient people exceedingly, and they need not to make a whole meal of them neither, and are fit to be planted in every garden. Caraway comfits once only dipped in sugar, and half a spoonful of them eaten in the morning fasting, and as many after each meal, is a most admirable remedy, for those that are troubled with wind.

MODERN USES: "It breaks wind," says Culpeper, who describes caraway seed's widespread traditional use to relieve digestive gas, dyspepsia, and diarrhea. Among its pharmacological activities include anti-inflammatory, antispasmodic, antimicrobial, antioxidant, carminative, and immunomodulatory effects. Up to 2 grams of seeds are chewed or crushed and made into tea. Traditional use as a diuretic is scientifically confirmed. **CAUTION:** Rare allergic reactions may occur. May be confused with poison hemlock (*Conium maculatum*) with fatal consequences.

....

CARNATIONS, CLOVE PINK

(DIANTHUS CARYOPHYLLUS)

Clove Gilliflowers

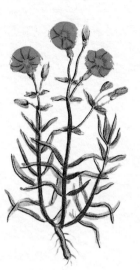

It is vain to describe an herb so well known. [Native to the Balkans, and introduced to European gardens and naturalized.]

GOVERNMENT AND VIRTUES: They are gallant, fine, temperate flowers, of the nature and under the dominion of Jupiter; yea, so temperate, that no excess, neither in heat, cold, dryness, nor moisture, can be perceived in them; they are great strengtheners both of the brain and heart, and will therefore serve either for cordials or cephalics, as your occasion will serve. There is both a syrup and a conserve made of them alone, commonly to be had at every apothecary's. To take now and then a little of either, strengthens nature much, in such as are in consumptions. They are also excellently good in hot pestilent fevers, and expel poison.

MODERN USES: Clove pink gets its name from the similarity of the flower's fragrance to cloves. Cultivated in England before the twelfth century, the "Clove Gillyflower" is the wild progenitor of the modern carnation, which has endless variations through hybridization and selection and is barely recognizeable as the plant of Culpeper's time. It was used to flavor ale and wine. Culpeper's contemporaries used the flowers to treat nervous complaints, as a spirit-lifting cordial, and to comfort the heart. By the late eighteenth century, it was used only for flavoring and coloring other medicines; use has fallen into obscurity except as a pleasantly fragranced ornamental flower. The essential oil is antibacterial, antiviral, and used as a traditional remedy for wound healing and to treat gum and throat infections. One study found that the essential oil is toxic to the larvae of the mosquito that carries West Nile virus. **CAUTION:** Some are allergic to carnations, an occupational hazard in the floral industry.

....

CARROTS

(DAUCUS CAROTA)

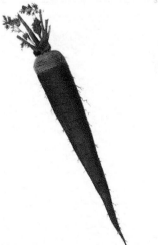

Garden Carrots are so well known, that they need no description; but they are of less physical use than the wild kind (as indeed almost in all herbs the wild are the most effectual in physic, as being more powerful in operation than the garden kinds).

PLACE: The wild kind grows in diverse parts of this land plentifully by the field-sides, and untilled places. [Native throughout Europe; widely naturalized in both eastern and western North America as well as parts of Africa.]

GOVERNMENT AND VIRTUES: Wild Carrots belong to Mercury, and therefore break wind, and remove stitches in the sides, provoke urine and women's courses, and helps to break and expel the stone; the seed also of the same works the like effect, and is good for the dropsy, and those whose bellies are swelling with wind; helps the cholic, the stone in the kidneys, and rising of the mother; being taken in wine, or boiled in wine and taken, it helps conception. The leaves being applied with honey to running sores or ulcers, do cleanse them.

I suppose the seeds of them perform this better than the roots; and though Galen commended garden Carrots highly to break wind, yet experience teaches they breed it first, and we may thank nature for expelling it, not they; the seeds of them expel wind indeed, and so mend what the root mars.

MODERN USES: Wild carrot root is used in herbal traditions as a diuretic, primarily to treat kidney and bladder conditions, particularly urinary calculi and difficulty urinating. The root of the cultivated carrot provides the benefit of high carotenoid content, which transforms into vitamin A when metabolized in the liver. **CAUTION:** Some individuals may be allergic to wild carrot. Given the similarity in the appearance of wild carrot and poison hemlock (*Conium maculatum*) leaves, there are many cases of poisoning.

....

CATNIP
(*NEPETA CATARIA*)
Nep, or Catmint

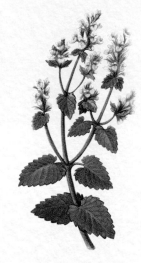

DESCRIPTION: Common Garden Catnip [has] four-square stalks, with a hoariness on them, a yard high or more, full of branches, bearing at every joint two broad leaves [with soft white hairs], and of a strong sweet scent. The flowers grow in large tufts at the tops of the branches.

PLACE: It is only nursed up in our gardens. [Found throughout most of Europe and western Asia; naturalized through North America and elsewhere.]

GOVERNMENT AND VIRTUES: It is an herb of Venus. Catnip is generally used for women to procure their courses, being taken inwardly or outwardly, either alone, or with other convenient herbs in a decoction to bathe them, or sit over the hot fumes thereof; and by the frequent use thereof, it takes away barrenness, and the wind, and pains of the mother. It is also used in pains of the head coming of any cold cause, catarrhs, rheums, and for swimming and giddiness thereof, and is of special use for the windiness of the stomach and belly. It is effectual for any cramp, or cold aches, to dissolve cold and wind that afflict the place, and is used for colds, coughs, and shortness of breath. The juice thereof drank in wine, is profitable for those that are bruised by an accident. The green herb bruised and applied to the fundament and lying there two or three hours, eases the pains of the piles; the juice also being made up into an ointment, is effectual for the same purpose. The head washed with a decoction thereof, it takes away scabs, and may be effectual for other parts of the body also.

MODERN USES: Bruised catnip leaves release essential oils and attract cats. This "catnip response" usually affects the approximately 70 percent of felines that have an inherited autosomal dominant gene, including house cats and large cats such as lions and tigers. Lasting for about fifteen minutes, it includes sniffing, licking, head-shaking, chin-rubbing and head-over rolling, but this effect is only produced by smelling the herb, not eating it. Catnip is not a human euphoric. The tea is used as a folk remedy for colds, flu, diarrhea, bronchitis, and menstrual disorders. It is antispasmodic, diaphoretic, carminative, and an emmenagogue.

....

CELANDINE

(CHELIDONIUM MAJUS)

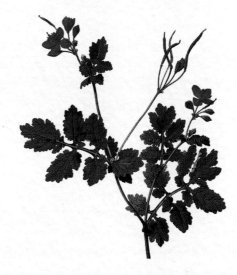

DESCRIPTION: This hath diverse tender, round stalks, very brittle and easy to break, with large tender broad leaves, of a dark blueish green colour, full of yellow sap, when any is broken, of a bitter taste, and strong scent. At the flowers [are] four [petals], after which come small long pods, with blackish seed therein.

PLACE: [Found in fields, wastelands, and near gardens throughout Europe. Widely naturalized in Asia, northwestern Africa, and cool, temperate areas of North America.]

GOVERNMENT AND VIRTUES: This is an herb of the Sun, and under the Celestial Lion, and is one of the best cures for the eyes; for, all that know anything in astrology, know that the eyes are subject to the luminaries; let it then be gathered when the Sun is in Leo, and the Moon in Aries, applying to this time; let Leo arise, then may you make into an oil or ointment, which you please, to anoint your sore eyes with. I can prove it doth both my own experience, and the experience of those to whom

I have taught it, that most desperate sore eyes have been cured by this only medicine; and then, I pray, is not this far better than endangering the eyes by the art of the needle? The herb or root boiled in white Wine and drank, a few Aniseeds being boiled therewith, opens obstructions of the liver and gall, helps the yellow jaundice; and often using it, helps the dropsy and the itch, and those who have old sores in their legs, or other parts of the body. The distilled water, with a little sugar and a little good treacle mixed therewith (the party upon the taking being laid down to sweat a little) has the same effect. The juice dropped into the eyes, cleanses them from films and cloudiness which darken the sight, but it is best to allay the sharpness of the juice with a little breast milk. It is good in all old filthy corroding creeping ulcers wheresoever, to stay their malignity of fretting and running, and to cause them to heal more speedily: The juice often applied to tetters, ring-worms, or other such like spreading cankers, will quickly heal them, and rubbed often upon warts, will take them away. The juice or decoction of the herb gargled between the teeth that ache, eases the pain, and the powder of the dried root laid upon any aching, hollow or loose tooth, will cause it to fall out. The juice mixed with some powder of brimstone is not only good against the itch, but takes away all discolourings of the skin whatsoever: and if it chance that in a tender body it causes any itchings or inflammations, by bathing the place with a little vinegar it is helped.

MODERN USES: A member of the poppy family (Papaveraceae), celandine has been evaluated for anti-inflammatory, choleretic, antimicrobial, antioxidant, antispasmodic, pain-relieving, and liver-protective properties. Various alkaloids and proteins in the plant's yellow exudate are believed to be responsible for the medicinal effects. Until recently (see Caution), preparations of celandine had been used in phytomedicine for the treatment of bile duct disorders, dyspepsia, flatulence, and irritable bowel syndrome. Externally it has been applied to warts and corns. Still widely used in Eastern Europe. **CAUTION:** At least fifty reports of liver toxicity associated with celandine have led to a recommendation by the European Medicines Agency that use of the herb should be discouraged. Culpeper describes celandine use for cataracts, a use which dates at least to the thirteenth century, but has no modern scientific basis.

....

CELANDINE, LESSER

(*FICARIA VERNA; SYN. RANUNCULUS FICARIA*)

Pilewort, Fogwort

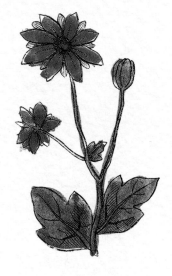

I wonder what ailed the ancients to give this the name Celandine, which resembles it neather in nature nor form; it acquired the name of Pilewort from its virtues, and it being no great matter where I set it down, so I set it down at all, I humoured Dr. Tradition so much, as to set him down here.

DESCRIPTION: This Celandine or Pilewort (which you please) doth spread many round pale green leaves, set on weak and trailing branches which lie upon the ground, and are flat, smooth, and somewhat shining, standing on a long foot-stalk, among which rise small yellow flowers.

PLACE: It grows for the most part in moist corners of fields and places that are near water sides, yet will abide in drier ground if they be a little shady. [Found throughout much of Europe and western Asia; naturalized and rapidly expanding its range in cool, moist woods and streamsides in North America.]

GOVERNMENT AND VIRTUES: It is under the dominion of Mars, and behold here another verification of the learning of the ancients, *viz.* that the virtue of an herb may be known by its signature; for if you dig up the root of it, you shall perceive the perfect image of the disease which they commonly call the piles. The decoction of the leaves and roots wonderfully helps piles and hemorrhoids, also kernels by the ears and throat, called the king's evil [unusual swelling of lymph nodes or scrofula], or any other hard wens or tumours.

Here's another secret for my countrymen and women: Pilewort made into an oil, ointment, or plaster, readily cures both the piles, or hemorrhoids, and the king's evil. The very herb borne about one's body next the skin helps in such diseases, though it never touch the place grieved; let poor people make much of it for those uses; with this I cured my own daughter of the king's evil, broke the sore, drew out a quarter of a pint of corruption, cured without any scar at all in one week's time.

MODERN USES: Lesser celandine has been used for centuries as a folk treatment for hemorrhoids. Pharmacological studies (mostly in Eastern Europe) suggest anti-inflammatory, astringent, antibiotic, and anti-hemorrhagic activity. The leaves, high in vitamin C, are harvested before the plant flowers in early spring and are traditionally eaten in small quantities. **CAUTION:** A 2015 case report attributed liver toxicity to the use of the plant.

....

CELERY
(*APIUM GRAVEOLENS*)
Smallage

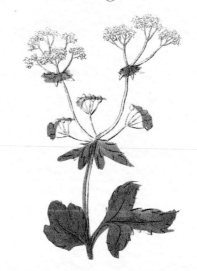

This is also very well-known, and therefore I shall not trouble the reader with any description thereof. [It is the wild source of the familiar vegetable celery.]

PLACE: It grows naturally in dry and marshy ground; but if it be sown in gardens, it there prospers very well.

GOVERNMENT AND VIRTUES: It is an herb of Mercury. [Celery] is hotter, drier, and much more medicinal than parsley, for it much more opens obstructions of the liver and spleen, rarefies thick phlegm, and cleanses it and the blood withal. It provokes urine and women's courses, and is singularly good against the yellow jaundice, tertian and quartan agues [malaria] if the juice thereof be taken, but especially made up into a syrup. The juice also put to honey of roses, and barley-water, is very good to gargle the mouth and throat of those that have sores and ulcers in them, and will quickly heal them. The same lotion also cleanses and heals all other foul ulcers and cankers elsewhere, if they be washed therewith. The seed is especially used to break and expel wind, to kill worms, and to help a stinking breath.

MODERN USES: Celery stems are best known as a familiar vegetable, but less appreciated are celery's traditional attributes as an aphrodisiac, diuretic, antispasmodic, and anti-inflammatory. Used as a folk medicine for the treatment of asthma, bronchitis, gout, and rheumatism. Celery seeds are used as a carminative to relieve gas and as a digestive stimulant, mild sedative, and anti-inflammatory for gout. **CAUTION:** Celery is known to cause severe allergic reactions in some individuals due to the high amounts of phototoxic compounds it contains.

....

CENTAURY

(*CENTAURIUM ERYTHRAEA;*
SYN. *EYRTHRAEA CENTAURIUM*)

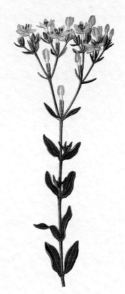

DESCRIPTION: This grows up most usually but with one round and somewhat crusted stalk, about a foot high or better; the flowers thus stand at the tops as it were in one umbel, are of a pale red. The whole plant is of an exceeding bitter taste.

PLACE: They grow ordinarily in fields, pastures, and woods. [Native to Europe, western Asia, northwestern Africa; naturalized in North America in the Pacific Northwest and Great Lakes region.]

GOVERNMENT AND VIRTUES: They are under the dominion of the Sun, as appears in that their flowers open and shut as the Sun, either shews or hides his face. This herb, boiled and drank, purges choleric and gross humours, and helps the sciatica; it opens obstructions of the liver, gall, and spleen, helps the jaundice, and eases the pains in the sides and hardness of the spleen, used outwardly, and is given with very good effect in agues. It helps those that have the dropsy, or the green-sickness, being much used by the Italians in powder for that purpose. It kill the worms in the belly, as is found by experience. The decoction thereof, *viz.* the tops of the stalks, with the leaves and flowers, is good against the cholic, and to bring down women's courses, and eases pains of the mother, and is very effectual in all pains of the joints, as the gout, cramps, or convulsions. A dram of the powder taken in wine is a wonderful good help against the biting and poison of an adder. It is singularly good both for green and fresh wounds, as also for old ulcers and sores, to close up the one and cleanse the other, and perfectly to cure them both, although they are hollow or fistulous; the green herb especially, being bruised and laid thereto. The decoction thereof dropped into the ears, cleanses them from worms, cleanses the foul ulcers and spreading scabs of the head, and takes away all freckles, spots, and marks in the skin, being washed with it; the herb is so safe you cannot fail in the using of it, only giving it inwardly for inward diseases. It is very wholesome, but not very toothsome.

MODERN USES: Centaury is widely regarded as a bitter tonic for the digestive system. It's a major ingredient in a proprietary combination phytomedicine—along with lovage (*Levisticum officinale*) and rosemary (*Rosmarinus officinalis*)—used for the prevention and treatment of urinary tract infections. The product is available in Belarus, Russia, and the Ukraine. Preparations of the plant, which contain the bitter component gentiopicrin, have been evaluated for antioxidant, antimicrobial, and anti-inflammatory activity, among other effects. Primarily used to treat dyspeptic discomfort by stimulating gastric secretions.

....

CHAMOMILE

(MATRICARIA CHAMOMILLA; SYN. MATRICARIA RECUTITA, CHAMOMILLA RECUTITA)

Camomile

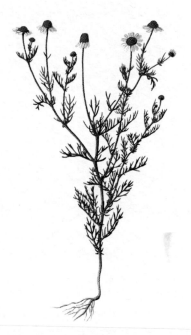

It is so well known everywhere, that it is but lost time and labour to describe it. [Native to the Mediterranean region and Eastern Europe, now widespread in Europe and East Asia, and naturalized in eastern North America. Widely cultivated elsewhere.]

GOVERNMENT AND VIRTUES: The virtues thereof are as follows. A decoction made of Chamomile, and drank, takes away all pains and stitches in the side. The flowers of Chamomile beaten, and made up into balls with Gill, drive away all sorts of agues, if the part grieved be anointed with that oil, taken from the flowers, from the crown of the head to the sole of the foot, and afterwards laid to sweat in his bed, and that he sweats well. This is Nechessor, an Egyptian's, medicine. It is profitable for all sorts of agues that come either from phlegm, or melancholy, or from an inflammation of the bowels, being applied when the humours causing them shall be concocted; and there is nothing more profitable to the sides and region of the liver and spleen than it. The bathing with a decoction of Chamomile takes away weariness, eases pains, to what part of the body so ever they be applied. It comforts the sinews that are over-strained, mollifies all swellings: It moderately comforts all parts that have need of warmth, digests and dissolves whatsoever has need thereof, by a wonderful speedy property. It eases all pains of the cholic and stone, and all pains and torments of the belly, and gently provokes urine. The flowers boiled in posset-drink provokes sweat, and helps to expel all colds, aches, and pains whatsoever, and is an excellent help to bring down women's courses. Syrup made of the juice of Chamomile, with the flowers, in white wine, is a remedy against the jaundice and dropsy. The oil made of the flowers of Chamomile, is much used against all hard swellings, pains or aches, shrinking of the sinews, or cramps, or pains in the joints, or any other part of the body. Being used in clysters, it helps to dissolve the wind and pains in the belly; anointed also, it helps stitches and pains in the sides.

MODERN USES: Chamomile is an herbal remedy that has stood the test of time. Dried chamomile flower heads are used in tea to relieve dyspepsia, gastritis, diarrhea, and mild anxiety. Although native to Europe, chamomile is used worldwide and is among the most commonly available herbal teas. It has antispasmodic, anti-inflammatory, and mild sedative actions, and is widely considered to be a gentle sleep aid. Chamomile extract (500 milligrams three times daily) has been evaluated in a clinical trial with positive outcomes for the treatment of generalized anxiety disorder. **CAUTION:** Rare allergic reactions have been linked to misidentification with other plant species.

....

CHESTNUT TREE
(CASTANEA SATIVA)
Chesnut Tree

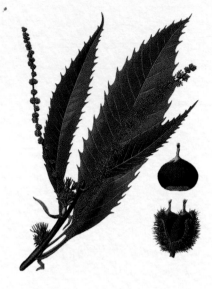

It were as needless to describe a tree so commonly known as to tell a man he had gotten a mouth.

PLACE: [Originating in deciduous mountain woodlands in southern Europe and western Asia, from Portugal to the Caspian Sea, the European sweet chestnut spread through Europe in ancient times, and was planted in woodlands and forests. By Roman times as many as eight different cultivated varieties were recognized.]

GOVERNMENT AND VIRTUES: The tree is abundantly under the dominion of Jupiter, and therefore the fruit must needs breed good blood, and yield commendable nourishment to the body; yet if eaten over-much, they make the blood thick, procure headache, and bind the body; the inner skin, that covers the nut, is of so binding a quality, that a scruple of it being taken by a man, or ten grains by a child, soon stops any flux whatsoever. The whole nut being dried and beaten into powder, and a dram taken at a time, is a good remedy to stop the terms in women. If you dry Chestnuts, (only the kernels I mean) both the barks being taken away, beat them into powder, and make the powder up into an electuary with honey, so have you an admirable remedy for the cough and spitting of blood.

MODERN USES: Though sweet chestnut nut is little used today medicinally, various by-products of its production, including the inner and outer husks and the leaves, are of research interest because of the potential antioxidant, antibacterial, anticarcinogenic, and heart-protective compounds that have been isolated from different plant parts. Traditionally the leaf tea was used to treat bronchitis, coughs, diarrhea, dyspepsia, and other conditions. The nuts of various species of *Castanea* have long been used for food in Europe, Asia, and North America. Billions of American chestnuts (*Castanea dentata*) died as the result of a blight in the early twentieth century; therefore, they are not as familiar a food as they once were to the American palate. **CAUTION:** Chestnut (*Castanea* spp.) should not be confused with the potentially toxic horse chestnut (*Aesculus* spp.).

....

CHICKPEA, GARBANZO BEAN
(CICER ARIETINUM)

Chick—Pease

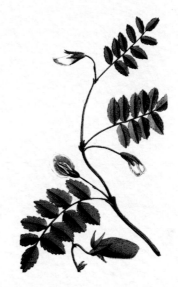

DESCRIPTION: The garden sorts whether red, black, or white, bring forth stalks a yard long, whereon do grow many small and almost round leaves. At the joints come forth one or two flowers, pea-fashion, either white or whitish, or purplish red.

PLACE AND TIME: They are sown in gardens, or fields as peas, being sown later than peas, and gathered at the same time with them, or presently after.

GOVERNMENT AND VIRTUES: They are both under the dominion of Venus. They are less windy than beans, but nourish more; they provoke urine, and are thought to increase sperm; they have a cleansing faculty, whereby they break the stone in the kidneys. To drink the cream of them, being boiled in water, is the best way. It moves the belly downwards, provokes women's courses and urine, increases both milk and seed. One ounce of Chickpeas, two ounces of French barley, and a small handful of Marshmallow roots, clean washed and cut, being boiled in the broth of a chicken, and four ounces taken in the morning, and fasting two hours after, is a good medicine for a pain in the sides. The white Chickpeas are used more for [food] than medicine, yet have the same effect, and are thought more powerful to increase milk and seed. The wild Chickpeas are so much more powerful than the garden kinds, by how much they exceed them in heat and dryness; whereby they do more open obstructions, break the stone, and have all the properties of cutting, opening, digesting, and dissolving; and this more speedily and certainly than the former.

MODERN USES: Chickpeas fall into the "your food should be your medicine" category. High in fiber, calcium, magnesium, proteins, and vitamin K, they're eaten in cultures around the world.

....

CHICKWEED

(*STELLARIA MEDIA*)

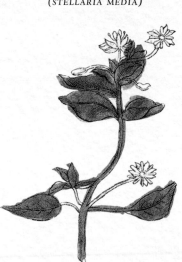

It is so generally known to most people, that I shall not trouble you with the description thereof,

nor myself with setting forth the several kinds, since but only two or three are considerable for their usefulness.

PLACE: They are usually found in moist and watery places, by wood sides, and elsewhere. [Chickweed is a cosmopolitan annual weed found throughout Europe, Asia, North America, and elsewhere.]

GOVERNMENT AND VIRTUES: It is a fine soft pleasing herb under the dominion of the Moon. It is found to be effectual as Purslane to all the purposes whereunto it serves, except for meat only. The herb bruised, or the juice applied (with cloths or sponges dipped therein) to the region of the liver, and as they dry, to have it fresh applied, doth wonderfully temperate the heat of the liver, and is effectual for all imposthumes [abscesses] and swellings whatsoever, for all redness in the face, wheals, pushes, itch, scabs; the juice either simply used, or boiled with hog's grease and applied, helps cramps, convulsions, and palsy. [It] is of good effect to ease pains from the heat and sharpness of the blood in the piles, and generally all pains in the body that arise of heat. Boil a handful of Chickweed, and a handful of red rose leaves dried, in a quart of muscadine, until a fourth part be consumed; then put to them a pint of oil of trotters or sheep's feet; let them boil a good while, still stirring them well; which being strained, anoint the grieved place therewith, warm against the fire, rubbing it well with one hand: and bind also some of the herb (if you will) to the place, and, with God's blessing, it will help it in three times dressing.

MODERN USES: Chickweed is a winter annual, usually emerging then going to seed early in the growing season. Fresh leaves are used as a salad green. Preparations of the fresh and dried leaf are widely used for skin conditions that cause redness or inflammation, much as Culpeper describes. It is believed to possess anti-inflammatory, diuretic, expectorant, cooling, and nutritional attributes. Its juice is a folk medicine to treat obesity. When evaluated in a laboratory model, it was found to prevent fat storage by inhibiting enzymes, resulting in a slowing of the absorption of fats and carbohydrates. More research is needed.

....

CHICORY

(*CICHORIUM INTYBUS*)

Succory

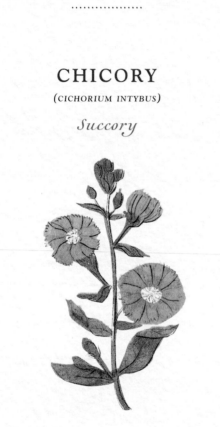

DESCRIPTION: [Chicory] bears blue flowers. The wild Chicory [has dandelion-like leaves at the base], from among which rises up a stalk, where stand the flowers, which are like [those of dandelions, only blue]. Take notice that the flowers are gone in on a sunny day, therefore delight in the shade. The whole plant is exceedingly bitter.

PLACE: This grows in many places [such as] untilled and barren fields [and roadsides]. [Native to Eurasia; a widespread weed elsewhere in North America, South America, and Australia.]

GOVERNMENT AND VIRTUES: It is an herb of Jupiter. Chicory is drier and less cold than Endive, so it opens more. A handful of the leaves, or roots boiled in wine or water, and a draught thereof drank fasting, drives forth choleric and phlegmatic humours, opens obstructions of the liver, gall and spleen; helps the yellow jaundice, the heat of the [kidneys], and of the urine; the dropsy also; and those that have an evil disposition in their bodies, by reason of long sickness, evil diet, &c. which the Greeks call Cachexia. A decoction thereof made with wine, and drank, is very effectual against long lingering ague [fevers]; and a dram of the seed in powder, drank in wine, before the fit of the ague [fever], helps to drive it away. The distilled water of the herb and flowers (if you can take them in time) hath the like properties, and is especially good for hot stomachs, and in [fevers], either pestilential or of long continuance; for swoonings and passions of the heart, for the heat and headache in children, and for the blood and liver. The said water, or the juice, or the bruised leaves applied outwardly, allay swellings, inflammations, St. Anthony's fire, pushes, wheals, and pimples, especially used with a little vinegar; as also to wash pestiferous sores. The said water is very effectual for nurses' breasts that are pained by the abundance of milk. The wild Succory, as it is more bitter, so it is more strengthening to the stomach and liver.

MODERN USES: Preparations of the bitter chicory root are used to stimulate digestion. Chicory is also a diuretic, laxative, and mild sedative. Used to relieve a feeling or fullness or bloating, slow digestion, and loss of appetite. Pharmacologically, it has anti-inflammatory, antidiabetic, antimicrobial, antioxidant, and immunostimulant effects;

liver-protective activity; and a low-density lipo-protein inhibiting effect. The leaves and flowers are used as vegetables, and the roasted root is a well-known additive to (or substitute for) coffee. The use of chicory root in coffee began as a means to stretch coffee supplies during wartime.

....

CHINESE LANTERN

(ALKEKENGI OFFICINARUM; SYN. PHYSALIS ALKEKENGI)

Winter–Cherries

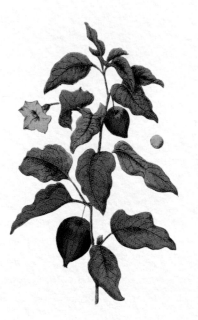

DESCRIPTION: The Chinese Lantern rises a yard high, [with] long green leaves, like nightshades, whitish flowers of five [petals], berries enclosed with thin skins, which change to reddish [and lantern-like with a red berry within].

PLACE: [Widespread and naturalized near gardens and field edges throughout most of Europe, western Asia, Japan, and China; widely cultivated and escaped from gardens.]

GOVERNMENT AND VIRTUES: This also is a plant of Venus. They are of great use in physic. The leaves being cooling, may be used in inflammations, but not opening as the berries and fruit are; which by drawing down the urine provoke it to be voided plentifully when it is stopped or grown hot, sharp, and painful in the passage; it is good also to expel the stone and gravel out of the kidneys and bladder, helping to dissolve the stone, and voiding it by grit or gravel sent forth in the urine; it also helps much to cleanse inward imposthumes [abscesses] or ulcers in the bladder, or in those that void a bloody or foul urine. The distilled water of the fruit, or the leaves together with them, or the berries, green or dry, distilled with a little milk and drank morning and evening with a little sugar, is effectual to all the purposes before specified, and especially against the heat and sharpness of the urine. I shall only mention one way, amongst many others, which might be used for ordering the berries, to be helpful for the urine and the stone; which is this. Take three or four good handfuls of the berries, either green or fresh, or dried, and having bruised them, put them into so many gallons of beer or ale when it is new tunned up. This drink taken daily, has been found to do much good to many, both to ease the pains, and expel urine and the stone, and to cause the stone not to engender. The decoction of the berries in wine and water is the most usual way; but the powder of them taken in drink is more effectual.

MODERN USES: Chinese lantern is a member of the nightshade family (Solanaceae) researched for possible anti-inflammatory, antibacterial, and antioxidant benefits. The fruits and seeds have been used in various herbal traditions (especially in China and India) for fevers, inflammation, difficulty urinating, and other urinary disorders. **CAUTION:** Green fruits contain solanine gly-coalkaloids, which may have an irritant effect on the gastrointestinal system.

....

CHIRON'S ALL-HEAL

(OPOPANAX CHIRONIUM)

All–Heal

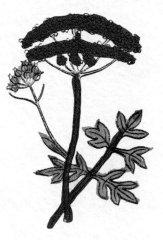

It is called All-heal, Hercules's All-heal, and Hercules's Woundwort. Some call it Panay, and others Opopane-wort.

DESCRIPTION: Its root is long, thick, and exceeding full of juice, of a hot and biting taste, the leaves are great and large, and winged almost like ash-tree leaves; towards the top come forth umbels of small yellow flowers.

PLACE: [A plant of well-drained, gravelly soils of the southern Mediterranean and Balkans.]

GOVERNMENT AND VIRTUES: It is under the dominion of Mars, hot, biting, and choleric; and remedies what evils Mars inflicts the body of man with, by sympathy, as vipers' flesh attracts poison, and the loadstone iron [magnetite]. It kills the worms, helps the gout, cramp, and convulsions, provokes urine, and helps all joint-aches. It helps all cold griefs of the head, the vertigo, falling-sickness, the lethargy, the wind cholic, obstructions of the liver and spleen, stone in the kidneys and bladder.

It provokes the terms [menstruation], expels the dead birth. It is excellent good for the griefs of the sinews, itch, stone, and tooth-ache, the biting of mad dogs and venomous beasts, and purges choler [bile] very gently.

MODERN USES: A gum resin from Chiron's all-heal was common in ancient pharmacies but fell into disuse by the mid-nineteenth century.

....

CHIVES

(ALLIUM SCHOENOPRASUM)

Cives

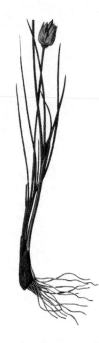

Called also Rush Leeks, Civet, and Sweth.

PLACE: [A familiar garden plant, chives grow wild in chalky, rocky soil throughout the colder regions of the Northern Hemisphere.]

GOVERNMENT AND VIRTUES: I confess I had not added these, had it not been for a country gentleman, who by a letter certified me, that amongst other herbs, I had left these out; they are indeed a kind of leek, hot and dry in the fourth degree as they are, and so under the dominion of Mars; If they be eaten raw, (I do not mean raw, opposite to roasted or boiled, but raw, opposite to chemical preparation) they send up very hurtful vapours to the brain, causing troublesome sleep, and spoiling the eye-sight, yet of them prepared by the art of the alchemist, may be made an excellent remedy for the stoppage of the urine.

MODERN USES: One of the most widely grown culinary herbs, chives are best described as healthful rather than medicinal, aiding in toning the digestive system. They have a tendency toward reducing blood pressure as well as antimicrobial and antioxidant effects. The fresh green hollow leaves or fresh flowers are used.

....

CINQUEFOIL
(POTENTILLA REPTANS)

Five–Leaved Grass

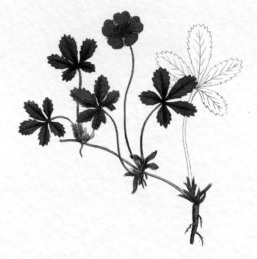

DESCRIPTION: It spreads and creeps, with long slender strings, and shoots forth many [five-parted] leaves, and bears many small yellow flowers.

PLACE: It grows by wood sides, hedges, the pathway in fields, and in the borders and corners of them almost through all this land. [A weed found in fields and wastelands in much of Europe, Asia, eastern North America, and Australia—in short, wherever Europeans have settled.]

GOVERNMENT AND VIRTUES: This is an herb of Jupiter, and therefore strengthens the part of the body it rules and if you give but a scruple (which is but twenty grains) of it at a time, either in white wine, or in white wine vinegar, you shall very seldom miss the cure of an ague, be it what ague soever, in three fits, It is an especial herb used in all inflammations and fevers, whether infectious or pestilential; or among other herbs to cool and temper the blood and humours in the body. As also for all lotions, gargles, infections, and the like, for sore mouths, ulcers, cancers, fistulas, and other corrupt, foul, or running sores. The juice hereof drank, about four ounces at a time, for certain days together, cures the quinsy and yellow jaundice; and taken for thirty days together, cures the falling sickness. The roots boiled in milk, and drank, is a most effectual remedy for all fluxes in man or woman, whether the white or red, as also the bloody flux [dysentery]. The roots boiled in vinegar, and the decoction thereof held in the mouth, eases the pains of the toothache. The juice or decoction taken with a little honey, helps the hoarseness of the throat, and is very good for the cough of the lungs. The distilled water of both roots and leaves, is also effectual to all the purposes aforesaid; and if the hands be often washed therein, and suffered at every time to dry in of itself without wiping, it will in a short time help the palsy, or shaking in them. The root boiled in vinegar, helps all knots, kernels, hard swellings, and lumps growing in any part of the flesh, being thereto applied; as also inflammations, and St. Anthony's fire, all imposthumes [abscesses], and painful sores with heat and putrefaction, the shingles also, and all other sorts of running and foul scabs, sores and itch. The same also boiled in wine, and applied to any joint full of pain, ache, or the gout in the hands or feet, or the hip gout, called the Sciatica, and the decoction thereof drank the while, doth cure them, and eases much pain in the bowels. The roots are likewise effectual to help ruptures or bursting, being used with other things available to that purpose, taken either inwardly or outwardly, or both; as also bruises or hurts by blows, falls, or the like, and to stay the bleeding of wounds in any parts inward or outward.

Some hold that one leaf cures a quotidian, three a tertian, and four a quartan ague [malaria] and a hundred to one if it be not Dioscorides; for he is full of whimsies. The truth is, I never stood so much upon the number of the leaves, nor whether I give it in powder or decoction. If Jupiter were strong, and the Moon applying to him, or his good aspect at the gathering, I never knew it miss the desired effect.

MODERN USES: The roots (and to a lesser extent the leaves) of this and other species of *Potentilla* have long been valued as astringents and anti-inflammatory herbs for the treatment of diarrhea, bleeding (internal and external), hemorrhoids (the powdered herb in appropriate topical formulations), and sore throat and bleeding gums (a tea is used as a rinse or gargle).

....

CLARY SAGE

(SALVIA SCLAREA)

Clear-Eye, Clary

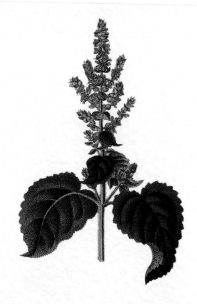

DESCRIPTION: Our ordinary garden Clary has four square stalks, with broad, rough, wrinkled, whitish, or hoary green leaves of a strong sweet scent.

The flowers grow somewhat like the flowers of Sage, but of a whitish blue colour.

PLACE: This grows in gardens.

GOVERNMENT AND VIRTUES: It is under the dominion of the Moon. The seed put into the eyes clears them from motes, and such like things gotten within the lids to offend them, as also clears them from white and red spots on them. The mucilage of the seed made with water, and applied to tumours, or swellings, disperses and takes them away; as also draws forth splinters, thorns, or other things gotten into the flesh. The leaves used with vinegar by itself, or with a little honey, doth help boils, felons, and the hot inflammation that are gathered by their pains, if applied before it be grown too great. The powder of the dried root put into the nose, provokes sneezing, and thereby purges the head and brain of much rheum [watery discharge] and corruption. The seed or leaves taken in wine, provokes to venery. It is of much use both for men and women that have weak backs, and helps to strengthen the kidneys: used either by itself, or with other herbs conducing to the same effect, and in tansies often. The fresh leaves dipped in a batter of flour, eggs, and a little milk, and fried in butter, and served to the table, is exceedingly profitable for those that are troubled with weak backs, and the effects thereof. The juice of the herb put into ale or beer, and drank, brings down women's courses, and expels the after-birth.

MODERN USES: A tea of fresh or dried clary sage leaves is a pleasant beverage used as a digestive tonic for relieving dyspepsia and gas. The essential oil is antibacterial, anti-inflammatory, antioxidant, and antiviral, and is also antifungal against *Candida albicans*. Grown commercially in France as a perfume ingredient. **CAUTION:** All essential oils are used in minute doses.

....

CLEAVERS
(*GALIUM APARINE*)

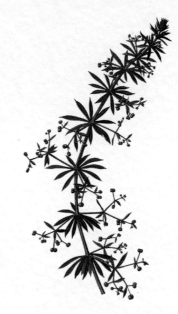

It is also called Aperine, Goose-shade, Goose-grass, and Cleavers.

DESCRIPTION: The common Cleavers have diverse very rough square stalks, rising up two or three yards high; the leaves are usually six, set in a round compass like a star, with very small white flowers. They will cleave to anything that will touch them.

PLACE: It grows by the hedge and ditch-sides in many places of this land, and is so troublesome an inhabitant in gardens, that it ramps upon, and is ready to choke whatever grows near it. [Widely distributed as a weed throughout the temperate regions of the world, including Europe, most of Asia, all of North America, and western South America.]

GOVERNMENT AND VIRTUES: It is under the dominion of the Moon. The juice of the herb and the seed together taken in wine, helps those bitten with an adder, by preserving the heart from the venom. It is familiarly taken in broth to keep them lean and lank, that are apt to grow fat. The distilled water drank twice a day, helps the yellow jaundice, and the decoction of the herb, in experience, is found to do the same, and stays lasks [diarrhea] and bloody-fluxes [dysentery]. The juice of the leaves, or they a little bruised, and applied to any bleeding wounds, stays the bleeding.

The juice also is very good to close up the lips of green wounds, and the powder of the dried herb strewed thereupon doth the same, and likewise helps old ulcers. Being boiled in hog's grease, it helps all sorts of hard swellings or kernels in the throat, being anointed therewith. The juice dropped into the ears, takes away the pain of them.

It is a good remedy in the Spring, eaten (being first chopped small, and boiled well) in water-gruel, to cleanse the blood, and strengthen the liver, thereby to keep the body in health, and fitting it for that change of season that is coming.

MODERN USES: A tea or tincture of the fresh or dried cleavers herb is used as a diuretic and for the treatment of skin disorders and high blood pressure; it also has antioxidant, anti-inflammatory, antimicrobial, and heart-protective effects. In traditional Chinese medicine the herb is used to detoxify tissue, treat irritated or blocked urinary passages and blood in the urine, and as a folk medicine in the treatment of leukemia. Cleavers is also being evaluated for anti-cancer activity.

CAUTION: Hooked hairs on stems may cause contact dermatitis.

....

COLTSFOOT
(*TUSSILAGO FARFARA*)

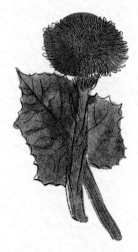

Called also Coughwort, Foal's-foot, Horse-hoof, and Bull's-foot.

DESCRIPTION: Yellowish flowers [appear before the rounded leaves shaped like the foot of a colt].

PLACE: It grows as well in wet grounds as in drier places. [Native to Europe, a widespread weed in cooler regions of North America and Asia.]

GOVERNMENT AND VIRTUES: The plant is under Venus, the fresh leaves or juice, or a syrup thereof is good for a hot dry cough, or wheezing, and shortness of breath. The dry leaves are best for those that have thin rheums and distillations upon their lungs, causing a cough, for which also the dried leaves taken as tobacco, or the root is good. The distilled water hereof simply, or with Elder flowers and Nightshade, is a singularly good remedy against hot agues, to drink two ounces at a time, and apply cloths wet therein to the head and stomach, which also does much good, being applied to any hot swellings and inflammations. It helps St. Anthony's fire, and burnings, and is good to take away wheals and small pushes that arise through heat; as also the burning heat of the piles, or privy parts, cloths wet therein being thereunto applied.

MODERN USES: Coltsfoot leaves and flowers are traditionally used as a demulcent, emollient, and expectorant, primarily in the treatment of coughs and upper respiratory tract infections. Used for pulmonary ailments such as bronchitis, laryngitis, asthma, and whooping cough; also for sore throat. **CAUTION:** Coltsfoot contains liver-toxic pyrrolizidine alkaloids, which can cause veno-occlusive disease of the liver. A small amount of the alkaloids has a cumulative effect over time, and the condition is only diagnosed with a liver biopsy. Acute poisoning can be caused by over-consumption of pyrrolidine alkaloid-containing plants. As a result, Germany banned the use of coltsfoot in 1992. The risks outweigh the benefits.

....

COMFREY

(SYMPHYTUM OFFICINALE)

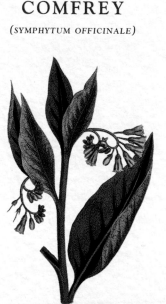

This is a very common but a very neglected plant. It contains very great virtues.

DESCRIPTION: The common Great Comfrey has diverse large hairy green leaves, so hairy or prickly, that if they touch any tender parts of the hands, face, or body, it will cause it to itch. At the ends stand many flowers one above another, which are somewhat long and hollow like the finger of a glove, of a pale whitish colour.

PLACE: They grow by ditches and water-sides, and in diverse fields that are moist, for therein they chiefly delight to grow. [Native to Europe; widely cultivated, naturalized, and persistent after cultivation (weedy) in North America and elsewhere.]

GOVERNMENT AND VIRTUES: This is an herb of Saturn, and I suppose under the sign Capricorn, cold, dry, and earthy in quality. What was spoken of Clown's Woundwort [Marsh Woundwort] may be said of this. The Great Comfrey helps those that spit blood, or make a bloody urine. The root boiled in water or wine, and the decoction drank, helps all inward hurts, bruises, wounds, and ulcer of the lungs, and causes the phlegm that oppresses them to be easily spit forth. It helps the defluction of rheum [watery discharge] from the head upon the lungs, the fluxes of blood or humours by the belly, women's immoderate courses, as well the reds as the whites, and the running of the kidneys happening by what cause soever. A decoction of the leaves hereof is available to all the purposes, though not so effectual as the roots. The roots being outwardly applied, help fresh wounds or cuts immediately, being bruised and laid thereto; and is special good for ruptures and broken bones; yea, it is said to be so powerful to consolidate and knit together, that if they be boiled with dissevered pieces of flesh in a pot, it will join them together again. It is good to be applied to women's breasts that grow sore by the abundance of milk coming into them; also to repress the over much bleeding of the hemorrhoids, to cool the inflammation of the parts thereabouts, and to give ease of pains. The roots of Comfrey taken fresh, beaten small, and spread upon leather, and laid upon any place troubled with the gout, doth presently give ease of the pains; and applied in the same manner, gives ease to pained joints, and profits very much for running and moist ulcers, gangrenes, mortifications, and the like, for which it hath by often experience been found helpful.

MODERN USES: Traditionally, comfrey leaves and root have been used as an expectorant, emollient, astrin- gent, and demulcent, both internally and externally. The root has been used to treat diarrhea, pharyngitis, tonsillitis, bronchitis, pneumonia, and coughs. It has anti-inflammatory, antioxidant, and wound-healing properties. Modern topical preparations (salves and creams)—with toxic pyrrolizidine alkaloids removed—have been evaluated with positive results in multiple clinical trials for the topical treatment of pain, inflammation, swelling of muscles and joints in degenerative arthritis, acute myalgia in the back, sprains, contusions, and strains after sports injuries and accidents. **CAUTION:** Like coltsfoot, comfrey contains liver-toxic pyrrolizidine alkaloids, which can cause veno-occlusive disease of the liver. A small amount of the alkaloids has a cumulative effect over time, and the condition is only diagnosed with a liver biopsy. Acute poisoning is caused by overconsumption of pyrrolidine alkaloid–containing plants. Only modern pyrrolizidine alkaloid–free preparations are considered safe for external use.

....

CORNFLOWER
(CYANUS SEGETUM; SYN. CENTAURIUM CYANUS)

Bachelor's Button, Blue—Bottle

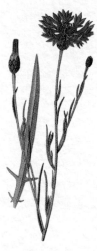

It is called Syanus, I suppose from the colour of it; Hurt-sickle, because it turns the edge of the sickles that reap the corn; Blue-blow, Corn-flower, and Blue-bottle.

DESCRIPTION: The flowers are of a bluish colour, consisting of an innumerable company of flowers set in a scaly head.

PLACE: They grow in cornfields, amongst all sorts of corn. If you take them up and transplant them in your garden, especially towards the full moon, they will grow more double than they are, and many times change colour. [Native to Europe and the Middle East; widely naturalized elsewhere.]

GOVERNMENT AND VIRTUES: As they are naturally cold, dry, and binding, so they are under the dominion of Saturn. The powder or dried leaves of the Blue-bottle, or Corn-flower, is given with good success to those that are bruised by a fall, or have broken a vein inwardly, and void much blood at the mouth; being taken in the water of Plantain, Horsetail, or the greater Comfrey, it is a remedy against the poison of the Scorpion, and resists all venoms and poison. The seed or leaves taken in wine, is very good against the plague, and all infectious diseases, and is very good in pestilential fevers. The juice put into fresh or green wounds, doth quickly solder up the lips of them together, and is very effectual to heal all ulcers and sores in the mouth. The distilled water of this herb has the same properties, and may be used for the effects aforesaid.

MODERN USES: Folkloric uses for cornflowers include a tea for fevers, menstrual disorders, and candida, as well as a bitter simulant for the liver and gallbladder. Seldom used.

....

COSTMARY

(TANACETUM BALSAMITA; SYN. BALSAMITA MAJOR, CHRYSANTHEMUM BALSAMITA)

Alcost, Balsam Herb

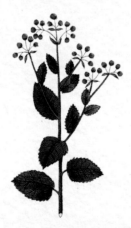

[A widespread native plant and/or weed of Eurasia, originating in southeastern Europe and southwest Asia.]

GOVERNMENT AND VIRTUES: It is under the dominion of Jupiter. The ordinary Costmary, as well as Maudlin, provokes urine abundantly, and moistens the hardness of the mother; it gently purges choler [bile] and phlegm, extenuating that which is gross, and cutting that which is tough and glutinous, cleanses that which is foul, and hinders putrefaction and corruption; it dissolves without attraction, opens obstructions, and helps their evil effects, and it is a wonderful help to all sorts of dry agues. It is astringent to the stomach, and strengthens the liver, and all the other inward parts; and taken in whey works more effectually. Taken fasting in the morning, it is very profitable for pains in the head that are continual, and to stay, dry up, and consume all thin rheums or distillations from the head into the stomach, and helps much to digest raw humours that are gathered therein. It is very profitable for those that are fallen into a continual evil disposition of the whole body, called Cachexia, but especially in the beginning of the disease. It is an especial friend and helps to evil, weak and cold livers. The seed is familiarly given to children for the worms, and so is the infusion of the flowers in white wine given them to the quantity of two ounces at a time; it makes an excellent salve to cleanse and heal old ulcers, being boiled with oil of olive, and Adder's tongue with it, and after it is strained, put a little wax, rosin, and turpentine, to bring it to a convenient body.

MODERN USES: Costmary is little used today. The leaves contain phenolic compounds with antioxidant activity. The essential oil from the leaves has been shown to have antimicrobial activity and experimental liver-protective effects. Costmary is used in folk medicine, particularly in Iran. Elsewhere in Asia Minor, it's a culinary herb, digestive carminative, and heart tonic. Also known as "Bible-leaf" because traditionally the leaves were dried flat and placed between book pages as a bookmark.

....

COTTON-THISTLE

(ONOPORDUM ACANTHIUM)

Down Thistle

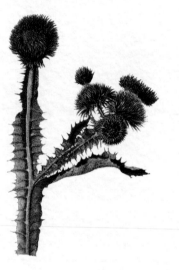

DESCRIPTION: This has large leaves covered with long hairy wool, or Cotton Down, set with most sharp and cruel spines, from the middle of whose head of flowers, thrust forth many purplish crimson [threadlike flowers].

PLACE: It grows in diverse ditches, banks, and highways, [generally everywhere where Britons have settled, including most of North America and elsewhere].

GOVERNMENT AND VIRTUES: Mars owns the plant, and manifest to the world, that though it may hurt your finger, it will help your body; for I fancy it much for the ensuing virtues. Pliny and Dioscorides write, That the leaves and roots thereof taken in drink, help those that have a crick in their neck; whereby they cannot turn their neck but their whole body must turn also (sure they do not mean those that have got a crick in their neck by being under the hangman's hand.) Galen saith, that the root and leaves hereof are of a healing quality, and good for such persons as have their bodies drawn together by some spasm or convulsion, as it is with children that have the rickets.

MODERN USES: Also known as Scotch thistle, cotton thistle has medicinal attributes that include fever-reducing, cough-suppressing, and expectorant activities; and diuretic and stomachic effects. Externally, the juice of the plant has been long used as a folk cancer remedy. In a study from 2016, potential anticancer activity was attributed to a class of chemical compounds known as sesquiterpene lactones found in the leaves. Leaf extracts contain a compound, onopordopicrin, which has mild antibacterial activity. The sesquiterpenes and additional compounds such as lignans and flavonoids have been linked to anti-inflammatory activity. Traditionally the young, peeled stalks were boiled and eaten as a wild food.

....

COUCH GRASS

(ELYMUS REPENS; SYN. ELYTRIGIA REPENS, AGROPYRON REPENS)

Dog's-Grass, or Cough Grass

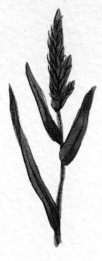

DESCRIPTION: It is well known, that the grass creeps far about underground, with long white joined roots, very sweet in taste. Watch the dogs when they are sick, and they will quickly lead you to it.

PLACE: It grows commonly through this land in diverse ploughed grounds to the no small trouble of the husbandmen, as also of the gardeners.

GOVERNMENT AND VIRTUES: 'Tis under the dominion of Jupiter, and is the most medicinal of all the Quick-grasses. Being boiled and drank, it opens obstructions of the liver and gall, and the stopping of urine, and eases the griping pains of the belly and inflammations; wastes the matter of the stone in the bladder, and the ulcers thereof also. The roots bruised and applied, do consolidate wounds. The seed doth more powerfully expel urine, and stays the lask [diarrhea] and vomiting. The distilled water alone, or with a little worm-seed, kills the worms in children. The way of use is to bruise the roots, and having well boiled them in white wine, drink the decoction. 'Tis opening but not purging, very safe. 'Tis a remedy against all diseases coming of stopping, and although a gardener be of another opinion, yet a physician holds half an acre of them to be worth five acres of Carrots twice told over.

MODERN USES: In phytomedicine the rhizome (underground stem) of couch grass is used in tea, tincture, and ethanolic extracts as a traditional mild diuretic in cases of minor urinary tract and bladder discomfort, especially when associated with low back pain, cystitis, urethritis, and kidney stones. It's also a folk medicine for rheumatism and arthritis. Lacking modern clinical studies, this herbal ingredient is approved in Europe based on long-standing and continued medicinal use.

....

COWSLIP

(PRIMULA VERIS)

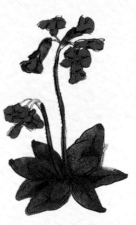

Both the wild and garden Cowslips are so well known, that I neither trouble myself nor the reader with a description of them. [Found in meadows and gardens throughout Europe; naturalized in North America.]

GOVERNMENT AND VIRTUES: Venus lays claim to this herb as her own, and it is under the sign Aries, and our city dames know well enough the ointment or distilled water of it adds beauty, or at least restores it when it is lost. The flowers are held to be more effectual than the leaves, and the roots of little use. An ointment made with them takes away spots and wrinkles of the skin, sun-burning, and freckles, and adds beauty exceedingly. They remedy all infirmities of the head coming of heat and wind, as vertigo, ephialtes [nightmares], false apparitions, phrensies, falling-sickness, palsies, convulsions, cramps, pains in the nerves. The roots ease pains in the back and bladder, and open the passages of urine. The leaves are good in wounds, and the flowers take away trembling. If the flowers be not well dried, and kept in a warm place, they will soon putrefy and look green: Have a special eye over them. If you let them see the Sun once a month, it will do neither the Sun nor them harm.

Because they strengthen the brain and nerves, and remedy palsies, Greeks gave them the name Paralysis. The flowers preserved or conserved, and the quantity of a nutmeg eaten every morning, is a sufficient dose for inward diseases; but for wounds, spots, wrinkles, and sunburns, an ointment is made of the leaves, and hog's grease.

MODERN USES: The dried flowering parts and dried roots of cowslip are used in modern phytomedicine preparations for the treatment of bronchitis, coughs, colds, and mucous discharges of the nose and throat. Contrary to Culpeper's belief that the "roots [are of] little use," the root is now the preferred plant part for mucous-resolving and expectorant activity. The dried flowers are traditionally used for nervousness and headaches.

....

CROSSWORT

(CRUCIATA LAEVIPES; SYN. GALIUM CRUCIATA)

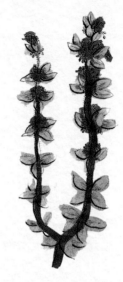

This herb receives its name from the situation of its leaves.

DESCRIPTION: Common Crosswort grows up with square hairy stalks a little above a foot high, having four small broad and pointed, hairy yet smooth thin leaves. Towards the tops of the stalks at the joints, stand small, pale yellow flowers.

PLACE: [Found in moist ground and meadows throughout Europe except Scandinavia; sporadically naturalized elsewhere.]

GOVERNMENT AND VIRTUES: It is under the dominion of Saturn. This is a singularly good wound herb, and is used inwardly, not only to stay bleeding of wounds, but to consolidate them, as it doth outwardly any green wound, which it quickly solders up, and heals. The decoction of the herb in wine, helps to expectorate the phlegm out of the chest, and is good for obstructions in the breast, stomach, or bowels, and helps a decayed appetite. It is also good to wash any wound or sore with, to cleanse and heal it. The herb bruised, and then boiled applied outwardly for certain days together, renewing it often; and in the meantime the decoction of the herb in wine, taken inwardly every day, doth certainly cure the rupture in any, so as it be not too inveterate; but very speedily, if it be fresh and lately taken.

MODERN USES: Crosswort is seldom used today except as a folk medicine in Eastern Europe, primarily as Culpeper describes, externally for the treatment of wounds. Contains coumarins and iridoid compounds that may be responsible for traditional claims; otherwise, it is little studied.

....

CUCKOO PINT

(*ARUM MACULATUM*)

Cuckow-Point, Lords-And-Ladies

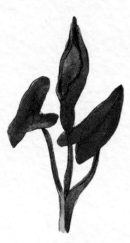

It is called Aron, Janus, Barba-aron, Calve's-foot, Ramp, Starchwort, Cuckow-point, and Wake Robin.

DESCRIPTION: [A member of the arum family with white-mottled or variegated arrow-shaped leaves and a flower spathe enveloping a club-like spadix, maturing to a cluster of bright red, berry-like fruits.] The whole plant is of a very sharp biting taste, pricking the tongue as nettles do the hands, and so abides for a great while without alteration. The root thereof was anciently used instead of starch to starch linen with.

PLACE: [It is widespread in northern temperate Europe and cultivated as an ornamental elsewhere.]

GOVERNMENT AND VIRTUES: It is under the dominion of Mars. The green leaves bruised, and laid upon any boil or plague sore, doth wonderfully help to draw forth the poison: A dram of the powder of the dried root taken with twice so much sugar in the form of a licking electuary, or the green root, doth wonderfully help those that are short-winded, as also those that have a cough; it breaks, digests, and rids away phlegm from the stomach, chest, and lungs. The milk wherein the root has been boiled is effectual also for the same purpose. The said powder taken in wine or other drink, or the juice of the berries, or the powder of them, or the wine wherein they have been boiled, provokes urine, and brings down women's courses and purges them effectually after child-bearing, to bring away the after-birth. Taken with sheep's milk, it heals the inward ulcers of the bowels. The distilled water thereof is effectual to all the purposes aforesaid. A spoonful taken at a time heals the itch; an ounce or more taken a time for some days together, doth help the rupture: The leaves either green or dry, or the juice of them, doth cleanse all manner of rotten and filthy ulcers, in what part of the body soever; and heals the stinking sores in the nose, called polypus. The root mixed with bean-flour, and applied to the throat or jaws that are inflamed, helps them. The berries or the roots beaten with the hot ox-dung, and applied, eases the pains of the gout. The leaves and roots boiled in wine with a little oil, and applied to the piles, eases them, and so doth sitting over the hot fumes thereof. The fresh roots bruised and distilled with a little milk, yields a most sovereign water to cleanse the skin from scurf, freckles, spots, or blemishes whatsoever therein.

Authors have left large commendations of this herb you see, but for my part, I have neither spoken with Dr. Reason nor Dr. Experience about it.

MODERN USES: It is no longer used medicinally. **CAUTION:** All plant parts contain needle-shaped sharp crystals of calcium oxalates, which cause severe irritation to the skin, mouth, mucous membranes, and throat, leading to swelling, possibly difficulty in breathing, and serious gastrointestinal irritation. It is called *lords and ladies* because of the supposed likeness of the flower parts to male and female sex organs.

....

CUCUMBERS

(*CUCUMIS SATIVUS*)

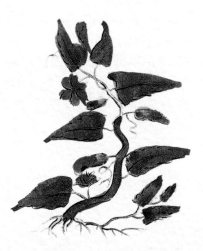

PLACE: [Cucumbers are believed to have originated in India, and were then cultivated over three thousand years ago, spreading to Europe more than two thousand years ago by the Greeks and Romans. Sometimes found growing wild at the site of old gardens.]

GOVERNMENT AND VIRTUES: There is no dispute to be made, but that they are under the dominion of the Moon, though they are so much cried out against for their coldness, and if they were but one degree colder they would be poison. The best of Galenists hold them to be cold and moist in the second degree, and then not so hot as either lettuce or purslane: They are excellently good for a hot stomach, and hot liver. The face being washed with their juice, cleanses the skin. The seed is excellent to provoke urine, and cleanses the passages thereof when they are stopped. There is not a better remedy for ulcers in the bladder, than are Cucumbers. The usual course is, to use the seeds in emulsions, as they make almond milk; but a far better way (in my opinion) is this: Take Cucumbers and bruise them well, and distil the water from them, and let such as are troubled with ulcers in the bladder drink no other drink. The face being washed with the same water, cures the reddest face that is; it is also excellently good for sun-burning, freckles, and abscesses.

MODERN USES: The cooling, soothing, and anti-inflammatory effects of cucumbers have made the vegetable, its juice, and extracts a favored anti-wrinkling and antiaging ingredient in cosmetics and skin lotions. High in potassium, antioxidants, and vitamin K, it is a vegetable valued for its nutritional and health benefits. Traditionally, cucumbers are considered diuretic.

....

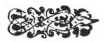

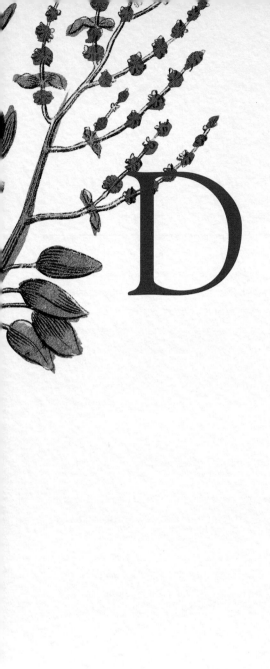

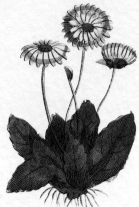

DAISIES

(LEUCANTHEMUM VULGARE; SYN.
CHRYSANTHEMUM LEUCANTHEMUM)

These are so well known almost to every child, that I suppose it needless to write any description of them. Take therefore the virtues of them as follows.

PLACE: [Native to and widespread in meadows, fields, and along roadsides throughout Europe; widespread in North America and designated a noxious weed in many states.]

GOVERNMENT AND VIRTUES: The herb is under the sign Cancer, and under the dominion of Venus, and therefore excellently good for wounds in the breast, and very fitting to be kept both in oils, ointments, and plasters, as also in syrup. The greater wild Daisy is a wound herb of good respect, often used in those drinks or salves that are for wounds, either inward or outward. A decoction made of them and drank, helps to cure the wounds made in the hollowness of the breast. The same also cures all ulcers and pustules in the mouth or tongue, or in the secret parts. The leaves bruised and applied to the private parts, or to any other parts that are swollen and hot, doth dissolve it, and temper the heat. A decoction made thereof, of Wallwort and

Agrimony, and the places fomented and bathed therewith warm, gives great ease to them that are troubled with the palsy, sciatica, or the gout. The same also disperses and dissolves the knots or kernels that grow in the flesh of any part of the body, and bruises and hurts that come of falls and blows; they are also used for ruptures, and other inward burnings, with very good success. An ointment made thereof doth wonderfully help all wounds that have inflammations about them, or by reason of moist humours having access unto them, are kept long from healing, and such are those, for the most part, that happen to joints of the arms or legs. The juice of them dropped into the running eyes of any, doth much help them.

MODERN USES: The common oxeye daisy is considered a serious weed in temperate regions worldwide. It has anti-inflammatory and antimicrobial activity, but is better known for causing contact dermatitis. Herbalists consider it antispasmodic, diuretic, and tonic, and it once was used for the treatment of bronchial coughs and catarrhs. Externally, it has been used in lotions for wounds, bruises, and inflammation. The young tender leaves were once used sparingly in salads. Forensic scientists suggest that the oxeye daisy may have been among the herbs used to embalm the heart of Richard the Lionheart in 1199 AD.

....

DANDELION
(TARAXACUM OFFICINALE)
Piss—a—Beds

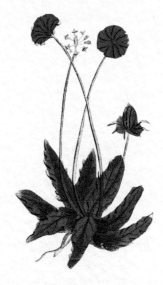

DESCRIPTION:. It is well known to have many long and deep gashed leaves, lying on the ground round about the head of the roots; the middle rib being white, which being broken, yields abundance of bitter milk, but the root much more. From among the leaves, arise many slender, weak, naked footstalks, every one of them bearing at the top one large yellow flower, consisting of many rows of yellow [petals].

PLACE: It grows frequently in all meadows and pasture-grounds.

GOVERNMENT AND VIRTUES: It is under the dominion of Jupiter. It is of an opening and cleansing quality, and therefore very effectual for the obstructions of the liver, gall, and spleen, and the diseases that arise from them, as the jaundice and hypochondriac; it opens the passages of the urine both in young and old; powerfully cleanses imposthumes [abscesses] and inward ulcers in the urinary passage, and by its drying and temperate quality doth afterwards heal them; for which purpose the decoction of the roots or leaves in white wine, or the leaves chopped as pot-herbs, with a few Alisanders, and boiled in their broth, are very effectual. And whoever is drawing towards a consumption or an evil disposition of the whole body, called cachexia, by the use hereof for some time together, shall find a wonderful help. It helps also to procure rest and sleep to bodies distempered by the heat of ague fits, or otherwise: The distilled water is effectual to drink in pestilential fevers, and to wash the sores.

You see here what virtues this common herb hath, and that is the reason the French and Dutch so often eat them in the Spring; and now if you look a little farther, you may see plainly without a pair of spectacles, that foreign physicians are not so selfish as ours are, but more communicative of the virtues of plants to people.

MODERN USES: Both dandelion leaves (the herb) and roots are used in modern herbal medicine. Dandelion leaf tea or extracts are diuretic and high in potassium. The leaf may help to replace potassium lost in urination. Older clinical case reports confirm diuretic activity. Leaf tea is used in phytotherapy for stimulating appetite and relieving dyspepsia. The root is also used for its diuretic properties and to stimulate bile flow, treat dyspepsia, and relieve gastrointestinal problems. It also has confirmed anti-inflammatory, antioxidant, and antibacterial activity and is suggested as a research subject for the prevention and treatment of type 2 diabetes. **CAUTION:** Contraindicated in obstructions of the bile duct and gallbladder.

. . . .

DEAD NETTLES

WHITE DEAD NETTLE
(LAMIUM ALBUM)
White Archangel

SPOTTED DEAD NETTLE
(LAMIUM MACULATUM)
Red Archangel

YELLOW ARCHANGEL
(LAMIUM GALEOBDOLON)

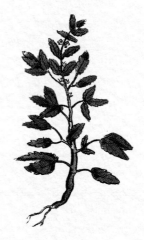

To put a gloss upon their practice, the physicians call an herb (which country people vulgarly know by the name of Dead Nettle) Archangel; whether they favour more of superstition or folly, I leave to the judicious reader. There is more curiosity than courtesy to my countrymen used by others in the explanation as well of the names, as description of this so well-known herb; which that I may not also be guilty of, take this short description, first, of the Red Archangel [*Lamium maculatum*].

DESCRIPTION: This [*Lamium maculatum*] has diverse square stalks, somewhat hairy, at the joints whereof grow two sad green leaves; [with] sundry gaping flowers of a pale reddish colour.

White Archangel [*Lamium album*] hath diverse square stalks, [with] two leaves at a joint, and greener also, more like unto Nettle leaves, but not stinging, yet hairy. [It has] more open gaping white flowers.

Yellow Archangel [*Lamium galeobdolon*] is like the White in the stalks and leaves; the flowers a little larger and more gaping, of a fair yellow colour in most, in some paler.

PLACE: They grow almost everywhere (unless it be in the middle of the street), the yellow most usually in the wet grounds of woods. [All grow throughout Europe and are naturalized in the United States. Yellow archangel is deemed a noxious weed in the state of Washington and the sale of live plants to gardeners is banned.]

GOVERNMENT AND VIRTUES: The Archangels are somewhat hot and drier than the stinging Nettles, and used with better success for the stopping and hardness of the spleen, than they, by using the decoction of the herb in wine, and afterwards applying the herb hot into the region of the spleen as a plaster, or the decoction with sponges. Flowers of the White Archangel are preserved or conserved to be used to stay the whites, and the flowers of the red to stay the reds in women. It makes the heart merry, drives away melancholy, quickens the spirits, is good against quartan agues [malaria recurring every four days], stancheth bleeding at mouth and nose, if it be stamped and applied to the nape of the neck; the herb also bruised, and with some salt and vinegar and hog's-grease, laid upon a hard tumour or swelling, or that vulgarly called the king's evil, do help to dissolve or discuss them; and being in like manner applied, doth much allay the pains, and give ease to the gout, sciatica, and other pains of the joints and sinews. It is also very effectual to heal green wounds, and old ulcers; also to stay their fretting, gnaw-

ing, and spreading. It draws forth splinters, and such like things gotten into the flesh, and is very good against bruises and burnings. But the Yellow Archangel is most commended for old, filthy, corrupt sores and ulcers, yea although they grow to be hollow, and to dissolve tumours. The chief use of them is for women, it being an herb of Venus.

MODERN USES: Here Culpeper has treated three separate plant species under a single entry. Research suggests white dead nettle has experimental anti-inflammatory and antimicrobial activity. Spotted dead nettle and Culpeper's "yellow archangel" (*Lamium galeobdolon*) are not used today. All are little researched.

·················

DEVIL'S BIT

(*SUCCISA PRATENSIS*)

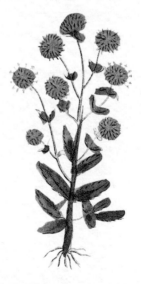

DESCRIPTION: This rises up with a round green smooth stalk, about two feet high. At the end of each branch stands a round head of many flowers set together of a bluish purple colour.

PLACE: The first grows as well in dry meadows and fields as moist, in many places of this land. [Found throughout Europe.]

GOVERNMENT AND VIRTUES: The plant is venereal, pleasing, and harmless. The herb or the root (all that the devil hath left of it) being boiled in wine, and drank, is very powerful against the plague, and all pestilential diseases or fevers, poisons also, and the biting of venomous beasts. It helps also those that are inwardly bruised by any causality, or outwardly by falls or blows, dissolving the clotted blood; and the herb or root beaten and outwardly applied, takes away the black and blue marks that remain in the skin. The decoction of the herb, with honey of roses put therein, is very effectual to help the inveterate tumours and swellings of the almonds [tonsils] and throat, by often gargling the mouth therewith. It helps also to procure women's courses, and eases all pains of the mother and to break and discuss wind therein, and in the bowels. The powder of the root taken in drink, drives forth the worms in the body. The juice or distilled water of the herb is effectual for green wounds, or old sores, and cleanses the body inwardly, and the seed outwardly, from sores, scurf, itch, pimples, freckles, morphew [blemishes], or other deformities thereof, especially if a little vitriol be dissolved therein.

MODERN USES: Devil's bit is little used today. The essential oil of the aboveground parts has antibacterial and antioxidant activity.

....

DILL
(ANETHUM GRAVEOLENS)

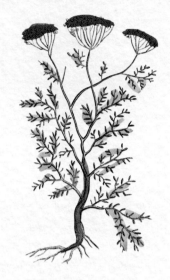

DESCRIPTION: The common Dill has four branches and smaller umbels of yellow flowers, which turn into small seed.

PLACE: It is most usually sown in gardens and grounds for the purpose, and is also found wild. [Thought to be native to the Mediterranean region of southern Europe and western Asia.]

GOVERNMENT AND VIRTUES: Mercury has the dominion of this plant, and therefore to be sure it strengthens the brain. The Dill being boiled and drank, is good to ease swellings and pains; it also stays the belly and stomach from casting. The decoction therefore helps women that are troubled with the pains and windiness of the mother, if they sit therein. It stays the hiccough, being boiled in wine, and but smelled unto being tied in a cloth. The seed is of more use than the leaves, and more effectual to digest raw and vicious humours, and is used in medicines that serve to expel wind, and the pains proceeding therefrom. The decoction of

Dill, be it herb or seed (only if you boil the seed you must bruise it) in white wine, being drank, it is a gallant expeller of wind, and provoker of the terms.

MODERN USES: Dillweed (leaves) are a familiar flavoring often associated with pickles. Dill seeds are used to relieve gas in the digestive system, stimulate digestion, and treat dyspepsia; also widely used in traditional medicine to stimulate milk flow, manage type 2 diabetes, treat urinary infections, and relieve gastrointestinal spasms. It has confirmed antispasmodic, carminative, anti-inflammatory, and analgesic activities. The seeds are eaten or crushed and taken in tea.

....

DOCK

(RUMEX CRISPUS, AND OTHER RUMEX SPECIES)

Yellow Dock

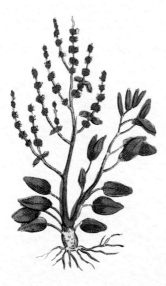

Many kinds of these are so well known, that I shall not trouble you with a description of them: My book grows big too fast.

GOVERNMENT AND VIRTUES: All Docks are under Jupiter, of which the Red Dock [*Rumex aquatica*], which is commonly called Bloodwort, cleanses the blood, and strengthens the liver; but the yellow Dock-root is best to be taken when either the blood or liver is affected by choler [bile]. All of them have a kind of cooling (but not all alike) drying quality, the sorrel [*Rumex acetosa*] being most cold, and the Bloodworts most drying. The roots boiled in vinegar help the itch, scabs, and breaking out of the skin, if it be bathed therewith. The distilled water of the herb and roots have the same virtue, and cleanses the skin from freckles, morphews [skin blemishes], and all other spots and discolourings therein.

All Docks being boiled with meat, make it boil the sooner: Besides Blood-wort is exceeding strengthening to the liver, and procures good blood, being as wholesome a pot herb as any growing in a garden; yet such is the nicety of our times, forsooth, that women will not put it into a pot, because it makes the pottage black; pride and ignorance (a couple of monsters in the creation) preferring nicety before health.

MODERN USES: The most commonly used dock in herbal practice is yellow dock (*Rumex crispus*), which is native to Europe and a widespread weed elsewhere. Yellow dock is used in Western herbal traditional as a "blood purifier," mild astringent, and treatment for enlarged lymph nodes, skin conditions, and dyspepsia. It has antioxidant and antibacterial activity. In Asian medicine systems, the root is used for the treatment of bleeding and loosening of the skin (dermatolysis) and to protect against osteoporosis. Extracts have experimental antimalarial activity. **CAUTION:** The fresh roots contain anthraquinones (which cause diarrhea) and the leaf contains liver-toxic oxalates.

....

DODDER

(CUSCUTA EPITHYMUM)

Clover Dodder, Odder-of-Thyme, Epithymum, and Other Dodders

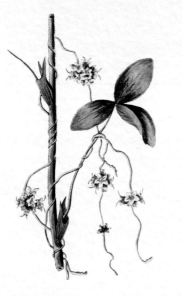

DESCRIPTION: [Usually yellow-orange throughout, dodders (*Cuscuta* spp.) are members of the morning-glory family. They are entirely without chlorophyll and wholly parasitic on their host plants.] It generally [takes on] the nature of the plant which it climbs upon.

PLACE: [At least 200 species of *Cuscuta* (dodder) grow worldwide. They are often associated as a weed with cultivated crops, but grow in a wide variety of habitats—from farmland to beaches and from temperate to tropical climates.]

GOVERNMENT AND VIRTUES: All Dodders are under Saturn. Tell not me of physicians crying up Epithymum, or that Dodder which grows upon Thyme, (most of which comes from Hemetius in Greece, or Hybla in Sicily, because those mountains abound with Thyme,) he is a physician indeed, that hath wit enough to choose the Dodder according to the nature of the disease and humour peccant. We confess, Thyme is the hottest herb it usually grows upon; and therefore that which grows upon Thyme is hotter than that which grows upon cold herbs; for it draws nourishment from what it grows upon, as well as from the earth where its root is, and thus you see old Saturn is wise enough to have two strings to his bow. This is accounted the most effectual for melancholy diseases, and to purge black or burnt choler [bile], which is the cause of many diseases of the head and brain, as also for the trembling of the heart, faintings and swoonings. It is helpful in all diseases and griefs of the spleen, and melancholy that arises from the windiness of the hypochondria. It purges also the kidneys by urine; it opens obstructions of the gall, whereby it profits them that have the jaundice; as also the leaves, the spleen.

The other Dodders do, as I said before, participate of the nature of those plants whereon they grow: As that which hath been found growing upon nettles in the west-country, hath by experience been found very effectual to procure plenty of urine where it hath been stopped or hindered. And so of the rest.

Sympathy and antipathy are two hinges upon which the whole mode of physic turns; and that physician who minds them not, is like a door off from the hooks, more like to do a man mischief, than to secure him. Then all the diseases Saturn causes, this helps by sympathy, and strengthens all the parts of the body he rules; such as be caused by Sol, it helps by antipathy. What those diseases are, see my judgment of diseases by astrology; and if you be pleased to look at the herb Wormwood, you shall find a rational way for it.

MODERN USES: Various species of dodder (there are upwards of 145 species worldwide) have been traditionally used as laxatives. Some have been studied for anti-inflammatory and mild central nervous system depressant activities. Seldom used today. **CAUTION:** Culpeper reminds us that this parasitic plant group may take on the "nature of those plants whereon they grow." This warning extends to dodder growing on toxic plants.

DOVESFOOT CRANESBILL

(GERANIUM MOLLE)

Dovefoot Geranium

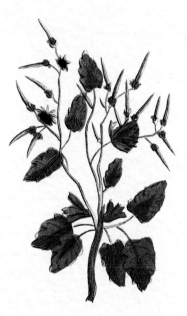

DESCRIPTION: This has diverse small, round, pale-green leaves, much like mallow [with slender reddish, weak, hairy stalks] where grow many very small bright red flowers of five [petals].

PLACE: It grows in pasture grounds, and by the path-sides in many places, and will also be in gardens. [Native from Europe to the Himalayas, it is a naturalized weed in both eastern and western North America and temperate South America.]

GOVERNMENT AND VIRTUES: It is a very gentle, though martial plant. It is found by experience to be singularly good for wind cholic, as also to expel the stone and gravel in the kidneys. The decoction thereof in wine, is an excellent good cure for those that have inward wounds, hurts, or bruises, both to stay the bleeding, to dissolve and expel the congealed blood, and to heal the parts, as also to cleanse and heal outward sores, ulcers, and fistulas; and for green wounds, many do only bruise the herb, and apply it to the places, and it heals them quickly. The same decoction in wine fomented to any place pained with the gout, or to joint-aches, or pains of the sinews, gives much ease. The powder or decoction of the herb taken for some time together, is found by experience to be singularly good for ruptures and burstings in people, either young or old.

MODERN USES: Dovesfoot cranesbill and other species of *Geranium* root and leaves contain compounds with styptic effects (ellagitannins). The root is used to stop bleeding, both internally and externally, and to promote healing. The tea is also used to treat diarrhea. In modern herbal medicine the most well-known geranium is the North American wild cranesbill (*Geranium maculatum*). Dovefoot cranesbill is little studied, but recent research on the chemistry of potentially active compounds was stimulated by its use in northern Portugal as a folk cancer remedy.

....

DYER'S BROOM

(GENISTA TINCTORIA)

Broom, Dyer's Greenweed

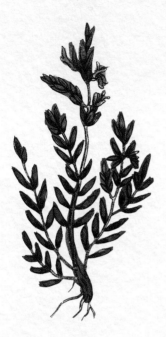

To spend time in writing a description hereof is altogether needless, it being so generally used by all the good housewives almost through this land to sweep their houses with, and therefore very well known to all sorts of people.

PLACE: They grow in many places of this land commonly, and as commonly spoil all the land they grow in. [Found throughout most of Europe; naturalized in Argentina.]

GOVERNMENT AND VIRTUES: The juice or decoction of the young branches, or seed, or the powder of the seed taken in drink purges downwards, and draws phlegmatic and watery humours from the joints; whereby it helps the dropsy, gout, sciatica, and pains of the hips and joints; it also provokes strong vomiting, and helps the pains of the sides, and swelling of the spleen, cleanses also the kidneys and bladder of the stone, provokes urine abundantly, and hinders the growing again of the stone in the body. The oil or water that is drawn from the end of the green sticks heated in the fire, helps the toothache. The juice of young branches made into an ointment of old hog's grease, and anointed, or the young branches bruised and heated in oil or hog's grease, and laid to the sides pained by wind, as in stitches, or the spleen, ease them in once or twice using it. The same boiled in oil is the safest and surest medicine to kill lice in the head or body of any; and is an especial remedy for joint aches, and swollen knees, that come by the falling down of humours.

MODERN USES: As the species name "tinctoria" suggests, dyer's broom was once widely used to produce a yellow dye. Considered a folk medicine as a diuretic and laxative. Traditionally, as Culpeper suggests, it also had a reputation as a treatment for rheumatism and gout. Primarily used to promote diuresis in cases when increased urination is indicated, such as to prevent urinary gravel or calculi. Like some other members of the pea family, such as soybeans, the herb contains the phytoestrogenic compound genistein. **CAUTION:** The herb is contraindicated in cases of high blood pressure.

....

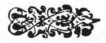

E

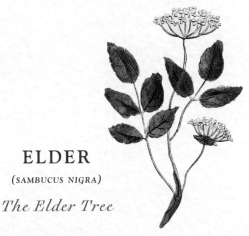

ELDER

(SAMBUCUS NIGRA)

The Elder Tree

I hold it needless to write any description of this, since every boy that plays with a pop-gun will not mistake another tree instead of Elder.

PLACE: The Elder-tree grows in hedges, being planted there to strengthen the fences and partitions of ground, and to hold the banks by ditches and water-courses. [Found throughout Europe, central Asia, North Africa, and naturalized in eastern South America. The North American *Sambucus canadensis* is also called *Sambucus nigra* subsp. *canadensis*.]

Government and virtues: [Elder is] under the dominion of Venus. The first shoots of the common Elder boiled like Asparagus, and the young leaves and stalks boiled in fat broth, doth mightily carry forth phlegm and choler [bile]. The middle or inward bark boiled in water, and given in drink, works much more violently; and the berries, either green or dry, expel the same humour, and are often given with good success to help the dropsy; the bark of the root boiled in wine, or the juice thereof drank, works the same effects, but more powerfully than either the leaves or fruit. The juice of the root taken, doth mightily procure vomiting, and purges the watery humours of the dropsy. The decoction of the root taken, cures the biting of an adder. It mollifies the hardness of the mother, if women sit thereon, and opens their veins, and brings down their courses: The berries boiled in wine perform the same effect; and the hair of the head washed therewith is made black. The juice of the green leaves applied to the hot inflammations of the eyes, assuages them. The decoction of the berries in wine, being drank, provokes urine; the distilled water of the flowers is of much use to clean the skin from sun-burning, freckles, morphew [blemishes], or the like; and takes away the headache, coming of a cold cause, the head being bathed therewith. The leaves or flowers distilled in the month of May, and the legs often washed with the said distilled water, it takes away the ulcers and sores of them. The eyes washed therewith, it takes away the redness and bloodshot; and the hands washed morning and evening therewith, helps the palsy, and shaking of them.

MODERN USES: Elder has been rehabilitated in modern phytomedicine. Taken in the form of extracts of the dried ripe elderberry fruit, it is one of the most widely used medicinal plants for the prevention and treatment of viral infections, particularly upper respiratory tract infections associated with colds and flu. Antiviral, antioxidant, and immunomodulatory activity are ascribed to the fruits. The dried fruits also have laxative effects. The dried flowers are traditionally used to treat colds, fever, and upper respiratory tract congestion. **CAUTION:** Avoid ingesting unripe berries or fresh plant parts as they contain cyanogenic glycosides that can cause symptoms of cyanide toxicity. Allergic reactions to elder are reported.

ELDER, DWARF

(SAMBUCUS EBULUS)

Danewort

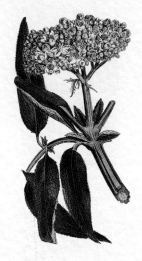

DESCRIPTION: This is but an herb every year, dying with his stalks to the ground, and rising afresh every Spring, and is like unto the Elder both in form and quality, rising up with square, rough, hairy stalks, four feet high, or more sometimes.

PLACE: [The Dwarf Elder grows wild in many places in Europe and North Africa.]

GOVERNMENT AND VIRTUES: Both Elder and Dwarf Tree are under the dominion of Venus.

The Dwarf Elder is more powerful than the common Elder in opening and purging choler [bile], phlegm, and water; in helping the gout, piles, and women's diseases, colours the hair black, helps the inflammations of the eyes, and pains in the ears, the biting of serpents, or mad dogs, burnings and scalding, the wind cholic, cholic, and stone, the difficulty of urine, the cure of old sores and fistulous ulcers. Either leaves or bark of Elder, stripped upwards as you gather it, causes vomiting.

MODERN USES: Dwarf elder is used far less than common elder. The dried flowers and dried fruits have a long history in traditional medicines, especially in southern Europe and central Asia. Preparations have been used in the treatment of inflammatory reactions from insect bites, sore throat, and hemorrhoids, among other uses. Components in the plant have been shown experimentally to have anti-inflammatory, antioxidant, and pain-relieving activity. A gel containing dwarf elder extract for the treatment of knee osteoarthritis showed positive results in a clinical study. **CAUTION:** Avoid ingesting unripe berries or fresh plant parts as they contain cyanogenic glycosides that can cause symptoms of cyanide toxicity. Allergic reactions to elder are reported.

....

ELECAMPANE

(*INULA HELENIUM*)

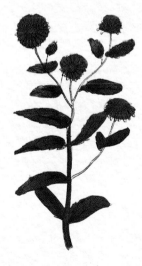

DESCRIPTION: It shoots forth many large leaves, long and broad, of a whitish green on the upper side, which arise up three or four feet high, bearing diverse great and large [yellow] flowers. The root is great and thick, of a very bitter taste, and strong, but good scent.

PLACE: It grows on moist grounds, and shady places and open borders of the fields, and in other waste places. [Native to most of temperate Asia and western Europe; escaped from gardens and found throughout Europe and much of eastern North America].

GOVERNMENT AND VIRTUES: It is a plant under the dominion of Mercury. The fresh roots of Elecampane preserved with sugar, or made into a syrup or conserve, are very effectual to warm a cold windy stomach, or the pricking therein, and sti[t]ches in the sides caused by the spleen; and to help the cough, shortness of breath, and wheezing in the lungs. The dried root made into powder, and mixed with sugar, and taken, serves to the same purpose, and is also profitable for those who have their urine stopped, or the stopping of women's courses, the pains of the mother and the stone in the kidneys, or bladder; it resists poison, and stays the spreading of the venom of serpents, as also putrid and pestilential fevers, and the plague itself. The roots and herbs beaten and put into new ale or beer, and daily drank, clears, strengthens, and quickens the sight of the eyes wonderfully. The decoction of the roots in wine, or the juice taken therein, kills and drives forth all manner of worms in the belly, stomach, and maw; and gargled in the mouth, or the root chewed, fastens loose teeth, and helps to keep them from putrefaction. And being drank is good for those that spit blood, helps to remove cramps or convulsions, gout, sciatica, pains in the joints, applied outwardly or inwardly, and is also good for those that [have hernias], or have any inward bruise. The root boiled well in vinegar beaten afterwards, and made into an ointment with hog's suet, or oil of trotters is an excellent remedy for scabs or itch in young or old; the places also bathed or washed with the decoction doth the same; it also helps all sorts of filthy old putrid sores or cankers whatsoever. The distilled water of the leaves and roots together, is very profitable to cleanse the skin of the face, or other parts, from any morphew [skin blemishes], spots, or blemishes therein, and make it clear.

MODERN USES: Elecampane root has been used for upper respiratory tract catarrhs, as an expectorant and cough suppressant in cases of bronchitis, dry cough, and pertussis. Traditionally, it has also been used for gastrointestinal tract conditions, as a worm expellant, and for the treatment of kidney and lower urinary tract infections. It has confirmed antimicrobial and antioxidant activity. **CAUTION:** The root contains a class of chemical components called sesquiterpene lactones, which are known to be irritating to the mucous membranes and may cause allergic reactions by binding to skin proteins and inducing hypersensitivity. Massage oil containing the root has produced allergic skin reactions.

....

ELM

(ULMUS SPP.)

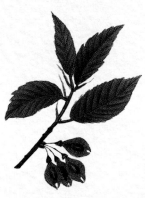

This tree is so well known, growing generally in all counties of this land, that it is needless to describe it.

PLACE: [Trees and shrubs in the genus *Ulmus*, elms are represented by twenty-five to thirty species found in temperate regions of the Northern Hemisphere. They tend to be common woodland species in Europe, temperate Asia, and North America. Elms can be challenging to identify as hybrids take on features of both parents.]

GOVERNMENT AND VIRTUES: It is a cold and saturnine plant. The leaves thereof bruised and applied, heal green wounds, being bound thereon with its own bark. The leaves or the bark used with vinegar, cures scurf and leprosy very effectually. The decoction of the leaves, bark, or root, being bathed, heals broken bones. The water that is found in the bladders on the leaves, while it is fresh, is very effectual to cleanse the skin, and make it fair; and if cloth be often wet therein, and applied to the ruptures of children, it heals them, if they be well bound-up with a truss. The decoction of the bark of the root, fomented, mollifies hard tumours, and the shrinking of the sinews. The roots of the Elm, boiled for a long time in water, and the fat arising on the top thereof, being clean skimmed off, and the place anointed therewith that is grown bald, and the hair fallen away, will quickly restore them again. The said bark ground with brine or pickle, until it come to the form of a poultice, and laid on the place pained with the gout, gives great ease. The decoction of the bark in water, is excellent to bathe such places as have been burnt with fire.

MODERN USES: Culpeper only treats elms in the generic sense, and it is not clear which species or hybrids he refers to. It is likely that in Culpeper's day, all elms were treated as a single entity. The North American species known as slippery elm (*Ulmus rubra*; syn. *Ulmus fulva*) is unique among elms in having high amounts of mucilage in the inner bark; therefore, it is used for the treatment of mucous membrane inflammations such as sore throat and is approved as a nonprescription drug (in lozenge form) in the United States.

....

ENDIVE

(*CICHORIUM ENDIVA*)

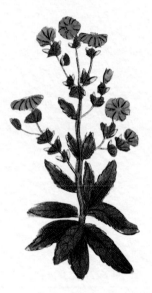

DESCRIPTION: Common garden Endive bears a longer and larger leaf than Succory [Chicory], and abides but one year; it has blue flowers.

PLACE: [Endive is essentially a garden plant of uncertain geographical origin, probably from southern Europe. Genetic selections likely evolved from wild chicory (*Cichorium intybus*). Endive differs from chicory in that it is an annual and less bitter in taste. It is an occasional waif at a garden's edge, a relic from cultivation.]

GOVERNMENT AND VIRTUES: It is a fine cooling, cleansing, jovial plant. The decoction of the leaves, or the juice, or the distilled water of Endive, serve well to cool the excessive heat of the liver and stomach, and in the hot fits of agues, and all other inflammations in any part of the body; it cools the heat and sharpness of the urine, and excoriation in the urinary parts. The seeds are of the same property, or rather more powerful, and besides are available for fainting, swoonings, and passions of the heart. Outwardly applied, they serve to temper the sharp humours of fretting ulcers, hot tumours, swellings, and pestilential sores; and wonderfully help not only the redness and inflammations of the eyes, but the dimness of the sight also; they are also used to allay the pains of the gout. You cannot use it amiss; a syrup of it is a fine cooling medicine for fevers.

MODERN USES: Endive leaves are a nutritious vegetable, but have no other use in modern herbal medicine. See chicory (page 55) for medicinal information.

....

ERYNGO

(ERYNGIUM MARITIMUM)

Eringo, or Sea–Holly

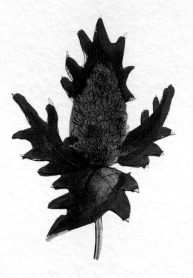

DESCRIPTION: The first leaves of our ordinary Sea-holly, are nothing so hard and prickly as when they grow old, being almost round, and deeply dented about the edges, hard and sharp pointed, and a little crumpled, of a bluish green colour. The root grows wonderfully long, even to eight or ten feet; of a pleasant taste, but much more, being artificially preserved, and candied with sugar.

PLACE: It is found about the sea coast in almost every [country of Europe and North Africa] which borders upon the sea.

GOVERNMENT AND VIRTUES: The plant is venereal, and breeds seed exceedingly, and strengthens the spirit procreative; it is hot and moist, and under the celestial Balance. The decoction of the root hereof in wine, is very effectual to open obstructions of the spleen and liver, and helps yellow jaundice, dropsy, pains of the loins, and wind cholic, provokes urine, and expels the stone, procures women's courses. The continued use of the decoction for fifteen days, taken fasting, and next to bedward, doth help the strangury, the difficulty and stoppage of urine, and the stone, as well as all defects of the lower back and kidneys; and if the said drink be continued longer, it is said that it cures the stone; it is found good against the French pox [syphilis]. The roots bruised and applied outwardly, help the kernels of the throat, commonly called the king's evil; or taking inwardly, and applied to the place stung or bitten by any serpent, heal it speedily. If the roots be bruised, and boiled in old hog's grease, or salted lard, and broken bones, thorns &c. remaining in the flesh, they do not only draw them forth, but heal up the place again, gathering new flesh where it was consumed. The distilled water of the whole herb, when the leaves and stalks are young, is profitable drank for all the purposes aforesaid; and helps the melancholy of the heart, as also for them that have their necks drawn awry, and cannot turn them without turning their whole body.

MODERN USES: In folk medicine in various traditions, especially in regions along the western Mediterranean coast, eryngo root is used for its anti-inflammatory and pain-relieving qualities in the treatment of inflammatory conditions of the urinary tract, such as urethritis, cystitis, and blockage or irritation of the bladder. It is also used as a cough suppressant. The essential oil of the seeds has antioxidant and antimicrobial activity.

CAUTION: Some *Eryngium* species are known to cause gastrointestinal irritation.

....

EYEBRIGHT

(EUPHRASIA OFFICINALIS AND RELATED SPECIES)

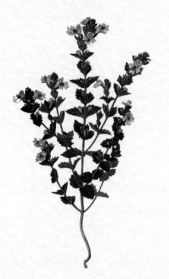

DESCRIPTION: Common Eyebright is a small, low herb. At the joints with the leaves, come forth small white flowers, marked with purple and yellow spots, or stripes.

PLACE: It grows in meadows, and grassy land. [Eyebright is a taxonomically complex plant group with over 350 microspecies collectively treated by herbalists as *Euphrasia officinalis*. It is found throughout cooler regions of the Northern Hemisphere.]

GOVERNMENT AND VIRTUES: It is under the sign of the Lion, and Sol claims dominion over it. If the herb was but as much used as it is neglected, it would half spoil the spectacle maker's trade; and a man would think, that reason should teach people to prefer the preservation of their natural before artificial spectacles; which that they may be instructed how to do, take the virtues of Eyebright as follows.

The juice or distilled water of Eyebright, taken inwardly in white wine or broth, or dropped into the eyes for diverse days together, helps all infirmities of the eyes that cause dimness of sight. Some make conserve of the flowers to the same effect. Being used any of the ways, it also helps a weak brain, or memory.

MODERN USES: Since before Culpeper's time, eyebright has been applied to the eyes either as a poultice or wash to treat conjunctivitis, eye fatigue, itchy irritated eyes, and other eye conditions. It has confirmed astringent and anti-inflammatory activity and possible protective effects against corneal-damaging ultraviolet B rays. **CAUTION:** Use only under the care and direct advice of a qualified medical practitioner.

....

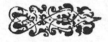

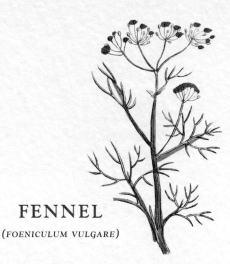

FENNEL
(FOENICULUM VULGARE)

Every garden affords this so plentifully, that it needs no description. [Found commonly in the Middle East, southern Europe, and much of Asia; naturalized in North America, particularly California.]

GOVERNMENT AND VIRTUES: One good old fashion is not yet left off, *viz.* to boil Fennel with fish; for it consumes that phlegmatic humour, which fish most plentifully afford and annoy the body with, though few that use it know wherefore they do it. I suppose the reason of its benefit this way is because it is an herb of Mercury, and under Virgo, and therefore bears antipathy to Pisces. Fennel is good to break wind, to provoke urine, and ease the pains of the stone, and helps to break it. The leaves or seed, boiled in barley water and drank are good for nurses, to increase their milk, and make it more wholesome for the child. The leaves, or rather the seeds, boiled in water, stays the hiccough, and takes away the loathings which oftentimes happen to the stomachs of sick and feverish persons and allays the heat thereof. The seed boiled in wine and drank, is good for those that are bitten with serpents, or have eaten poisonous herbs, or mushrooms. The seed and the roots much more, help to open obstructions of the liver, spleen, and gall, and thereby help the painful and windy swellings of the spleen, and the yellow jaundice; as also the gout and cramps. The seed is of good use in medicines to help shortness of breath and wheezing by stopping of the lungs. Both leaves, seeds, and roots thereof are much used in drink or broth, to make people more lean that are too fat. The sweet Fennel is much weaker in physical uses than the common Fennel. The wild Fennel is stronger and hotter than the tame, and therefore most powerful against the stone, but not so effectual to increase milk, because of its dryness.

MODERN USES: Fennel seed is widely used in traditional medicine systems throughout the world for dyspepsia and mild gastrointestinal upset accompanied by a feeling of fullness and flatulence. It is also used for congestion of the upper respiratory tract. The seeds are chewed, or the ground seeds are made into tea or syrup. **CAUTION:** Some individuals may be sensitive or allergic to fennel seed.

....

FERNS, MALE FERN
(DRYOPTERIS FILIX-MAS)

AND LADY FERN
(ATHYRIUM FILIX-FEMINA)

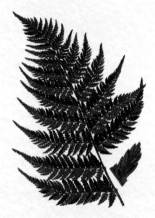

DESCRIPTION: Of this there are two kinds principally to be treated of, *viz.* the Male [*Dryopteris filix-mas*] and Female [Lady Fern (*Athyrium filix-femina*)]. The Female grows higher than the Male, but the leaves thereof are smaller, and more divided and dented, and of as strong a smell as the male; the virtue of them are both alike.

PLACE: They grow both in heaths and in shady places near hedge-sides. [Male fern is native to most of Europe, northern Asia, and the Rocky Mountains, and is naturalized elsewhere. Lady fern is found throughout North America and Europe.]

GOVERNMENT AND VIRTUES: It is under the dominion of Mercury, both Male and Female. The roots of both these sorts of Fern being bruised and boiled in Mead, or honeyed water, and drank, kills both the broad and long worms in the body, and abates the swelling and hardness of the spleen. They are dangerous for women with child to meddle with, by reason they cause abortions. The roots bruised and boiled in oil, or hog's grease, make a very profitable ointment to heal wounds, or pricks gotten in the flesh. The powder of them used in foul ulcers, dries up their malignant moisture, and causes their speedier healing. These ferns being burned, the smoke thereof drives away serpents, gnats, and other noisome creatures.

MODERN USES: Traditionally, the oil or preparations of the oleoresin of male fern root are used under practitioner supervision as a single-dose worm expellant for tapeworms. However, the fern is considered toxic and has largely been replaced by safer modern drugs. Considered milder than male fern, lady fern is also traditionally used as a worm-expellant but, as Culpeper warns, it too is considered toxic. **CAUTION:** Avoid use.

....

FEVERFEW

(*TANACETUM PARTHENIUM*)

Featherfew

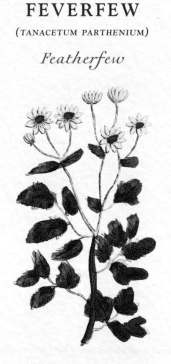

DESCRIPTION: Common Feverfew has large, fresh, green leaves, much torn or cut on the edges. It has many single flowers, consisting of many small white [petals] standing round about a yellow thrum in the middle. The scent of the whole plant is very strong, and the taste is very bitter.

PLACE: This grows wild in many places, but is for the most part nourished in gardens, [having been naturalized after cultivation].

GOVERNMENT AND VIRTUES: Venus commands this herb, and has commended it to succor her sisters (women) and to be a general strengthener of their wombs, and remedy such infirmities as a careless midwife hath there caused if they will but be pleased to make use of her herb boiled in white wine, and drink the decoction; it cleanses the womb, expels the after-birth, and doth a woman all the good she can desire of an herb. And if any grumble because they cannot get the herb in winter, tell them, if they please, they may make a syrup of it in summer; it is chiefly used for the disease of the mother, whether it be the strangling or rising of the mother, or hardness, or inflammation of the same, applied outwardly thereunto. The decoction thereof made with some sugar, or honey put thereto, is used by many with good success to help the cough and stuffing of the chest, by colds, as also to cleanse the kidneys and bladder, and helps to expel the stone in them. It is very effectual for all pains in the head coming of a cold cause, the herb being bruised and applied to the crown of the head; also for the vertigo, that is a running or swimming in the head.

The distilled water takes away freckles, and other spots and deformities in the face. The herb bruised and heated on a tile, with some wine to moisten it, or fried with a little wine and oil in a frying-pan, and applied warm outwardly to the places, helps the wind and cholic in the lower part of the belly. It is an especial remedy against opium taken too liberally.

MODERN USES: Culpeper hints at today's primary use of the herb and its preparations, "for all pains in the head." Feverfew has a long tradition of use in the prevention or treatment of migraine. Starting in the 1980s, various pharmacological and clinical studies showed that anti-inflammatory and antisecretory activity of the leaf provided temporary relief from or prevented migraine, tension headaches, and related symptoms such as nausea. **CAUTION:** Chewing the fresh leaves or ingesting them internally caused mouth ulcerations in about 17 percent of individuals. This effect is systemic and not the result of contact dermatitis. Allergic reactions are also reported.

....

FIELD PENNYCRESS

(THLASPI ARVENSE)

Treacle Mustard

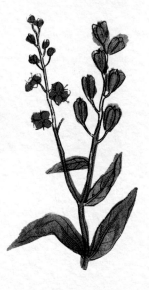

DESCRIPTION: It rises up, about a foot high, having soft green leaves, wavy, but not cut into the edges, broadest towards the ends; the flowers are white that grow at the tops of the branches, [in a] spike-fashion. [It is] somewhat sharp in taste, and smelling of garlick, especially in the fields where it is natural.

PLACE: [Found in fields and waysides throughout all of Europe and Asia; naturalized as a weed elsewhere.]

GOVERNMENT AND VIRTUES: The Mustards are said to purge the body both upwards and downwards, and procure women's courses so abundantly, that it suffocates the birth. It breaks inward imposthumes, being taken inwardly; and used in clysters, helps the sciatica. The seed applied, doth the same. It is an especial ingredient in mithridate and treacle, being of itself an antidote resisting poison, venom and putrefaction.

MODERN USES: Also known as "stinkweed" for its strong garlic-like odor, field pennycress is little used as a medicinal plant, but it has been used topically as an embrocation to stimulate circulation in cases of rheumatism. It is also suggested as an oilseed-producing cover crop for farmlands that are fallow throughout the winter months. **CAUTION:** Topical use for rheumatism suggests the plant is an irritant.

....

FIELD PEPPERWORT

(*LEPIDIUM CAMPESTRE*)

Mithridate Mustard

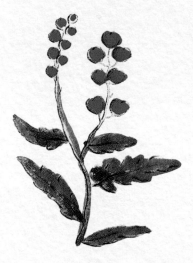

DESCRIPTION: This grows higher than [field pennycress (*Thlaspi arvense*) (see page 89)], spreading more, [and the] leaves are smaller and narrower. The flowers are small and white, growing on long branches.

PLACE: [Common in grasslands and most of Europe; naturalized as a weed in North America.]

GOVERNMENT AND VIRTUES: Both of them are herbs of Mars. The Mustards are said to purge the body both upwards and downwards, and procure women's courses so abundantly, that it suffocates the birth. It breaks inward imposthumes [abscesses], being taken inwardly; and used in clysters, helps the sciatica. It is also available in many cases for which the common Mustard is used, but somewhat weaker.

MODERN USES: Field pepperwort is seldom used medicinally. Of research interest as a possible oilseed crop. Flowering tops and seed heads used topically for rheumatism like field pennycress.

FIG TREE

(*FICUS CARICA*)

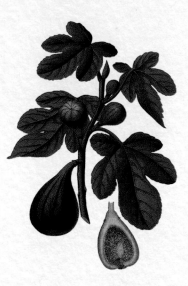

To give a description of a tree so well known to everybody that keep it in a garden, is needless. They prosper very well in English gardens, yet are fitter for medicine than for any other profit which is gotten by the fruit of them.

PLACE: [Native to the Middle East and western Asia; cultivated for at least twelve thousand years and widely naturalized.]

GOVERNMENT AND VIRTUES: The tree is under the dominion of Jupiter. The milk that issues out from the leaves or branches where they are broken off, being dropped upon warts, takes them away. The decoction of the leaves is excellently good to wash sore heads with: and there is scarcely a better remedy for the leprosy than it is. It clears the face also of morphew [skin blemishes], and the body of white scurf, scabs, and running sores. If it be dropped into old fretting ulcers, it cleanses out the moisture, and brings up the flesh; because you cannot have the leaves green all the year, you may make an ointment of them whilst you can. A decoction of the leaves being drank inwardly, or rather a syrup made of them, dissolves congealed blood caused by bruises or falls, and helps the bloody flux [dysentery]. The ashes of the wood made into an ointment with hog's grease, helps kibes and chilblains. The juice being put into a hollow tooth, eases pain. A syrup made of the leaves, or green fruit, is excellently good for coughs, hoarseness, or shortness of breath, and all diseases of the breast and lungs; it is also extremely good for the dropsy and falling sickness. They say that the Fig Tree, as well as the Bay Tree, is never hurt by lightning; as also, if you tie a bull, be he ever so mad, to a Fig Tree, he will quickly become tame and gentle. As for such figs as come from beyond sea, I have little to say, because I write not of exotics.

MODERN USES: Figs are grown in warm temperate and subtropical climates and used globally. In addition to their food value, they are known for having a laxative effect. Most modern research has focused on the medicinal effects of the leaves, to which antioxidant, antimicrobial, experimental anticancer, antispasmodic, blood-thinning, and antiparasitic effects are attributed. Figs or fig leaves are used as folk remedies for abscesses, cancer, corns, cough, flu, hemorrhoids, pimples (or skin blemishes, as Culpeper describes), and warts. **CAUTION:** Some individuals may be allergic to both the leaves (including leaf preparations) and the fruits.

....

FIGWORT

(SCROPHULARIA NODOSA)

Throat–Wort

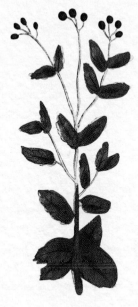

DESCRIPTION: Common great Figwort sends square stalks, three or four feet high; at the tops of the stalks stand many purple flowers, which are sometimes gaping and open.

PLACE: It grows frequently in moist and shadowy woods, and in the lower parts of the fields and meadows. [Native to most of Europe and sporadically naturalized in North America.]

GOVERNMENT AND VIRTUES: Some Latin authors call it Cervicaria, because it is appropriated to the neck; and we Throatwort, because it is appropriated to the throat. Venus owns the herb, and the Celestial Bull will not deny it; therefore a better remedy cannot be for the king's evil [unusual swelling of lymph nodes or scrofula], because the Moon that rules the disease, is exalted there. The decoction of the herb taken inwardly, and the bruised herb applied outwardly, dissolves clotted and congealed blood within the body, coming by any wounds, bruise, or fall; and is no less effectual for the king's evil, or any other knobs, kernel, bunches, or wens growing in the flesh wheresoever; and for the hemorrhoids, or piles. An ointment made hereof may be used at all times when the fresh herb is not to be had. The distilled water of the whole plant, roots and all, is used for the same purposes, and dries up the superfluous, virulent moisture of hollow and corroding ulcers; it takes away all redness, spots, and freckles in the face, as also the scurf, and any foul deformity therein, and the leprosy likewise.

MODERN USES: Figwort has significant antifungal and antibacterial effects with analgesic and wound-healing activity. These pharmacological effects support traditional external use of the herb as a poultice for bruises, sprains, swelling, inflammation, wounds, and skins eruptions, such as those associated with scrofula (or king's evil)—lymph node swellings historically associated with tuberculosis. It is also used for chronic skin conditions such as eczema, psoriasis, and pruritus.

....

FLEAWORT

(*PULICARIA VULGARIS, PULICARIA DYSENTERICA*)

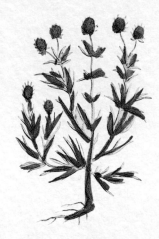

DESCRIPTION: Ordinary Fleawort [*Pulicaria vulgaris*] rises up with a stalk two feet high or more, [with] long and narrow whitish green leaves somewhat hairy. At the top of every branch come forth small whitish yellow threads, like to those of the Plantain herbs. The whole plant [smells] somewhat like rosin.

There is another sort [*Pulicaria dysenterica*], differing not from the former in the manner of growing, but only that the stalk and branches being somewhat greater.

PLACE: [Native to Europe, extending to Iran and North Africa; declining in northern Europe due to habitat loss.]

GOVERNMENT AND VIRTUES: The herb is cold, and dry, and saturnine. I suppose it obtained the name of Fleawort, because the seeds are so like Fleas. The seeds fried, and taken, stays the flux or lask [diarrhea] of the belly, and the corrosions that come by reason of hot choleric, or sharp and malignant humours, or by too much purging of any violent medicine. The mucilage of the seed made with Rose-water, and a little sugar-candy put thereto, is very good in all hot agues and burning fevers, and other inflammations, to cool the thirst, and lenify the dryness and roughness of the tongue and throat. It helps also hoarseness of the voice, and diseases of the breast and lungs, caused by heat, or sharp salt humours, and the pleurisy also. The mucilage of the seed made with Plantain water, whereunto the yoke of an egg or two, and a little Populeon [ointment of poplar buds] are put, is a most safe and sure remedy to ease the sharpness, pricking, and pains of the hemorrhoids or piles, if it be laid on a cloth, and bound thereto. It helps all inflammations in any part of the body, and the pains that come thereby, as the headache and megrims [depression], and all hot imposthumes [abscesses], swellings, or breaking out of the skin, as blains, wheals, pushes, purples, and the like, as also the joints of those that are out of joint, the pains of the gout and sciatica, the burstings of young children, and the swellings of the navel, applied with oil of roses and vinegar. It is also good to heal the nipples and sore breasts of women, being often applied thereunto. The juice of the herb with a little honey put into the ears helps the running of them, and the worms breeding in them: The same also mixed with hog's grease, and applied to corrupt and filthy ulcers, cleanses them and heals them.

MODERN USES: Fleawort is seldom used today, but this aromatic plant is of interest to scientists who study essential oils for potential antibacterial and antiviral use. It has potential as a treatment for the protozoal disease leishmaniasis.

....

FLIXWEED

(*DESCURAINIA SOPHIA; SYN. SISYMBRIUM SOPHIA*)

Fluxweed

DESCRIPTION: It rises up with a round upright hard stalk, four or five feet high, spread into sundry branches, whereon grow many greyish green leaves, very finely cut and severed into a number of short and almost round parts.

PLACE: They flower wild in the fields. [A weed of wastelands throughout Europe, Asia, North Africa, and much of western North America.]

GOVERNMENT AND VIRTUES: This herb is saturnine also. Both the herb and seed of Fluxweed is of excellent use to stay the flux or lask of the belly, being drank in water wherein gads of steel heated have been often quenched; and is no less effectual for the same purpose than Plantain or Comfrey, and to restrain any other flux of blood in man or woman, as also to consolidate bones broken or out of joint. The juice thereof drank in wine, or the decoction of the herb drank, doth kill the worms in the stomach or belly, or the worms that grow in putrid and filthy ulcers, and made into a salve doth quickly heal all old sores, how foul or malignant so ever they be. The distilled water of the herb works the same effect, although somewhat weaker, yet it is a fair medicine, and more acceptable to be taken. It is called Fluxweed because it cures the flux, and for its uniting broken bones, &c. Paracelsus extols it to the skies. It is fitting that syrup, ointment, and plasters of it were kept in your house.

MODERN USES: Flixweed is little used in Western herbalism, but the seeds are used in preparations in traditional Chinese medicine to relieve asthma and cough, as a diuretic, and to enhance cardiac function (by reducing edema). Also used in Persian traditional medicine; in modern Iran it is used for fevers, constipation, as a digestive tonic and cardiotonic, and for its astringent and expectorant effects—an example of how one culture's weed is another's herbal medicine. Experimental studies confirm anti-inflammatory, analgesic, antioxidant, and fever-reducing effects.

....

FLUELLIN, ROUND-LEAVED
(KICKXIA SPURIA; SYN. LINARIA SPURIA)
Lluellin

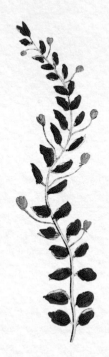

DESCRIPTION: It shoots forth many long branches, set with almost red leaves; at the joints all along the stalks, come forth small flowers, gaping somewhat like Snapdragons, with the upper jaw of a yellow colour, and the lower of a purplish, with a small heel or spur behind.

There is another sort of Lluellin [sharp-pointed fluellin or toadflax (*Kickxia elatine*; syn. *Linaria elatine*)] which has longer branches wholly trailing upon the ground, two or three feet long, and somewhat thinner. The flowers are more white than yellow, and the purple not so far.

PLACE: They grow in diverse fields, and borders. [Found in various parts of Europe and the United Kingdom; naturalized in eastern and western North America.]

GOVERNMENT AND VIRTUES: It is a Lunar herb. The leaves bruised and applied with barley meal to watering eyes that are hot and inflamed by defluxions from the head, do very much help them, as also the fluxes of blood or humours, as the lask [diarrhea], bloody flux [dysentery], women's courses, and stays all manner of bleeding at the nose, mouth, or any other place, or that comes by any bruise or hurt, or bursting a vein; it wonderfully helps all those inward parts that need consolidating or strengthening, and is no less effectual both to heal and close green wounds, than to cleanse and heal all foul or old ulcers, fretting or spreading cankers or the like. This herb is of a fine cooling, drying quality, and an ointment or plaster of it might do a man a courtesy that hath any hot virulent sores: 'Tis admirable for the ulcers of the French pox [syphilis]; if taken inwardly, may cure the disease.

MODERN USES: Culpeper's "Lluellin" has been erroneously confused in various editions of the *English Physician* with speedwell (*Veronica officinalis*), which shares the same common name "fluellein," a word of Welsh or possibly of Dutch origin. Culpeper clearly describes the snapdragon-like *Kickxia* species, which are types of toadflax with spurred yellow and purple flowers. They contain compounds called iridoids that have been associated with possible antidiabetic and antimicrobial activity. The expressed juice has been used as a folk cancer remedy. Scarcely researched and seldom used today.

....

FOXGLOVE

(DIGITALIS PURPUREA)

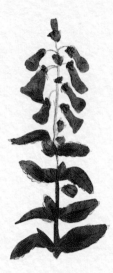

DESCRIPTION: It has many long and broad leaves, a little soft or woolly, and of a hoary green colour, among which rise up stalks, from whence to the top [are] large and long hollow reddish-purple flowers, with some white spots within them.

PLACE: It grows on dry sandy ground [in fields, flower gardens, and wastelands throughout Europe; naturalized elsewhere].

GOVERNMENT AND VIRTUES: The plant is under the dominion of Venus, being of a gentle cleansing nature. The herb is frequently used by the Italians to heal any fresh or green wound, the leaves being but bruised and bound thereon; and the juice thereof is also used in old sores, to cleanse, dry, and heal them. The decoction hereof made up with some sugar or honey, is available to cleanse and purge the body both upwards and downwards, sometimes of tough phlegm and clammy humours, and to open obstructions of the liver and spleen. An ointment of it is one of the best remedies for scabby head that is.

MODERN USES: English physician William Withering (1741–99) revealed the use of foxglove as a cardiac stimulant in 1785, based on a secret family recipe that "an old woman in Shropshire" held for the treatment of dropsy (swollen legs due to fluid accumulation). Dropsy or edema is a telltale sign of cardiac insufficiency. Since that time, well-controlled, pharmacentically synthesized doses of this toxic plant or mixtures of its pure glycosides, including digoxin and digitoxin, adjusted to the needs of individual patients, have been used in the management of cardiac insufficiency, hypertonia, and heart rhythm abnormalities. **CAUTION:** Avoid use. All parts of foxglove are toxic and ingesting any plant part could be fatal. Notice that Culpeper primarily limits his list of uses to external applications.

....

FUMITORY

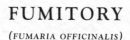

(*FUMARIA OFFICINALIS*)

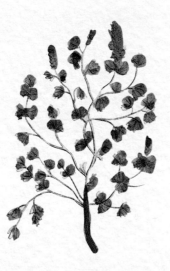

DESCRIPTION: Our common Fumitory is a tender sappy herb, with finely cut and jagged leaves of a whitish-blueish sea green colour. At the tops of the branches stand many small flowers, made like little birds, of a reddish purple colour, with whitish bellies.

PLACE: [Found in fields and gardens from Europe to central Asia and naturalized sporadically in North and South America.]

GOVERNMENT AND VIRTUES: Saturn owns the herb, and presents it to the world as a cure for his own disease, and a strengthener of the parts of the body he rules. If by my astrological judgment of diseases, from the decumbiture (horoscope at the onset of confinement to sick bed), you find Saturn author of the disease, or if by direction from a nativity you fear a saturnine disease approaching, you may by this herb prevent it in the one, and cure it in the other, and therefore it is fit you keep a syrup of it always by you. The juice or syrup made thereof, or the decoction made in whey by itself, with some other purging or opening herbs and roots to cause it to work the better (itself being but weak) is very effectual for the liver and spleen, opening the obstructions thereof, and clarifying the blood from saltish, choleric, and adust humours, which cause leprosy, scabs, tetters, itches, and such like breakings-out of the skin, and after the purgings doth strengthen all the inwards parts. It is also good against the yellow-jaundice, and spends it by urine, which it procures in abundance.

The powder of the dried herb given for some time together, cures melancholy, but the seed is strongest in operation for all the former diseases. The distilled water of the herb is also of good effect in the former diseases, and conduces much against the plague and pestilence, being taken with good treacle. The distilled water also, with a little water and honey of roses, helps all sores of the mouth or throat, being gargled often therewith. The juice dropped into the eyes, clears the sight and takes away redness and other defects in them, although it procure some pain for the present, and cause tears. The juice of the Fumitory and Docks mingled with vinegar, and the places gently washed therewith, cures all sorts of scabs, pimples, blotches, wheals, and pushes which arise on the face or hands or any other parts of the body.

MODERN USES: Dried fumitory has been used in tea for the treatment of spasms or colicky pain affecting the gastrointestinal tract, gallbladder, and bile ducts. Herbalists traditionally use it in the treatment of irritable bowel syndrome. Historically, the herb has been used internally as a diuretic and laxative and externally for the treatment of eczema, psoriasis, and scabies.

....

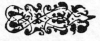

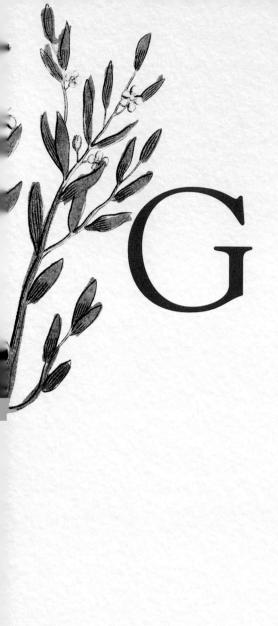

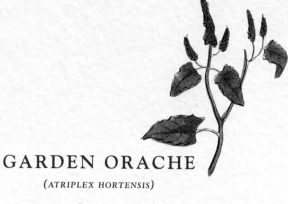

GARDEN ORACHE

(ATRIPLEX HORTENSIS)

Garden Arrach

Called also Orach, and Arage; it is cultivated for domestic uses.

PLACE: [Native to Central Asia and the Caucasus. Now grown as an ornamental.]

GOVERNMENT AND VIRTUES: It is under the government of the Moon; in quality cold and moist like unto her. [If eaten] it softens and loosens the [stool], and fortifies the expulsive faculty. The herb, whether it be bruised and applied to the throat, or boiled, and in like manner applied, it matters not much, it is excellently good for swellings in the throat: the best way, I suppose, is to boil it, apply the herb outwardly: the decoction of it, besides, is an excellent remedy for the yellow jaundice.

MODERN USES: Perhaps well-known in the English kitchen garden in Culpeper's day, garden orache was introduced to Europe from western Asia by 1548, but was seldom used two hundred years later, as it had been replaced by spinach. Garden orache is sometimes grown as an ornamental, or the seed is used in birdseed mixes. It has escaped, becoming a weed. Not used in herbal medicine.

....

GARLIC

(ALLIUM SATIVUM)

Garlick

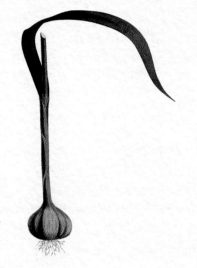

The offensiveness of the breath of him that hath eaten Garlick, will lead you by the nose to the knowledge hereof, and (instead of a description) direct you to the place where it grows in gardens, which kinds are the best, and most physical.

PLACE: [Only known in gardens, garlic has evolved over seven thousand years of cultivation and does not occur in the wild. Its closest wild relatives are found in Central Asia, where garlic may have originated.]

GOVERNMENT AND VIRTUES: Mars owns this herb. This was anciently accounted the poor man's treacle, it being a remedy for all diseases and hurts (except those which itself breed). It provokes urine, and women's courses, helps the biting of mad dogs and other venomous creatures, kills worms in children, cuts and voids tough phlegm, purges the head, helps the lethargy, is a good preservative against, and a remedy for any plague, sore, or foul ulcers; takes away spots and blemishes in the skin, eases pains in the ears, ripens and breaks imposthumes [abscesses], or other swellings. And for all those diseases the onions are as effectual. But the Garlick hath some more peculiar virtues besides the former, *viz.* it hath a special quality to discuss inconveniences coming by corrupt agues or mineral vapours; or by drinking corrupt and stinking waters; as also by taking wolf-bane, henbane, hemlock, or other poisonous and dangerous herbs. It is also held good in hydropick diseases, the jaundice, falling sickness, cramps, convulsions, the piles or hemorrhoids, or other cold diseases. Many authors quote many diseases this is good for; but conceal its vices. Its heat is very vehement, and all vehement hot things send up but ill-favored vapours to the brain. In choleric men it will add fuel to the fire; in men oppressed by melancholy, it will attenuate the humour, and send up strong fancies, and as many strange visions to the head; therefore let it be taken inwardly with great moderation; outwardly you may make bolder with it.

MODERN USES: Today garlic is used to reduce the risks associated with cardiovascular disease including lowering low-density lipoproteins, cholesterol, blood pressure, and blood sugar. It is considered a blood thinner, thereby increasing blood flow. Various garlic preparations have been evaluated in dozens of controlled clinical studies with positive results. Garlic is used for the supportive management and prevention of age-dependent vascular disease such as atherosclerosis. **CAUTION:** Due to its blood-thinning effects, garlic should not be consumed before surgery, or with certain medications. Consult your medical professional.

. . . .

GARLIC MUSTARD

(ALLIARIA PETIOLATA)

Sauce–Alone, Jack–by–the–Hedge–Side

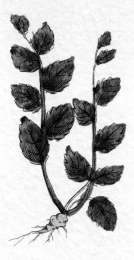

DESCRIPTION: The lower leaves of this are rounder than those that grow towards the top. The flowers are white. The plant, or any part thereof, being bruised, smells of garlic, but more pleasantly, and tastes somewhat hot and sharp, almost like unto rocket.

PLACE: It grows in fields in many places. [Found throughout Europe. Naturalized and rapidly spreading in North America, where it is becoming a serious invasive alien, choking out both native prairies in the West and those in open wood in the eastern United States. Global warming increases its spread because its seeds germinate earlier than native plants, thus crowding out natives before they have a chance to grow.]

GOVERNMENT AND VIRTUES: It is an herb of Mercury. This is eaten by many country people as a sauce to their salt fish, and helps well to digest the crudities and other corrupt humours engendered thereby. It warms also the stomach, and causes digestion. The juice thereof boiled with honey is accounted to be as good as hedge mustard for the cough, to cut and expectorate the tough phlegm. The seed bruised and boiled in wine, is a singularly good remedy for the wind colic, or the stone, being drank warm: It is also given to women troubled with the mother, both to drink, and the seed put into a cloth, and applied while it is warm, is of singularly good use. The leaves also, or the seed boiled, is good to be used in clysters to ease the pains of the stone. The green leaves are held to be good to heal the ulcers in the legs.

MODERN USES: Used as a folk medicine as described by Culpeper. As the name "garlic mustard" implies, this member of the mustard family combines chemical constituents found in both garlic and mustards, leading to a peppery, strong garlic flavor. This chemical combination defends the plant against a broad range of enemies, even killing soil bacteria and fungi beneficial to native plants. Garlic mustard is a one-species wrecking crew for native plants in open fields and woodlands. It is built to survive and multiply. Used in small amounts as flavoring, or in times of famine as a broth. **CAUTION:** Contains cyanide; avoid eating uncooked leaves or consuming large quantities.

....

GENTIAN

(GENTIANELLA AMARELLA; SYN. GENTIANA AMARELLA)

Felwort, or Baldmony

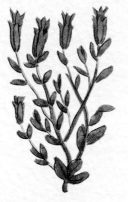

It is confessed that Gentian, which is most used amongst us, is brought over from beyond sea, yet we have two sorts of it growing frequently in our nation, which, besides the reasons so frequently alleged why English herbs should be fittest for English bodies, has been proved by the experience of diverse physicians, to be not a wit inferior in virtue to that which comes from beyond sea, therefore be pleased to take the description of them as follows.

DESCRIPTION: The greater of the two [felwort (*Gentianella amarella*)] hath many small long roots thrust down deep into the ground, and abiding all the Winter. The stalks are sometimes two feet high; the flowers are long and hollow, of a purple colour, ending in fine corners. The smaller sort [field gentian (*Gentianella campestris*)], grows up, not a foot high; on the tops of these stalks grow diverse perfect blue flowers.

PLACE: [*Gentianella amarella* occurs in diverse habitats throughout most of Europe. *Gentianella campestris* is widespread in central and northern Europe.]

GOVERNMENT AND VIRTUES: They are under the dominion of Mars, and one of the principal herbs he is ruler of. They resist putrefactions, poison, and a surer remedy cannot be found to prevent the pestilence than it is; it strengthens the stomach exceedingly, helps digestion, comforts the heart, and preserves it against faintings and swoonings. The powder of the dry roots helps the biting of mad dogs and venomous beasts, opens obstructions of the liver, and restores an appetite for their meat to such as have lost it. The herb steeped in wine, and the wine drank, refreshes such as be over-weary with traveling, and grow lame in their joints, either by cold or evil lodgings; it helps stitches, and griping pains in the sides. It is an admirable remedy to kill the worms, by taking half a dram of the powder in a morning in any convenient liquor; the same is excellently good to be taken inwardly for the king's evil [unusual swelling of lymph nodes or scrofula]. It helps agues of all sorts, and the yellow jaundice, as also the bots in cattle; when kine [cows] are bitten on the udder by any venomous beast, do but stroke the place with the decoction of any of these, and it will instantly heal them.

MODERN USES: In keeping with his purpose to promote herbs of the English countryside for English readers, Culpeper dismisses gentian "from beyond the sea"—the yellow gentian (*Gentiana lutea*) of the Alps—in favor of the five blue-flowered English species of *Gentiana*. The roots of many, if not all, *Gentiana* species contain compounds such as gentipicroside and amarogentin, which set the standard for extreme bitterness taste values. Thus, the roots of various gentians stimulate saliva and gastric juice and are used as a bitter digestive stimulant for lack of appetite, anorexia, and dyspepsia, and as a tonic to the gastrointestinal system.

....

GERMANDER

(TEUCRIUM CHAMAEDRYS)

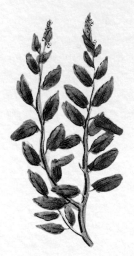

DESCRIPTION: Common Germander has small and somewhat round leaves. The flowers stand[ing] at the tops [are] of a deep purple colour. [Commonly grown in herb gardens as a short evergreen woody hedge, it originates from and is found throughout much of north-central Europe to south-central Russia.]

GOVERNMENT AND VIRTUES: It is a most prevalent herb of Mercury, and strengthens the brain and apprehension exceedingly when weak, and relieves them when drooping. It is most effectual against the poison of all serpents, being drank in wine, and the bruised herb outwardly applied; used with honey, it cleanses old and foul ulcers. It is likewise good for the pains in the sides and cramps. It is also good against all diseases of the brain, as continual head-ache, falling-sickness, melancholy, drowsiness and dullness of the spirits, convulsions and palsies. A dram of the seed taken in powder purges by urine, and is good against the yellow jaundice. The juice of the leaves dropped into the ears kills the worms in them. The tops thereof, when they are in flowers, steeped twenty-four hours in a draught of white wine, and drank, kills the worms in the belly.

MODERN USES: A longtime folk use of germander was to treat obesity. It was even approved for that purpose in France until the early 1990s, when over two dozen cases of acute hepatitis, including one fatality, occurred in women who had used germander products for weight loss. This incident resulted in a ban on the sale of the herb in France and elsewhere. It was also used as a traditional remedy for mild diarrhea and as an oral analgesic. **CAUTION:** Don't ingest due to confirmed liver toxicity. Avoid.

....

GOLDENROD

(SOLIDAGO VIRGAUREA)

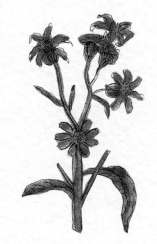

DESCRIPTION: This rises up two feet high, and sometimes more, having thereon many narrow and long dark green leaves, with diverse small yellow flowers.

PLACE: [Found in open woodlands, fields, meadows, rocky cliffs, and hedgerows throughout most of Europe, extending into East Asia.]

GOVERNMENT AND VIRTUES: Venus claims the herb, and therefore to be sure it respects beauty lost. Arnoldus de Villa Nova commends it much against the stone in the kidneys, and to provoke urine in abundance, whereby also the gravel and stone may be voided. The decoction of the herb, green or dry, or the distilled water thereof, is very effectual for inward bruises, as also to be outwardly applied, it stays bleeding in any part of the body, and of wounds. It is a sovereign wound herb, inferior to none, both for the inward and outward hurts; green wounds, old sores and ulcers, are quickly cured therewith. It also is of especial use in all lotions for sores or ulcers in the mouth, throat, or private parts of man or woman. The decoction also helps to fasten the teeth that are loose in the gums.

MODERN USES: European goldenrod increases diuresis and blood flow to the kidneys without stimulating the loss of sodium and chloride. Used in modern phytomedicine in the treatment of kidney and bladder inflammation, urinary calculi, and kidney gravel, and in the supportive treatment of urinary tract infections. It is considered diuretic, antispasmodic, and anti-inflammatory. **CAUTION:** Topical products may cause contact dermatitis. Other allergies are possible.

....

GOOSEBERRY

(RIBES UVA-CRISPA; SYN. RIBES GROSSULARIA)

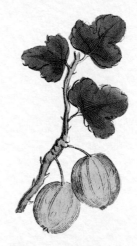

PLACE: [Found in hedges, open woods, and scrubland. Native to most of Europe; naturalized in the northeastern United States and the Canadian Maritime Provinces.]

GOVERNMENT AND VIRTUES: They are under the dominion of Venus. The berries, while they are unripe, being scalded or baked, are good to stir up a fainting or decayed appetite, especially such whose stomachs are afflicted by choleric humours. They are excellently good to stay longings of women with child. You may keep them preserved with sugar all the yearlong. The decoction of the leaves cools hot swellings and inflammations; as also St. Anthony's fire. The ripe Gooseberries being eaten, are an excellent remedy to allay the violent heat both of the stomach and liver. The young and tender leaves break the stone, and expel gravel both from the kidneys and bladder.

MODERN USES: Gooseberries are mostly eaten as a food. The seed oil of the related shrub black currant (*Ribes nigrum*) is a rich source of gamma-linolenic acid (GLA), an essential fatty acid from dietary sources. GLA-containing seed oils have been suggested for possible clinical use in treating premenstrual syndrome (PMS), atopic eczema, cardiovascular disease, rheumatoid arthritis, and various problems associated with diabetes, among other conditions.

....

GOOSEFOOT, STINKING

(CHENOPODIUM VULVARIA)

Arrach, Wild and Stinking

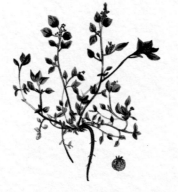

DESCRIPTION: This has small, almost round leaves, a little pointed and, of a dusky mealy colour, growing on the slender stalks and branches that spread on the ground, with small flowers set with the leaves. It smells like rotten fish, or something worse.

PLACE: It grows usually upon dunghills, [disturbed soils, and wastelands. Native in most of Europe and naturalized in North America.]

GOVERNMENT AND VIRTUES: Stinking Arrach is used as a remedy to women pained, and almost strangled with the mother, by smelling to it; but inwardly taken there is no better remedy under the moon for that disease. I would be large in commendation of this herb, were I but eloquent. It is an herb under the dominion of Venus, and under the sign Scorpio; it is common almost upon every dunghill. The works of God are freely given to man, his medicines are common and cheap, and easily found. I commend it for a universal medicine for the womb, and such a medicine as will easily, safely, and speedily cure any disease thereof, as the fits of the mother, dislocation, or falling out thereof; cools the womb being over-heated. And let me tell you this, and I will tell you the truth, heat of the womb is one of the greatest causes of hard labour in child-birth. It makes barren women fruitful. It cleanseth the womb if it be foul, and strengthens it exceedingly; it provokes the terms if they be stopped, and stops them if they flow immoderately; you can desire no good to your womb, but this herb will affect it; therefore if you love children, if you love health, if you love ease, keep a syrup always by you, made of the juice of this herb, and sugar (or honey, if it be to cleanse the womb), and let such as be rich keep it for their poor neighbors; and bestow it as freely as I bestow my studies upon them, or else let them look to answer it another day, when the Lord shall come to make inquisition for blood.

MODERN USES: A quaint historical relic. Useful for the entertainment value of Culpeper's charm of phrase.

Writing in 1777, English botanist William Curtis (1746–99) states: "There is some difficulty in ascertaining several of the plants of this genus, but that difficulty cannot be alleged against the present species, as it is at all times, both fresh and dried, discoverable by its smell alone; the whole plant, if ever so slightly bruised betwixt the thumb and fingers, communicating a very permanently disagreeable odor, resembling, in the opinion of most person, stale salt fish" (*Flora Londinensis* Vol. 5).

GORSE

(ULEX EUROPAEUS)

The Furze Bush

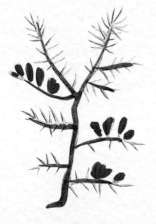

It is as well known by this name, as it is in some counties by the name of Gorz or Whins, that I shall not need to write any description thereof, my intent being to teach my countrymen what they know not, rather than to tell them again of that which is generally known before.

PLACE: They are known to grow on dry barren heaths, and other waste, gravelly or sandy grounds. [Native to western Europe; naturalized in western North America and temperate South America, and considered a noxious weed that is prone to catch fire.]

GOVERNMENT AND VIRTUES: Mars owns the herb. They are hot and dry, and open obstructions of the liver and spleen. A decoction made with the flowers thereof hath been found effectual against the jaundice, as also to provoke urine, and cleanse the kidneys from gravel or stone.

MODERN USES: Gorse itself is rarely used as a medicinal plant. However, a specific lectin extracted from the seeds is used as a diagnostic tool in blood tests to identify antigens on human red blood cells, serving as a biomarker for screening the presence of cancer cells.

....

GRAPE VINE

(VITIS VINIFERA)

PLACE: [Wine is believed to have originated in the Caucasus, the ancestral home of the grapevine, at least seven thousand years ago. Over thousands of years, grapes spread throughout Europe and wherever they would grow in the world. There are more than eight thousand varieties of grapes.]

GOVERNMENT AND VIRTUES: The leaves of the English vine being boiled, makes a good lotion for sore mouths; being boiled with barley meal into a poultice, it cools inflammations of wounds; the dropping of the vine, when it is cut in the Spring, which country people call Tears, being boiled in a syrup, with sugar, and taken inwardly, is excellent to stay women's longings after everything they see, which is a disease many women with child are subject to. The decoction of Vine leaves in white wine doth the like. Also the tears of the Vine, drank two or three spoonfuls at a time, breaks the stone in the bladder. This is a good remedy, and it is discreetly done, to kill a Vine to cure a man, but the salt of the leaves are held to be better. The ashes of the burnt branches will make teeth that are as black as a coal, to be as white as snow, if you but every morning rub them with it. It is a most gallant Tree of the Sun, very sympathetically with the body of men, and that is the reason spirit of wine is the greatest cordial among all vegetables.

MODERN USES: Culpeper celebrates the spirit of wine as the greatest cordial. Little has changed in attitudes toward wine. Aside from the well-known antioxidant benefits of red wine, an extract of grapeseed has also been shown to have strong antioxidant activity. The extracts are used to prevent or treat peripheral venous insufficiency, reducing a tendency to bruising and varicosities. The extract is anti-inflammatory and of potential value in improving skin damage due to ultraviolet radiation.

....

GROMWELL

(LITHOSPERMUM OFFICINALE)

Gromel

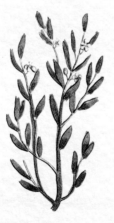

DESCRIPTION: The greater Gromwell [*Lithospermum purpureocaeruleum*] grows up with slender hard and hairy stalks, with hairy dark green leaves thereon. At the joints, come forth blue flowers.

The smaller wild Gromwell [*Lithospermum arvense*] sends forth diverse upright hard branched stalks, two or three feet high, at every one of which grow small, long, hard, and rough leaves; among which come forth small white flowers. The garden or common Gromwell [*Lithospermum officinale*] has diverse upright, slender, woody, hairy stalks, and white flowers.

PLACE: The two first grow wild in barren or untilled places, and by the wayside in many places [in Europe and Asia; occasionally naturalized in eastern North America].

GOVERNMENT AND VIRTUES: The herb belongs to Dame Venus; thus if Mars cause the cholic or stone, as usually he doth, if in Virgo, this is your cure. These are accounted to be of as singular force as any herb or seed whatsoever, to break the stone and to void it, and the gravel either in the kidneys or bladder, as also to provoke urine being stopped, and to help strangury [painful, frequent urination]. The seed is of greatest use, being bruised and boiled in white wine or in broth, or the like, or the powder of the seed taken therein. The herb itself, (when the seed is not to be had) either boiled, or the juice thereof drank, is effectual to all the purposes aforesaid, but is not so powerful or speedy.

MODERN USES: As gromwell seeds were thought to resemble kidney stones, the doctrine of signatures—in which a plant part was thought to resemble an organ of the body—dictated that the herb be used to treat urinary calculi and gravel. Not used today. **CAUTION:** Like coltsfoot, gromwell contains liver-toxic pyrrolizidine alkaloids, which can cause veno-occlusive disease of the liver; therefore, the herb is no longer considered safe to use.

....

GROUND ELDER

(AEGOPODIUM PODAGRARIA)

Gout–Wort, or Herb Gerrard

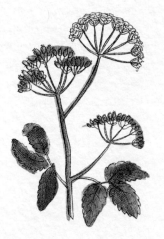

DESCRIPTION: It is a low herb, seldom rising half a yard high, having sundry leaves standing on brownish green stalks by three, snipped about, and of a strong unpleasant savour: The umbels of the flowers are white.

PLACE: It grows by hedge and wall-sides, and often in the border and corner of fields, and in gardens also. [Originally brought to monasteries from the European continent, ground elder is now a widespread weed of wastelands in eastern North America and Australia.]

GOVERNMENT AND VIRTUES: Saturn rules it. Neither is it to be supposed Goutwort hath its name for nothing but upon experiment to heal the gout and sciatica; as also joint-aches, and other cold griefs. The very bearing of it about one eases the pains of the gout, and defends him that bears it from the disease.

MODERN USES: Young ground elder leaves have been used as a vegetable. Considered diuretic, mildly sedative, and anti-inflammatory, the fresh roots and leaves have long been used in traditional medicine for the treatment of gout, both internally as a tincture and externally as a poultice. The herb has also been used for sciatica. One laboratory study evaluated the potential of the tincture to potentiate the effect of the prescription drug metformin in type 2 diabetes. Laboratory models from another study show a tendency to reduce low-density lipoprotein cholesterol, but the results are preliminary and inconclusive. The species name *podagraria* honors its use for treatment of podagra—gout pain in the big toe.

....

GROUND IVY

(GLECHOMA HEDERACEA)

Alehoof

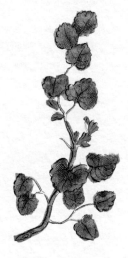

DESCRIPTION: This well-known herb lies, spreads and creeps upon the ground, shoots forth roots, at the corners of tender jointed stalks, set with two round leaves at every joint somewhat hairy, crumpled and unevenly dented about the edges [from which] come, long flowers of a blueish purple colour, with small white spots upon the lips.

PLACE: It is commonly found [in lawns, edges of fields, and hedges], and other waste grounds, [throughout Europe and North America].

GOVERNMENT AND VIRTUES: It is an herb of Venus, and therefore cures the diseases she causes by sympathy, and those of Mars by antipathy; you may usually find it all the yearlong except the year be extremely frosty; it is quick, sharp, and bitter in taste, and is thereby found to be hot and dry; a singular herb for all inward wounds, exulcerated [sore, inflamed] lungs, or other parts, either by itself, or boiled with other the like herbs; and being drank, in a short time it eases all griping pains, windy and choleric humours in the stomach, spleen or belly; helps the yellow jaundice, by opening the stoppings of the gall and liver, and melancholy, by opening the stoppings of the spleen; expels venom or poison, and also the plague; it provokes urine and women's courses; the decoction of it in wine drank for some time together, procures ease to them that are troubled with the sciatica, or hip-gout: as also the gout in hands, knees or feet; if you put to the decoction some honey and a little burnt alum, it is excellently good to gargle any sore mouth or throat, and to wash the sores and ulcers in the private parts of man or woman; it speedily helps fresh wounds, being bruised and bound thereto. The juice of it boiled with a little honey and verdigris, doth wonderfully cleanse fistulas, ulcers, and stays the spreading or eating of cancers and ulcers; it helps the itch, scabs, wheals, and other breakings out in any part of the body. The juice dropped into the ears helps the noise and singing of them, and helps the hearing which is decayed. It is good to [add to a barrel of] new drink, for it will clarify it in a night, that it will be the fitter to be drank the next morning; or if any drink be thick with removing, or any other accident, it will do the like in a few hours.

MODERN USE: Ground ivy leaves were traditionally used to flavor and clarify beer, hence the name "alehoof." In traditional Chinese medicine, ground ivy is used in prescriptions for gallstones, edema, abscesses, diabetes, inflammation, and jaundice. Used for chronic bronchial catarrh as a mild expectorant and astringent. CAUTION: May cause labored breathing and throat irritation in livestock; similar side effects are also reported for humans, along with gastrointestinal or kidney irritation. Little used today. Lack of clinical and safety data but well-studied chemistry.

....

GROUND PINE
(AJUGA CHAMAEPITYS)

Chamepitys

DESCRIPTION: Our common Ground Pine grows low, with slender, small, long, narrow, greyish, or whitish leaves, smelling somewhat strong, like unto rosin: The flowers are small, and of a pale yellow colour.

PLACE: [Found in chalky soils throughout most of Europe, North Africa, and the Middle East.]

GOVERNMENT AND VIRTUES: Mars owns the herb. The decoction of Ground Pine drank, doth wonderfully prevail against the strangury, or any inward pains arising from the diseases of the kidneys and urine, and is especially good for all obstructions of the liver and spleen, and gently opens the body; for which purpose they were wont in former times to make pills with the powder thereof, and the pulp of figs. It marvelously helps all the diseases of the mother, inwardly or outwardly applied, procuring women's courses, and expelling the dead child and after-birth; yea, it is so powerful upon those feminine parts, that it is utterly forbidden for women with child, for it will cause abortion or delivery before the time. The decoction of the herb in wine taken inwardly, or applied outwardly, or both, for some time together, is also effectual in all pains and diseases of the joints, as gouts, cramps, palsies, sciatica, and aches. It helps also all diseases of the brain, proceeding of cold and phlegmatic humours and distillations, as also for the falling sickness. It is a special remedy for the poison of the aconites, and other poisonous herbs, as also against the stinging of any venomous creature. It is a good remedy for a cold cough, especially in the beginning. For all the purposes aforesaid, the herb being tunned up in new drink and drank, is almost as effectual, but far more acceptable to weak and dainty stomachs. The distilled water of the herb hath the same effects, but more weakly. The green herb, or the decoction thereof, being applied, dissolves the hardness of women's breasts, and all other hard swellings in any other part of the body. The green herb also applied, or the juice thereof with some honey, not only cleanses putrid, stinking, foul, and malignant ulcers and sores of all sorts, but heals and solders up the lips of green wounds in any part also. Let pregnant women forbear, for it works violently upon the feminine part.

MODERN USES: Ground pine is traditionally used as a diuretic and emmenagogue for the treatment of urinary disease. In the Middle East, it has been used for rheumatism, gout, jaundice, inflammation, fever, and joint pain. It has confirmed antioxidant activity and possibly toxic effects against cancer cells from the iridoids contained in the leaves and flowers. **CAUTION:** As Culpeper warns, avoid during pregnancy, as well as during breastfeeding. A little-used herb of unknown toxicity; best to avoid use.

....

GROUNDSEL

(*SENECIO VULGARIS*)

DESCRIPTION: Our common Groundsel [is] set with long and somewhat narrow green leaves, cut in on the edges, somewhat like the oak-leaves. At the tops of the branches stand many small green heads, out of which grow several small, yellow threads or thumbs, which are the flowers.

PLACE: They grow almost everywhere, as well on tops of walls, as at the foot amongst rubbish and untilled grounds, but especially in gardens. [In so many words, Culpeper tells us it's a weed. An annual weed throughout Europe, Asia, and North America.]

GOVERNMENT AND VIRTUES: [Groundsel] is Venus's mistress-piece, and is as gallant and universal a medicine for all diseases coming of heat, in what part of the body so ever they be, as the sun shines upon; it is very safe and friendly to the body of man: yet causes vomiting if the stomach be afflicted; if not, purging: and it doth it with more gentleness than can be expected; it is moist, and something cold withal, thereby causing expulsion, and repressing the heat caused by the motion of the internal parts in purges and vomits. Lay by our learned receipts; take so much Senna, so much Scammony, so much Colocynthis, so much infusion of Crocus Metallorum, &c. this herb alone preserved in a syrup, in a distilled water, or in an ointment, shall do the deed for you in all hot diseases, and, shall do it, 1, Safely; 2, Speedily.

The decoction of this herb (saith Dioscorides) made with wine, and drank, helps the pains of the stomach, proceeding of choler [bile], (which it may well do by a vomit) as daily experience shews. The juice thereof taken in drink, or the decoction of it in ale, gently performs the same. It is good against the jaundice and falling sickness, being taken in wine; as also against difficulty of making water. It provokes urine, expels gravel in the kidneys; a dram thereof given in oxymel, after some walking or stirring of the body. It helps also the sciatica, griping of the belly, the cholic, defects of the liver, and provokes women's courses. The fresh herb boiled and made into a poultice, applied to the breasts of women that are swollen with pain and heat, as also the private parts of man or woman, the seat or fundament, or the arteries, joints, and sinews, when they are inflamed and swollen, doth much ease

them; and used with some salt, helps to dissolve knots or kernels in any part of the body. The juice of the herb, or as (Dioscorides saith) the leaves and flowers, with some fine Frankincense in powder, used in wounds of the body, nerves or sinews, doth singularly help to heal them. The distilled water of the herb performs well all the aforesaid cures, but especially for inflammations or watering of the eyes, by reason of the defluxion of rheum [watery discharge] unto them.

MODERN USES: As a successful invasive weed, common groundsel has evolved a chemical defense against predation: liver-toxic pyrrolizidine alkaloids, which are found throughout the plant. It was formerly used by herbalists to expel worms, induce sweating for fevers, and as a diuretic. It was also considered purgative, and the young leaves were eaten for scurvy. Despite the virtues extolled by Culpepper, it is no longer used in herbal treatments. **CAUTION:** Like coltsfoot and comfrey, groundsel contains liver-toxic pyrrolizidine alkaloids, which can cause veno-occlusive disease of the liver; therefore, the herb is no longer considered safe for use. Avoid.

....

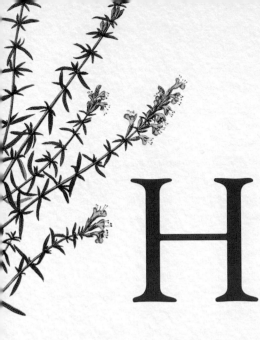

H

HART'S-TONGUE

(*ASPLENIUM SCOLOPENDRIUM*;
SYN. *PHYLLITIS SCOLOPENDRIUM*)

DESCRIPTION: This has [strap-like, simple] leaves arising from the root, about a foot long, smooth and green above [with a prominent brown mid-rib beneath]. [A perennial fern native to much of northern Europe and temperate North America in the Great Lakes region.]

GOVERNMENT AND VIRTUES: Jupiter claims dominion over this herb, therefore it is a singular remedy for the liver, both to strengthen it when weak, and ease it when afflicted, you shall do well to keep it in a syrup all the year; For though authors say it is green all the year, I scarcely believe it. Hart's Tongue is much commended against the hardness and stoppings of the spleen and liver, and against the heat of the liver and stomach, and against lasks [diarrhea], and the bloody-flux [dysentery]. The distilled water thereof is also very good against the passions of the heart, and to stay the hiccough, to help the falling of the palate, and to stay the bleeding of the gums, being gargled in the mouth. Dioscorides saith, it is good against the stinging or biting of serpents. As for the use of it, my direction at the latter end will be sufficient, and enough for those that are studious in physic, to whet their brains upon for one year or two.

MODERN USES: Rarely used and little researched. The powdered leaves were traditionally used in folk medicine as an antispasmodic and to treat external wounds. Also once used as an astringent and diuretic; considered a demulcent and an expectorant.

....

HAWKWEED

(*HIERACIUM SPP.*)

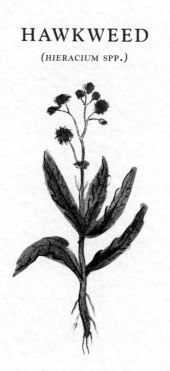

There are several sorts of Hawk-weed, but they are similar in virtues.

DESCRIPTION: It has many large leaves lying upon the ground, much rent or torn on the sides into gashes like Dandelion, but with greater parts, more like the smooth Sow Thistle, from among which rises a hollow, rough stalk, two or three feet high, bearing on them sundry pale, yellow flowers. The whole plant is full of bitter-milk.

PLACE: It grows in diverse places about the field sides, and the path-ways in dry grounds [Found throughout Eurasia; widely naturalized in North America and elsewhere.]

GOVERNMENT AND VIRTUES: Saturn owns it. Hawkweed (saith Dioscorides) is cooling, somewhat drying and binding, and therefore good for the heat of the stomach, and gnawings therein; for inflammations and the hot fits of agues. The juice thereof in wine, helps digestion, discusses wind, hinders crudities abiding in the stomach, and helps the difficulty of making water, the biting of venomous serpents, and stinging of the scorpion, if the herb be also outwardly applied to the place, and is very good against all other poisons. A scruple of the dried root given in wine and vinegar, is profitable for those that have the dropsy. The decoction of the herb taken in honey, digests the phlegm in the chest or lungs, and with Hyssop helps the cough. The decoction thereof, and of Chicory, made with wine, and taken, helps the wind cholic and hardness of the spleen; it procures rest and sleep, hinders venery and venerous dreams, cooling heats, purges the stomach, increases blood, and helps the diseases of the kidneys and bladder. Outwardly applied, it is used with good success in fretting or creeping ulcers, especially in the beginning. The green leaves bruised, and with a little salt applied to any place burnt with fire, before blisters do rise, helps them; as also inflammations, St. Anthony's fire, and all pushes and eruptions, hot and salt phlegm. The same applied with meal and fair water in manner of a poultice, to any place affected with convulsions, the cramp, and such as are out of joint, doth give help and ease. The distilled water cleanses the skin, and takes away freckles, spots, morphew [skin blemishes], or wrinkles in the face.

MODERN USES: This dandelion-like weed is little used today. It gets the name hawkweed from the ancient folk belief that hawks sharpened their eyesight by nibbling on the plant. Generally, this taxonomically complex group of weeds has been used as a tonic—it has astringent and expectorant properties—mostly to stop bleeding or coughs.

....

HAWTHORN

(CRATAEGUS LAEVIGATA, CRATAEGUS MONOGYNA)

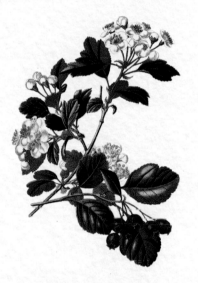

It is not my intention to trouble you with a description of this tree, which is so well-known that it needs none. It is ordinarily but a hedge bush, although being pruned and dressed, it grows to a tree of a reasonable height.

As for the Hawthorn Tree at Glastonbury, which is said to flower yearly on Christmas-day, it rather shews the superstition of those that observe it for the time of its flowering, than any great wonder, since the like may be found in diverse other places of this land. If the weather be frosty, it flowers not until January, or that the hard weather be over.

PLACE: [English hawthorn (*Crataegus laevigata*) is native to England and other parts of northern Europe in woods and along hedgerows. One-seed hawthorn (*Crataegus monogyna*) is native to England and grows throughout Europe at the border of forests, scrublands, and along hedges.]

GOVERNMENT AND VIRTUES: It is a tree of Mars. The seeds in the berries beaten to powder being drank in wine, are held singularly good against the stone, and are good for the dropsy. The distilled water of the flowers stay the lask [diarrhea]. If cloths or sponges be wet in the distilled water, and applied to any place wherein thorns and splinters, or the like, do abide in the flesh, it will notably draw them forth. And thus you see the thorn gives a medicine for its own pricking, and so doth almost everything else.

MODERN USES: The leaf and flower of English hawthorn and one-seed hawthorn are used for the clinical support of cardiovascular activity, especially as a cardiotonic for the treatment of cardiac output at the beginning stages of heart disease when physical activity is not limited. Hawthorn berries have also been traditionally used as a cardiotonic, but recent science confirms that the pharmacological and clinical usefulness depends upon a combination of the components in the flowers and leaves. Little science supports the use of berry extracts. Hawthorn preparations are standardized to a certain percentage of a combination of compounds including oligomeric proanthocyanidins and flavonoids. **CAUTION:** Heart conditions can only be diagnosed and treated by a qualified medical practitioner.

....

HAZELNUT

(CORYLUS AVELLANA)

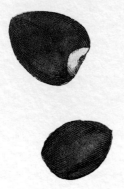

Hazel Nuts are so well known to everybody, that they need no description.

PLACE: [Native to England and most of Europe, growing in woods, scrublands, along hedgerows, and at the edge of meadows.]

GOVERNMENT AND VIRTUES: They are under the dominion of Mercury. The parted kernels made into an electuary, or the milk drawn from the kernels with mead or honeyed water, is very good to help an old cough; and being parched, and a little pepper put to them and drank, digests the distillations of rheum [watery discharge] from the head. The dried husks and shells, to the weight of two drams, taken in red wine, stays lasks [diarrhea] and women's courses, and so doth the red skin that covers the kernels, which is more effectual to stay women's courses.

And if this be true, as it is, then why should the vulgar so familiarly affirm, that eating nuts causes shortness of breath, when nothing is more false? For, how can that which strengthens the lungs, cause shortness of breath? I confess, the opinion is far older than I am. If any part of the Hazel Nut be stopping, it is the husks and shells, and no one is so mad as to eat them. And the red skin which covers the kernel, you may easily pull off. Thus I have made an apology for Nuts, which cannot speak for themselves.

MODERN USES: Hazelnuts are much better known as a food than a medicinal herb. Filberts are another species of hazelnut (*Corylus maxima*), grown since ancient times. American hazelnut (*Corylus americana*) seed oil was used to treat coughs. The seed oil, as well as the seed husks, have been suggested as possible sources of antioxidant compounds. **CAUTION:** Some individuals may be allergic to hazelnut and hazelnut products.

....

HEART'S EASE

(VIOLA TRICOLOR)

This is that herb which such physicians as are licensed to blaspheme by authority, without danger of having their tongues burned through with a hot iron, called an herb of the Trinity. It is also called by those that are more moderate, Three Faces in a Hood, Live in Idleness, Cull me to you; and in Sussex we call them Pansies.

PLACE: Besides those which are brought up in gardens, they grow commonly wild in the fields. [Found throughout Europe and Asia; sporadically naturalized in North and South America.]

GOVERNMENT AND VIRTUES: The herb is really saturnine, something cold, viscous, and slimy. A strong decoction of the herbs and flowers (if you will, you may make it into syrup) is an excellent cure for the French pox [syphilis], the herb being a gallant antivenereal: and that antivenereals are the best cure for that disease, far better and safer than to torment them with the flux, diverse foreign physicians have confessed. The spirit of it is excellently good for the convulsions in children, as also for the falling sickness, and a gallant remedy for the inflammation of the lungs and breasts, pleurisy, scabs, itch, etc. It is under the celestial sign Cancer.

MODERN USES: Heart's ease is traditionally used in the treatment of inflammatory disease, including atopic dermatitis and psoriasis. Recent research suggests that the antioxidant activity of the herb may have a protective effect in the treatment of neurodegenerative diseases (suggesting it could be a future research subject in the treatment of Alzheimer's disease). Heart's ease also has anti-inflammatory, antimicrobial, and mild sedative activity, and has been traditionally used to treat anxiety, insomnia, and hypertension.

....

HEDGE HYSSOP
(GRATIOLA OFFICINALIS)

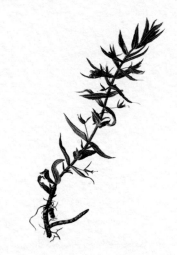

DESCRIPTION: A smooth, low plant, not a foot high, very bitter in taste, with many square stalks, and two small leaves at each joint. The flowers stand being of a fair purple colour, with some white spots in them.

PLACE: It grows in wet low grounds, and by the water-sides [originating in western Europe and extending to western Siberia and western Asia].

GOVERNMENT AND VIRTUES: It is an herb of Mars, and as choleric and churlish as he is, being a most violent purge, especially of choler [bile] and phlegm. It is not safe taking it inwardly, unless it be well rectified by the art of the alchemist, and only the purity of it given; so used it may be very helpful both for the dropsy, gout, and sciatica; outwardly used in ointments it kill worms, the belly anointed with it, and is excellently good to cleanse old and filthy ulcers.

MODERN USES: Seldom used today. The juice of hedge hyssop is considered a strong purgative and diuretic. Various species of Gratiola in North

America and elsewhere were traditionally used. Anti-inflammatory, antioxidant, and antimicrobial activity have been attributed to flavonoids in the plant. **CAUTION:** Hedge hyssop is a potentially dangerous plant that contains a cucurbitacin glycoside called elatericide, which is responsible for the strong purgative effects. Herbalists no longer recommend it for use.

....

HEDGE MUSTARD

(*SISYMBRIUM OFFICINALE*)

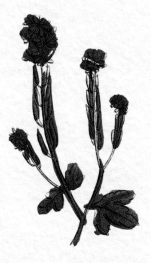

DESCRIPTION: This grows up usually but with one blackish green stalk, tough, easy to bend, but not to break, whereon grow long, rough, or hard rugged [ragged] leaves. The flowers are small and yellow.

PLACE: [This grows frequently in wastelands, fields, and roadsides. Native and common throughout much of Europe and North Africa; naturalized and weedy in Asia, much of South America, and parts of North America.]

GOVERNMENT AND VIRTUES: Mars owns this herb also. It is singularly good in all the diseases of the chest and lungs, hoarseness of voice: and by the use of the decoction thereof for a little space, those have been recovered who had utterly lost their voice, and almost their spirits also. The juice thereof made into a syrup, or licking medicine, with honey or sugar, is no less effectual for the same purpose, and for all other coughs, wheezing, and shortness of breath. The same is also profitable for those that have the jaundice, pleurisy, pains in the back and loins. The seed is held to be a special remedy against poison and venom. It is singularly good for the sciatica, and in joint-aches, ulcers, and cankers in the mouth, throat, or behind the ears, and no less for the hardness and swelling of the testicles, or of women's breasts.

MODERN USES: Historically, hedge mustard has had a very specific traditional use for chronic coughs, hoarseness, and throat irritation (due to voice strain). It is used in a syrup or the expressed juice is mixed in honey. Also considered diuretic and expectorant. One study confirms that a dry water extract of hedge mustard may help repair damage to the vocal cords of smokers, due to an antioxidant effect. Science confirms skeletal muscle-relaxant effects, antimicrobial activity, and antimutagenic effects (which are being researched for cancer prevention).

....

HEMP

(CANNABIS SATIVA)

Marijuana

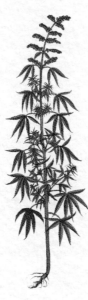

This is so well known to every good housewife in the country, that I shall not need to write any description of it.

PLACE: [Hemp is one of the oldest known cultivated plants, grown for at least eight thousand years. A form of *Cannabis sativa* with low levels of psychoactive compounds, it has been primarily used historically for fiber or seed production. The earliest evidence suggests it may have originated in central Asia (northwest China). Cultivated worldwide.]

GOVERNMENT AND VIRTUES: It is a plant of Saturn, and good for something else, you see, than to make rope only. The seed of Hemp consumes wind, and by too much use thereof disperses it so much that it dries up the natural seed for procreation; yet, being boiled in milk and taken, helps such as have a hot dry cough. The Dutch make an emulsion out of the seed, and give it with good success to those that have the jaundice, especially in the beginning of the disease, if there be no [fever] accompanying it, for it opens obstructions of the gall, and causes digestion of choler [bile]. The emulsion or decoction of the seed stays lasks [diarrhea] and continual fluxes, eases the cholic, and allays the troublesome humours in the bowels, and stays bleeding at the mouth, nose, or other places. It is held very good to kill the worms in men or beasts. The decoction of the root allays inflammations of the head, or any other parts. The herb itself, or the distilled water thereof doth the like. The decoction of the root eases the pains of the gout, the hard humours of knots in the joints, the pains and shrinking of the sinews, and the pains of the hips. The fresh juice mixed with a little oil and butter, is good for any place that hath been burnt with fire, being thereto applied.

MODERN USES: If Culpeper were alive today, he would write a book on hemp. The seed oil of various *Cannabis* genetic selections is extremely low in tetrahydrocannabinol (THC), the component responsible for the euphoric effect of marijuana, and widely available today as "CBD oils." These oils, which contain other non-euphoric cannabidiols, have gained popularity in the treatment of pain, anxiety, and depression. They're also used supportively in cancer patients undergoing conventional treatments, and for other purposes. **CAUTION:** Legality of use is determined by various regional and national governmental regulations.

....

HENBANE

(HYOSCYAMUS NIGER)

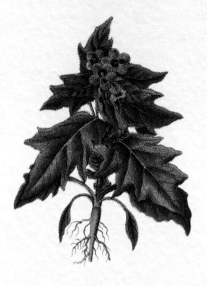

DESCRIPTION: Our common Henbane has very large, thick, soft, woolly leaves, lying on the ground, much cut in, or torn on the edges, of a dark, ill greyish green colour; [the flowers are] a deadish yellowish colour, paler towards the edges, with many purplish veins therein, and of a dark, yellowish purple in the center of the flower. The whole plant, has a very heavy, ill, soporiferous smell, somewhat offensive.

PLACE: It commonly grows by the waysides, under hedges and walls [originating in Europe, western Asia, and northern Africa].

GOVERNMENT AND VIRTUES: I wonder how astrologers could take on them to make this an herb of Jupiter; and yet Mizaldus, a man of a penetrating brain, was of that opinion as well as the rest; the herb is indeed under the dominion of Saturn, and I prove it by this argument: All the herbs which delight most to grow in saturnine places, are saturnine herbs. Henbane delights most to grow in saturnine places, and whole cart loads of it may be found near the places where they empty the common Jakes [privies], and scarce a ditch [is] to be found without it growing by it. Ergo, it is an herb of Saturn.

The leaves of Henbane do cool all hot inflammations in the eyes, or any other part of the body; and are good to assuage all manner of swellings of the privities, or women's breast, or elsewhere, if they be boiled in wine, and either applied themselves, or the fomentation warm; it also assuages the pain of the gout, the sciatica, and other pains in the joints which arise from a hot cause. And applied with vinegar to the forehead and temples, helps the headache and want of sleep in hot fevers. The juice of the herb or seed, or the oil drawn from the seed, does the like. The decoction of the herb or seed, or both, kills lice in man or beast. The fume of the dried herb, stalks and seed, burned, quickly heals swellings, chilblains or kibes in the hands or feet, by holding them in the fume thereof.

Take notice, that this herb must never be taken inwardly; outwardly, an oil ointment, or plaster of it, is most admirable for the gout, to cool the venereal heat of the kidneys in the French pox [syphilis]; to stop the toothache, being applied to the aching side: to allay all inflammations, and to help the diseases before premised.

MODERN USES: Henbane is a highly toxic plant that contains a mixture of alkaloids including atropine, hyoscyamine, scopolamine, and other bioactive compounds. **CAUTION:** Although some of these alkaloids in purified form are used in minute, highly controlled dosages in modern medicine, henbane is relegated to the realm of deadly plants. Avoid use.

....

HERB ROBERT
(GERANIUM ROBERTIANUM)

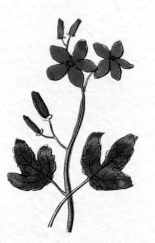

The Herb Robert is held in great estimation by farmers, who use it in diseases of their cattle.

DESCRIPTION: It rises up with a reddish stalk two feet high. At the tops of the stalks come forth diverse flowers made of five [petals] of a reddish colour. The root is small and thready, and smells, as the whole plant, very strong, almost stinking.

PLACE: This grows frequently [at field edges in open woods, throughout Europe, western Asia, and northern Africa. It is naturalized in temperate North America and South America].

GOVERNMENT AND VIRTUES: It is under the dominion of Venus. Herb Robert is commended not only against the stone, but to stay blood, where or howsoever flowing, it speedily heals all green wounds, and is effectual in old ulcers in the private parts, or elsewhere. You may persuade yourself this is true, and also conceive a good reason for it, do but consider it is an herb of Venus, for all it hath a man's name.

MODERN USES: Considered astringent and rich in phenolic and flavonoid compounds, herb Robert is used externally as a folk medicine to treat wounds. Science confirms its antioxidant and anti-inflammatory activity. A tea of the plant has been used in folk medicine to treat hypertension. **CAUTION:** May cause contact dermatitis in some individuals.

....

HOG'S FENNEL
(PEUCEDANUM OFFICINALE)
Sow Fennel

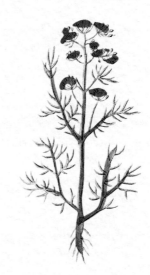

DESCRIPTION: Common Hog's-Fennel has branched stalks of thick and long leaves, three for the most part joined together, among which arises a straight stalk, [with umbels] of yellow flowers, [with] flat, thin, and yellowish seed, bigger than Fennel seed. The roots grow great and deep, and yields a yellowish milk, or clammy juice, almost like a gum.

PLACE: [Plentiful in grasslands throughout Europe.]

GOVERNMENT AND VIRTUES: This is also an herb of Mercury. The juice of Hog's-Fennel (saith Dioscorides and Galen) used with vinegar and rose water, or the juice with a little Euphorbium put to the nose, helps those that are troubled with the lethargy, frenzy, giddiness of the head, the falling sickness, long and inveterate headaches, the palsy, sciatica, and the cramp, and generally all the diseases of the sinews, used with oil and vinegar. The juice dissolved in wine, or put into an egg, is good for a cough, or shortness of breath, and for those that are troubled with wind in the body. It purges the belly gently, expels the hardness of the spleen, gives ease to women that have sore travail in child-birth, and eases the pains of the kidneys and bladder, and also the womb. A little of the juice dissolved in wine, and put into a hollow tooth, eases the pain. The root is less effectual to all the aforesaid disorders; yet the powder of the root cleanses foul ulcers, being put into them, and takes out splinters of broken bones, or other things in the flesh, and heals them up perfectly, as also, dries up old and inveterate running sores, and is of admirable virtue in all green wounds.

MODERN USES: The essential oil of hog's fennel has been shown to have mild antibacterial activity. Seldom used today, the root and its preparations were formerly used topically to treat skin ulcers and toothache, and internally to treat dyspepsia, colic, flatulence, fevers, cough, and colds. The gummy substance in the root is used in folk medicine as a diuretic and is considered anti-inflammatory. **CAUTION:** May cause allergic reactions.

....

HONEYSUCKLE

(LONICERA PERICLYMENUM)

Woodbine

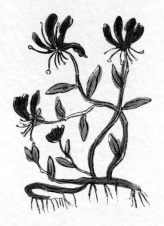

It is a common [deciduous climber in western Europe, growing along hedges, fence rows, and woods].

GOVERNMENT AND VIRTUES: Doctor Tradition, that grand introducer of errors, that hater of truth, lover of folly, and the mortal foe to Dr. Reason, hath taught the common people to use the leaves or flowers of this plant in mouth-water, and by long continuance of time, hath so grounded it in the brains of the vulgar, that you cannot beat it out with a beetle. All mouth-waters ought to be cooling and drying, but Honeysuckles are cleansing, consuming and digesting, and therefore fit for inflammations; thus Dr. Reason. Again if you please, we will leave Dr. Reason a while, and come to Dr. Experience, a learned gentleman, and his brother. Take a leaf and chew it in your mouth, and you will quickly find it likelier to cause a sore mouth and throat than to cure it. Well then, if it be not good for this, what is it good for? It is good for something, for God and nature made nothing in vain. It is an herb of Mercury, and appropriated to the lungs. Crab claims dominion over it; neither is it a foe to the Lion. If the lungs be afflicted by Jupiter, this is your cure. It is fitting a conserve made of the flowers were kept in every gentlewoman's house. I know no better cure for an asthma than this. Besides, it takes away the evil of the spleen, provokes urine, helps cramps, convulsions, and palsies, and whatsoever griefs come of cold or stopping. If you please to make use of it as an ointment, it will clear your skin of morphew [blemishes], freckles, and sun-burns, or whatsoever else discolors it, and then the maids will love it. Authors say, the flowers are of more effect than the leaves, and that is true; but they say the seeds are least effectual of all. But Dr. Reason told me, that there was a vital spirit in every seed to beget its like; and Dr. Experience told me, that there was a greater heat in the seed than there was in any other part of the plant. That heat was the mother of action, and then judge if old Dr. Tradition (who may well be honored for his age, but not for his goodness) hath not so poisoned the world with errors before I was born, that it was never well in its wits since, and there is a great fear it will die mad.

MODERN USES: More valued in poetry than medicine, the common honeysuckle of the British Isles and Europe is little used today. Decoctions of the tops of the stems were formerly used as a gargle for sore throat and a cleansing wash for wounds. Japanese honeysuckle (*Lonicera japonica*) leaves and stems, and separately the flowers, are used in traditional Chinese medicine as a treatment for upper respiratory tract infections—"appropriate to the lungs," just as Culpeper describes. **CAUTION:** Honeysuckle leaves can be irritating. The berries of this and other honeysuckles may cause gastrointestinal distress.

....

HOPS
(*HUMULUS LUPULUS*)

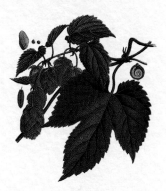

These are so well known that they need no description; I mean the manured kind, which every good husband or housewife knows.

PLACE: They delight to grow in low moist grounds, and are found in all parts of this land. [Native from Great Britain to Siberia; widely naturalized in North America.]

GOVERNMENT AND VIRTUES: It is under the dominion of Mars. [It works] to open obstructions of the liver and spleen, to cleanse the blood, to loosen the belly, to cleanse the kidneys from gravel, and provoke urine. The decoction of the tops of Hops, works the same effects. In cleansing the blood they help to cure the French diseases [syphilis], and all manner of scabs, itch, and other breakings-out of the body; as also all tetters, ringworms, and spreading sores, the morphew [skin blemishes] and all discolouring of the skin. The decoction of the flowers and hops do help to expel poison that any one hath drank. Half a dram of the seed in powder taken in drink, kills worms in the body, brings down women's courses, and expels urine. A syrup made of the juice and sugar, cures the yellow jaundice, eases the headache that comes of heat, and tempers the heat of the liver and stomach, and is profitably given in long and hot fevers that rise in choler [bile] and blood. Both the wild and the manured are alike effectual in all the aforesaid diseases. By all these testimonies beer appears to be better than ale.

MODERN USES: Hops are best known as the bitter, aromatic, soporific flavoring of beer. Hops and their preparations are used in modern phytomedicine for mood disturbances including unrest, anxiety, and sleeplessness. Hops are antispasmodic, antibacterial, and mildly sedative. They also contain phytoestrogenic compounds and have been traditionally used for the relief of menopausal symptoms. **CAUTION:** May cause allergies in some individuals. An occupational hazard is "hop-picker fatigue," which occurs when workers in hop fields are exposed to the crystalline resin released by the seedpods.

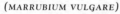

HOREHOUND

(MARRUBIUM VULGARE)

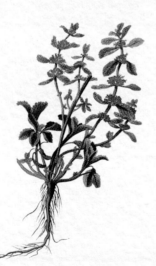

DESCRIPTION: Common Horehound grows up with square hairy stalks, two feet high, with two round

crumpled rough leaves of a sullen hoary green colour, and a very bitter taste. The flowers are small, white, and gaping, set in a rough, hard prickly husk round about the joints.

PLACE: It is found in many parts of this land, in dry grounds, and waste green places. [Widespread throughout Eurasia; commonly cultivated in herb gardens and naturalized in North America, South America, and Australia.]

GOVERNMENT AND VIRTUES: It is an herb of Mercury. A decoction of the dried herb, with the seed, or the juice of the green herb taken with honey, is a remedy for those that are short-winded, have a cough, or are fallen into a consumption, either through long sickness, or thin distillations of rheum [watery discharge] upon the lungs. It helps to expectorate tough phlegm from the chest, being taken from the roots of Iris or Orris. It is given to them that have taken poison, or are stung or bitten by venomous serpents. The leaves used with honey, purge foul ulcers, stay running or creeping sores, and the growing of the flesh over the nails. It also helps pains of the sides. The juice with wine and honey, helps to clear the eyesight, and snuffed up into the nostrils, purges away the yellow-jaundice, and with a little oil of roses dropped into the ears, eases the pains of them. Galen saith, it opens obstructions both of the liver and spleen, and purges the breast and lungs of phlegm: and used outwardly it both cleanses and digests. A decoction of Horehound (saith Matthiolus) is available for those that have hard livers, and for such as have itches and running tetters. The powder hereof taken, or the decoction, kills worms. The green leaves bruised, and boiled in old hog's grease into an ointment, heals the biting of dogs, abates the swellings and pains that come by any pricking of thorns, or such like means; and used with vinegar, cleanses and heals tetters. There is a syrup made of Horehound to be had at the apothecaries, very good for old coughs, to rid the tough phlegm; as also to void cold rheums from the lungs of old folks, and for those that are asthmatic or short-winded.

MODERN USES: Horehound is traditionally used in folk medicine worldwide for the treatment of respiratory conditions including colds, asthma, and bronchitis, and for the symptomatic relief of sore throat; it is also used for hypertension and type 2 diabetes. A bitter herb used to stimulate appetite, horehound is considered analgesic, antispasmodic, antihypertensive, anti-inflammatory, cardioprotective, and immunomodulating. Marrubiin, a component in the leaves, has expectorant and pain-inhibiting effects.

....

HORSERADISH

(ARMORACIA RUSTICANA)

Horse–Raddish

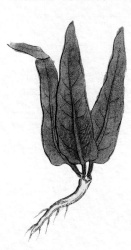

DESCRIPTION: The Horseradish hath its first leaves, that rise before Winter, about a foot and a half long, very much cut in or torn on the edges into many parts. The root is great, long, white and rug-ged, shooting up heads of leaves, and of a strong, sharp, and bitter taste almost like mustard.

PLACE: It is found wild in some places, but is chiefly planted in gardens. [Native to the Caucasus; cultivated and naturalized in most of Europe by the Middle Ages; also found in Asia and much of North America.]

GOVERNMENT AND VIRTUES: It is under Mars. The juice of Horseradish given to drink, is held to be very effectual for the scurvy. It kills the worms in children, being drank, and also laid upon the belly. The root bruised and laid to the place grieved with the sciatica, joint-ache, or the hard swellings of the liver and spleen, doth wonderfully help them all. The distilled water of the herb and root is more familiar to be taken with a little sugar for all the purposes aforesaid.

MODERN USES: Horseradish is best known as a flavoring and is used in small amounts as a pungent, mustard-like condiment. Its preparations are used for the supportive treatment of catarrhs of the upper respiratory tract and urinary tract infections. Traditionally, both the root and leaves were used to prevent or treat scurvy. The root contains similar antioxidant, antimicrobial, antispasmodic, and anti-inflammatory compounds as mustard (including the glucosinolate sinigrin, which is primarily responsible for horseradish's pungency). **CAUTION:** Fresh horseradish root or its products may cause allergies in sensitive individuals. Freshly grated roots may irritate mucosal and gastrointestinal tissue.

....

HORSETAIL

(EQUISETUM SPP.)

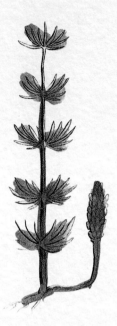

Of that there are many kinds [there are eight species of *Equisetum* in England as well as some hybrids], but I shall not trouble you nor myself with any large description of them, which to do, were but, as the proverb is, to find a knot in a rush, all the kinds thereof being nothing else but knotted rushes, some with leaves, and some without. Take the description of the most eminent sort as follows.

DESCRIPTION: The great Horsetail [*Equisetum telmateia*] at the first springing has heads somewhat like those of asparagus, and afterwards grow to be hard, rough, hollow stalks, jointed at sundry places up to the top, a foot high, where grow on each side a bush of small long rush-like hard leaves, each part resembling a horsetail, from whence it is so called.

PLACE: This (as most of the other sorts hereof) grows in wet grounds [throughout most the world].

GOVERNMENT AND VIRTUES: The herb belongs to Saturn, yet is very harmless, and excellently good for the things following: Horsetail, the smoother rather than the rough, and the leaves rather than the bare, is most physical. It is very powerful to staunch bleeding either inward or outward, the juice or the decoction thereof being drank, or the juice, decoction, or distilled water applied outwardly. It also stays all sorts of lasks [diarrhea] and fluxes in man or woman, and bloody urine; and heals also not only the inward ulcers, and the excoriation of the entrails, bladder, &c. but all other sorts of foul, moist and running ulcers, and soon solders together the tops of green wounds. It cures all ruptures in children. The decoction thereof in wine being drank, provokes urine, and helps the stone and strangury; and the distilled water thereof drank two or three times in a day, and a small quantity at a time, also eases the bowels, and is effectual against a cough that comes by distillations from the head. The juice or distilled water being warmed, and hot inflammations, pustules or red wheals, and other breakings-out in the skin, being bathed therewith, doth help them, and doth no less the swelling heat and inflammation of the lower parts in men and women.

MODERN USES: Traditionally, a tea of the stems of this primitive plant was used as a folk remedy for bloody urine and sour stomach ailments. As a diuretic, it was thought to increase urine flow without electrolyte loss. Horsetail contains up to 15 percent silica and is known as scouring rush, since the stems were used to clean cooking pots and as sandpaper. Today it is mostly used as a diuretic for edema and as an antibacterial for inflammatory urinary conditions. It has a styptic effect, helping to staunch bleeding, and is also used for osteoporosis and rheumatism. **CAUTION:** Some species, such as *Equisetum palustre* (marsh horsetail), contain toxic alkaloids and should be avoided.

....

HOUND'S-TONGUE

(CYNOGLOSSUM OFFICINALE)

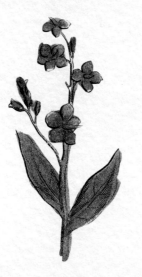

DESCRIPTION: The great ordinary Hound's Tongue has many long and somewhat narrow, soft, hairy, darkish green leaves, from among which rises up a rough hairy stalk about two feet high, with some smaller leaves thereon, and branched at the tops with many flowers set along the same, which branch is crooked or turned inwards before it flowers, which consist of small purplish red [petals] of a dead colour [though] sometimes a white flower.

PLACE: It grows in moist places of this land, in waste grounds, and untilled places, by highway sides, lanes, and hedge-sides [throughout Europe and western Asia. Naturalized in North America and considered a noxious weed in the western United States and Canada].

GOVERNMENT AND VIRTUES: It is a plant under the dominion of Mercury. The root is very effectually used in pills, as well as the decoction, or otherwise, to stay all sharp and thin defluxions of rheum [watery discharge] from the head into the eyes or nose, or upon the stomach or lungs, as also for coughs and shortness of breath. The leaves bruised, or the juice of them boiled in hog's lard, and applied, helps falling away of the hair, as also for any place that is scalded or burnt. The leaves bruised and laid to any green wound doth heal it up quickly. The root baked under the embers, wrapped in paste or wet paper, or in a wet double cloth, and thereof a suppository made, doth very effectually help the painful piles or hemorrhoids. The distilled water of the herbs and roots is very good to all the purposes aforesaid, to be used as well inwardly to drink, as outwardly to wash any sore place, for it heals all manner of wounds and punctures, and those foul ulcers that arise by the French pox [syphilis]. Mizaldus adds that the leaves laid under the feet, will keep the dogs from barking at you. It is called Hound's-tongue, because it ties the tongues of hounds; whether true, or not, I never tried, yet I cured the biting of a mad dog with this only medicine.

MODERN USES: Hound's-tongue is little used today, but it has been used externally as folk remedy for hemorrhoids. **CAUTION:** Like coltsfoot and comfrey, hound's-tongue contains liver-toxic pyrrolizidine alkaloids, which can cause veno-occlusive disease of the liver. A small amount of the alkaloids has a cumulative effect over time, and the condition is only diagnosed with a liver biopsy. Acute poisoning can be caused by over-consumption of pyrrolidine alkaloid-containing plants. Also causes acute poisoning in horses or cattle. Best to avoid.

....

HOUSELEEK

(*SEMPERVIVUM TECTORUM*)

Sengreen

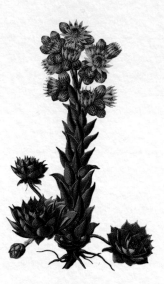

[It is] so well known to my countrymen, that I shall not need to write any description.

PLACE: It grows commonly upon walls and house-sides, and flowers in July. [Native to rocky fields in the Pyrenees and western Balkans, houseleek has been cultivated for centuries throughout Europe.]

GOVERNMENT AND VIRTUES: It is an herb of Jupiter, and it is reported by Mezaldus, to preserve what it grows upon from fire and lightning. Our ordinary Houseleek is good for all inward heats as well as outward, and in the eyes or other parts of the body; a posset made with the juice of Houseleek, is singularly good in all hot agues, for it cools and tempers the blood and spirits, and quenches the thirst; and also good to stay all hot defluctions or sharp and salt rheums in the eyes, the juice being dropped into them, or into the ears. It helps also other fluxes of humours in the bowels, and the immoderate courses of women. It cools and restrains all other hot inflammations, St. Anthony's fire, scaldings and burnings, the shingles, fretting ulcers, cankers, tetters, ringworms, and the like; and much eases the pains of gout proceeding from any hot cause. The juice also takes away warts and corns in the hands or feet, being often bathed therewith, and the skin and leaves being laid on them afterwards. It eases also the headache, and distempered heat of the brain in frenzies, or through want of sleep, being applied to the temples and forehead. The leaves bruised and laid upon the crown or seam of the head, stays bleeding at the nose very quickly. The distilled water of the herb is profitable for all the purposes aforesaid. The leaves being gently rubbed on any place stung with nettles or bees, doth quickly take away the pain.

MODERN USES: The juice or cooled tea of this succulent herb is used in the western Balkans for the treatment of earache, hemorrhoids, stomachache, warts, skin cancers, ulcers, and high blood sugar. Antioxidant, anti-inflammatory, antimicrobial, and pain-relieving flavonols and phenolic compounds in houseleek leaf juice have been linked to effectiveness in treating earache. Traditionally considered cooling and astringent.

....

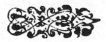

HYSSOP

(HYSSOPUS OFFICINALIS)

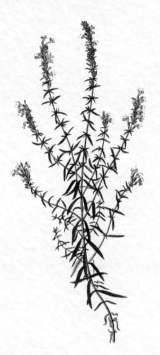

Hyssop is so well known to be an inhabitant in every garden, that it will save me labour in writing a description thereof. [Found in dry, gravelly soils in the Mediterranean region in southern Europe and northern Africa; widely cultivated in herb gardens.]

GOVERNMENT AND VIRTUES: The herb is Jupiter's, and the sign Cancer. It strengthens all the parts of the body under Cancer and Jupiter; which what they may be, is found amply described in my astrological judgment of diseases. Dioscorides saith, that Hyssop boiled with Rue and honey, and drank, helps those that are troubled with coughs, shortness of breath, wheezing and rheumatic distillation upon the lungs; taken also with oxymel [simple syrup made with honey and vinegar], it purges gross humours by stool; and with honey, kills worms in the belly; and with fresh and new figs bruised, helps

to loosen the belly, and more forcibly if the root of Iris and cresses be added thereto. It amends and cherishes the native colour of the body, spoiled by the yellow jaundice; and being taken with figs, helps the dropsy and spleen; being boiled with wine, it is good to wash inflammations, and takes away the black and blue spots and marks that come by strokes, bruises, or falls, being applied with warm water. It is an excellent medicine for the quinsy, or swellings in the throat, to wash and gargle it, being boiled in figs; it helps the toothache, being boiled in vinegar and gargled therewith. Being bruised, and salt, honey, and cumin seed put to it, helps those that are stung by serpents. The oil thereof (the head being anointed) kills lice, and takes away itching of the head. It helps those that have the falling sickness, which way so ever it be applied. It helps to expectorate tough phlegm, and is effectual in all cold griefs or diseases of the chests or lungs, being taken either in syrup or licking medicine. The green herb bruised, and a little sugar put thereto, doth quickly heal any cut or green wounds, being thereunto applied.

MODERN USES: Read between Culpeper's lines and you can see that hyssop and its preparations have been in continuous use from ancient times until today. Hyssop is traditionally used as a carminative and expectorant. Also used as a respiratory spasmolytic for treating tight, nonproductive coughing, wheezing, and other symptoms associated with asthma. The leaf tea is a gargle for sore throat. Externally, a poultice of the herb is used for bruises and pain relief. Hyssop is considered anti-inflammatory, antimicrobial, antiviral, and antioxidant. Experimentally, a 50 percent ethanolic extract of hyssop has been found to inhibit the HIV-1 virus in laboratory experiments. **CAUTION:** Not to be confused with potentially toxic hedge hyssop.

....

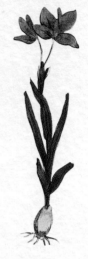

IRIS

(IRIS GERMANICA)

Flower-de-Luce

It is so well known, being nourished up in most gardens, that I shall not need to spent time in writing a description thereof. [Found throughout Europe. Widely grown as a garden ornamental and naturalized in many parts of the world.]

GOVERNMENT AND VIRTUES: The herb is Lunar. The juice or decoction of the green root of the flaggy kind of Iris, with a little honey drank, doth purge and cleanse the stomach of gross and tough phlegm, and choler [bile] therein. It helps the jaundice and the dropsy, evacuating those humours both upwards and downwards; and because it some-what hurts the stomach, is not to be taken without honey and spikenard. The same being drank, doth ease the pains and torments of the belly and sides, the shaking of agues, the diseases of the liver and spleen, the worms of the belly, the stone in the kidneys, convulsions and cramps that come of old humours; it also helps those whose seed passes from them unawares. It is a remedy against the bitings and stinging of venomous creatures, being boiled in water and vinegar and drank. Boiled in water and drank, it provokes urine, helps the cholic, brings down women's courses. It is much commended against the cough, to expectorate rough phlegm. It much eases pains in the head, and procures sleep; being put into the nostrils it procures sneezing, and thereby purges the head of phlegm. The juice of the root applied to the piles or hemorrhoids, gives much ease. The decoction of the roots gargled in the mouth, eases the toothache, and helps the stinking breath. The root itself, either green or in powder, helps to cleanse, heal, and incarnate wounds, and to cover the naked bones with flesh again, that ulcers have made bare; and is also very good to cleanse and heal up fistulas and cankers that are hard to be cured.

MODERN USES: The common garden iris and its many hybrids, especially the dried root of *Iris germanica* var. *florentina* (Orris root), are used as a fixative in potpourris for their violet-like fragrance. Garden iris is traditionally used in cough suppressant and bronchial teas and is considered strongly laxative. **CAUTION:** The dried root is typically not used because of potential toxicity; such effects are revealed in detail by Culpeper as "virtues."

....

IVY

(HEDERA HELIX)

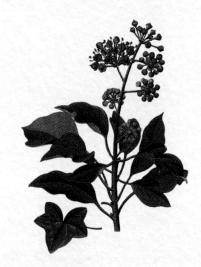

It is so well known to every child almost, to grow in woods upon the trees, and upon the stone walls of churches, houses, &c. and sometimes to grow alone of itself, though but seldom.

PLACE: [An evergreen woody vine native to most of Europe; grown as an ornamental and widely naturalized in Asia and North America.]

GOVERNMENT AND VIRTUES: It is under the dominion of Saturn. A pinch of the flowers, which may be about a dram, (saith Dioscorides) drank twice a day in red wine, helps the lask [diarrhea], and bloody flux [dysentery]. It is an enemy to the nerves and sinews, being much taken inwardly, but very helpful to them, being outwardly applied. Pliny saith, the yellow berries are good against the jaundice; and taken before one be set to drink hard, preserves from drunkenness, and helps those that spit blood. The berries are a singular remedy to prevent the plague, as also to free them from it that have got it, by drinking the berries thereof made into a powder, for two or three days together. They being taken in wine, do certainly help to break the stone, provoke urine, and women's courses. The fresh leaves of Ivy, boiled in vinegar, and applied warm to the sides of those that are troubled with the spleen, ache, or stitch in the sides, do give much ease. The same applied with some Rosewater, and oil of Roses, to the temples and forehead, eases the headache, though it be of long continuance. The fresh leaves boiled in wine, and old filthy ulcers hard to be cured washed therewith, do wonderfully help to cleanse them. It also quickly heals green wounds, and is effectual to heal all burnings and scaldings, and all kinds of ulcerations coming thereby, or by salt phlegm or humours in other parts of the body. The juice of the berries or leaves snuffed up into the nose, purges the head and brain of thin rheum [watery discharge] that makes defluxions into the eyes and nose, and curing the ulcers and stench therein. Those that are troubled with the spleen, shall find much ease by continual drinking out of a cup made of Ivy, so as the drink may stand some small time therein before it be drank. Cato saith, that wine put into such a cup, will soak through it, by reason of the antipathy that is between them. There seems to be a very great antipathy between wine and Ivy; for if one hath got a surfeit by drinking of wine, his speediest cure is to drink a draught of the same wine wherein a handful of Ivy leaves, being first bruised, have been boiled.

MODERN USES: Ivy is a folk medicine for gout and rheumatism and is used externally for burns and wounds. Components of the leaves have anti-bacterial, anti-inflammatory, and analgesic effects, among others. Extracts of ivy leaf are used in modern phytomedicine as an expectorant and antispasmodic for catarrhs of the upper respiratory tract and in the treatment of inflammatory bronchial conditions. Mostly used in prepared, standardized extracts, rarely as a home remedy. CAUTION: The fresh leaves are known to cause contact dermatitis. The berries are considered potentially toxic; avoid.

....

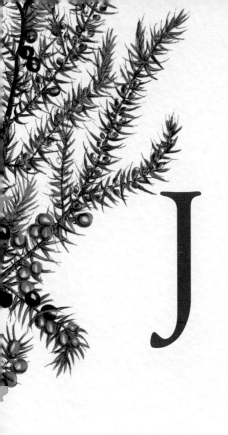

J

JUNIPER
(JUNIPERUS COMMUNIS)
Juniper Bush

For to give a description of a bush so commonly known is needless.

PLACE: They grow plentifully [in fields, wood edges, and rocky outcrops in most of Europe, northern North America, and Asia]. The berries are not ripe the first year, but continue green two Summers and one Winter before they are ripe; at which time they are all of a black colour.

GOVERNMENT AND VIRTUES: This admirable solar shrub is scarce to be paralleled for its virtues. The berries are hot in the third degree, and dry but in the first, being a most admirable counter-poison, and as great a resister of the pestilence, as any growing; they are excellent good against the biting of venomous beasts, they provoke urine exceedingly, and therefore are very available to dysuria and stranguries. It provokes the terms, helps the fits of the mother, strengthens the stomach exceedingly, and expels the wind. Indeed there is scarce a better remedy for wind in any part of the body, or the cholic, then by eating ten or a dozen of the ripe berries every morning fasting. They are admirably good for a cough, shortness of breath, and consumption, pains in the belly, ruptures, cramps, and convulsions. They strengthen the brain exceedingly, help the memory, and fortify the sight by strengthening the optic nerves; are excellently good in all sorts of agues; help the gout and sciatica, and strengthen the limbs of the body. The berries stay all fluxes, help the hemorrhoids or piles, and kill worms in children. The berries break the stone, procure appetite when it is lost, and are excellently good for all palsies, and falling-sickness.

MODERN USES: A widely used folk medicine by different world cultures. Traditionally juniper fruits or berries (technically cones) are used as a carminative, urinary antiseptic, diuretic, and anti-inflammatory for cystitis and bladder problems (such as bladder infections) as well as a treatment for rheumatic pain and hemorrhoids. Described activities include anti-inflammatory, antioxidant, antidiabetic, and antimicrobial effects, among others.

In phytomedicine, juniper is used for dyspeptic complaints and in combination with other herbs for bladder and kidney problems. **CAUTION:** Typically used for no longer than one week, as prolonged use can irritate the kidneys.

....

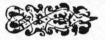

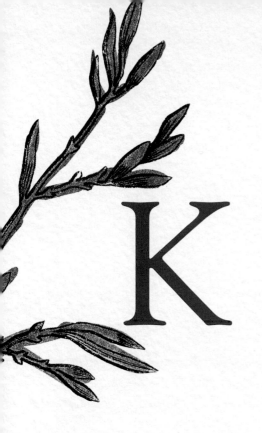

K

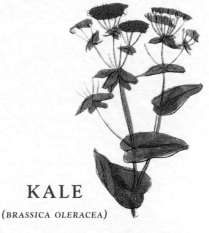

KALE

(BRASSICA OLERACEA)

Thoroughwax, or Thorough Leaf

DESCRIPTION: Kale, whose lower leaves [are] of a bluish colour. The flowers are small and yellow, standing in tufts at the heads of the branches.

PLACE: [Mostly cultivated.]

GOVERNMENT AND VIRTUES: [It is] under the influence of Saturn. Kale is of singular good use for all sorts of bruises and wounds either inward or outward; and old ulcers and sores likewise, if the decoction of the herb with water and wine be drank, and the place washed therewith, or the juice of the green herb bruised, or boiled, either by itself, or with other herbs, in oil or hog's grease, to be made into an ointment to serve all the year. The decoction of the herb, or powder of the dried herb, taken inwardly, and the same, or the leaves bruised, and applied outwardly, is singularly good for all ruptures and burstings, especially in [young] children. Being applied with a little flour and wax to children's navels that stick forth, it helps them.

MODERN USES: There is no doubt that the many varieties and genetic variations of this large group of mustard family members have evolved greatly in cultivation since Culpeper's time. *Brassica oleracea*, from which kale derives, includes cabbages, cauliflower, broccoli, and Brussels sprouts, among others. Aside from the obvious nutritional benefits, these vegetables contain compounds that are believed to prevent or control cancer over the long term.

....

KIDNEYWORT

(UMBILICUS RUPESTRIS)

Wall Pennyroyal, Wall Pennywort

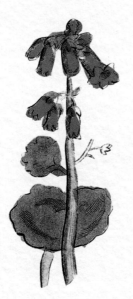

DESCRIPTION: It has many thick, flat, and round leaves growing from the root, every one having a long footstalk, fastened underneath, from among which arise tender, smooth, hollow stalks half a foot high, bearing a number of flowers, set round about a long spike one above another, which are hollow and like a little bell of a whitish green colour.

PLACE: It grows plentifully upon stone and mud walls, upon rocks also, and in stony places upon the ground. [Native from Greece to the United Kingdom, and from the Iberian Peninsula to North Africa.]

GOVERNMENT AND VIRTUES: Venus challenges the herb under Libra. The juice or the distilled water being drank, is very effectual for all inflammations and unnatural heats, to cool a fainting hot stomach, a hot liver, or the bowels: the herb, juice, or distilled water thereof, outwardly applied, heals pimples. The said juice or water helps to heal sore kidneys, torn or fretted by the stone, or exulcerated [sore, inflamed] within; it also provokes urine, is available for the dropsy, and helps to break the stone. Being used as a bath, or made into an ointment, it cools the painful piles or hemorrhoidal veins. It is no less effectual to give ease to the pains of the gout, the sciatica, and helps the kernels or knots in the neck or throat, called the king's evil [unusual swelling of lymph nodes or scrofula]: healing kibes and chilblains if they be bathed with the juice, or anointed with ointment made thereof, and some of the skin of the leaf upon them: it is also used in green wounds to stay the blood, and to heal them quickly.

MODERN USES: Little if ever used today. Formerly, fresh bruised kidneywort leaves were applied to wounds. Between 1849 and 1855, several English practitioners extolled the herb for the treatment of epilepsy, but it was then found to be of no value and the treatment was discredited.

....

KNAPWEED

(CENTAUREA NIGRA)

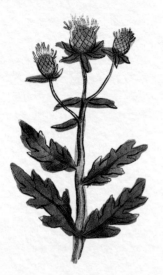

DESCRIPTION: The common sort hereof has many long and somewhat dark green leaves, sometimes a little rent or torn on both sides in two or three places, and somewhat hairy; amongst which arises a long round stalk, four or five feet high, whereof stand great scaly green heads, and from the middle of them [a head of] dark purplish red [flowers].

PLACE: It grows in most fields and meadows, and about their borders and hedges, and in many waste grounds. [Native to Europe, elsewhere naturalized and weedy.]

GOVERNMENT AND VIRTUES: Saturn challenges the herb for his own. This Knapweed helps to stay fluxes, both of blood at the mouth or nose, or other outward parts, and those veins that are inwardly broken, or inward wounds, as also the fluxes of the belly. It stays distillation of thin and sharp humours from the head upon the stomach and lungs. It is good for those that are bruised by any fall, blows or otherwise, and is profitable for those that are bursten, and have ruptures, by drinking the decoction of the herb and roots in wine, and applying the same outwardly to the place. It is singularly good in all running sores, cancerous and fistulous, drying up of the moisture, and healing them up so gently, without sharpness. It doth the like to running sores or scabs of the head or other parts. It is of special use for the soreness of the throat, swelling of the uvula and jaws, and excellently good to stay bleeding, and heals up all green wounds.

MODERN USES: The root and seeds of this and other *Centaurea* species (such as *Centaurea scabiosa*) were used as diuretics and diaphoretics (to break fevers). The leaves were used to treat wounds. Knapweed is seldom used today, though antibacterial activity has been described.

KNOTGRASS

(POLYGONUM AVICULARE)

Prostrate Knotweed

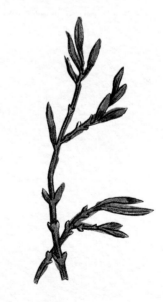

It is generally known so well that it needs no description.

PLACE: It grows in by the highway sides, and by foot-paths in fields; as also by the sides of old walls. [A weed native to Europe and found throughout North America, temperate South America, and cooler regions of southern Africa].

GOVERNMENT AND VIRTUES: Saturn seems to me to own the herb, and yet some hold the Sun; out of doubt 'tis Saturn. The juice of the common kind of Knotgrass is most effectual to stay bleeding of the mouth, being drank in steeled or red wine; and the bleeding at the nose, to be applied to the forehead or temples, or to be squirted up into the nostrils. It is no less effectual to cool and temper the heat of the blood and stomach, and to stay any flux of the blood and humours, as lasks [diarrhea], bloody-flux [dysentery], and women's courses. It is singularly good to provoke urine, help the strangury [painful, frequnt urination], and allays the heat that comes thereby; and is powerful by urine to expel the gravel or stone in the kidneys and bladder, a dram of the powder of the herb being taken in wine for many days together. Being boiled in wine and drank, it is profitable to those that are stung or bitten by venomous creatures, and very effectual to stay all defluxions of rheumatic humours upon the stomach, and kills worms in the belly or stomach, quiets inward pains that arise from the heat, sharpness and corruption of blood and choler [bile]. The distilled water hereof taken by itself or with the powder of the herb or seed, is very effectual to all the purposes aforesaid, and is accounted one of the most sovereign remedies to cool all manner of inflammations, breaking out through heat, hot swellings and imposthumes [abscesses], gangrene and fistulous cankers, or foul filthy ulcers, being applied or put into them; but especially for all sorts of ulcers and sores happening in the private parts of men and women. It helps all fresh and green wounds, and speedily heals them. It is very prevalent for broken joints and ruptures.

MODERN USES: Knotgrass was historically used as an astringent for diarrhea, dysentery, and hemorrhaging (such as nosebleeds), but it is little used today. However, as it is a widespread weed in Asia, Korean and Chinese scientists have explored bioactive compounds in the plant and its potential to treat arthritis and gout. Other studies described pharmacological effects including antiobesity, antioxidant, anticancer, antihypertensive, bronchodilation, and diuretic activity effects.

....

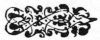

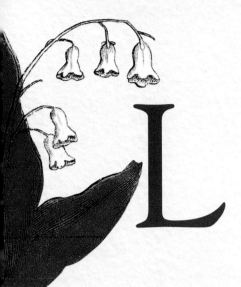

L

LADY'S BEDSTRAW
(GALIUM VERUM)

Ladies' Bed-Straw

Besides the common name above written, it is called Cheese-Rennet, because it performs the same office.

DESCRIPTION: This rises up with diverse small brown, and square upright stalks, a yard high or more; at the tops of the branches grow many long tufts or branches of yellow flowers.

PLACE: They grow in meadow and pastures both wet and dry, and by the hedges. [Found in fields throughout Europe, most of Asia, and northwest Africa. Sporadically naturalized in North America.]

GOVERNMENT AND VIRTUES: An herb of Venus, and therefore strengthening the parts both internal and external, which she rules. The decoction of the herb, is good to fret and break the stone, provoke the urine, stays inward bleeding, and heals inward wounds. The herb or flower bruised and put into the nostrils, stays their bleeding likewise. The flowers and herbs being made into an oil, by being set in the sun, and changed after it has stood ten or twelve days; or into an ointment being boiled in *Axunga* [lard], or salad oil, with some wax melted therein, after it is strained; either the oil made thereof, or the ointment, do help burnings with fire, or scalding with water. The same also, or the decoction of the herb and flower, is good to bathe the feet of travelers, whose long running causes stiffness in the sinews and joints. If the decoction be used warm, and the joints afterwards anointed with ointment, it helps the dry scab, and the itch in children; and the herb is also very good for the sinews, arteries, and joints, to comfort and strengthen them after travel, cold, and pains.

MODERN USES: Seldom used and little researched, lady's bedstraw contains components with antioxidant and antimicrobial effects.

....

LADY'S MANTLE

(ALCHEMILLA XANTHOCHLORA; SYN. ALCHEMILLA VULGARIS)

Ladies' Mantle

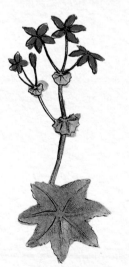

DESCRIPTION: It has many leaves rising from the root standing upon long hairy foot-stalks, being almost round, and a little cut on the edges, folded or plaited at first, and then crumpled and a little hairy, as the stalk is also, with small yellowish green heads, and flowers of a whitish colour breaking out of them.

PLACE: It grows naturally in many pastures and wood sides in [most of Western and northern Europe. Naturalized in northeastern North America].

GOVERNMENT AND VIRTUES: Venus claims the herb as her own. Ladies' Mantle is very proper for those wounds that have inflammations, and is very effectual to stay bleeding, vomiting, fluxes of all sorts, bruises by falls or otherwise, and helps ruptures; and such women as have large breasts, causing them to grow less and hard, being both drank and outwardly applied. The distilled water drank for 20 days together helps conception, and to retain the birth; if the women do sometimes also sit in a bath made of the decoction of the herb. It is one of the most singular wound herbs that is, and therefore highly prized and praised by the Germans, who use it in all wounds inward and outward, to drink a decoction thereof, and wash the wounds therewith, or dip tents therein, and put them into the wounds, which wonderfully dries up all humidity of the sores, and abates inflammations therein. It quickly heals all green wounds, not suffering any corruption to remain behind, and cures all old sores, though fistulous and hollow.

MODERN USES: A folk medicine to stop bleeding both internally and externally. Lady's mantle is used for wound healing, diarrhea, dysentery, and excessive menstrual bleeding. Scientists have confirmed anti-inflammatory, antioxidant, antimicrobial, antimutagenic, antiviral, hemostatic, and blood pressure–lowering effects from leaf extracts. Contains phenolic compounds, primarily ellagitannins, which are associated with medicinal effects.

....

LAVENDER

(LAVANDULA ANGUSTIFOLIA; SYN. LAVANDULA VERA)

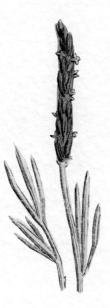

Being an inhabitant almost in every garden, it is so well known, that it needs no description. [Native to dry soils of the Mediterranean region; widely grown in herb gardens since ancient times.]

GOVERNMENT AND VIRTUES: Mercury owns the herb; and it carries his effects very potently. Lavender is of a special good use for all the griefs and pains of the head and brain that proceed of a cold cause, as the apoplexy, falling-sickness, the dropsy, or sluggish malady, cramps, convulsions, palsies, and often faintings. It strengthens the stomach, and frees the liver and spleen from obstructions, provokes women's courses. The flowers of Lavender steeped in wine, helps them to make water that are stopped, or are troubled with the wind or cholic, if the place be bathed therewith. A decoction made with the flowers of Lavender, Horehound, Fennel and Asparagus root, and a little Cinnamon, is very profitably used to help the falling-sickness, and the giddiness or turning of the brain: to gargle the mouth with the decoction thereof is good against the toothache. Two spoonfuls of the distilled water of the flowers taken, helps them that have lost their voice, as also the tremblings and passions of the heart, and faintings and swooning, not only being drank, but applied to the temples, or nostrils to be smelled unto; but it is not safe to use it where the body is replete with blood and humours, because of the hot and subtle spirits wherewith it is possessed. The essential oil drawn from Lavender, usually called Oil of Spike, is of so fierce and piercing a quality, that it is cautiously to be used, some few drops being sufficient, to be given with other things, either for inward or outward griefs.

MODERN USES: Lavender flowers are mildly sedative and used for restlessness, insomnia, nervous stomach, nervous intestinal discomfort, and other conditions. Lavender preparations have claimed tonic, stimulant, antispasmodic, carminative, sedative, stomachic, and diuretic qualities. In folk traditions, lavender has been used for nervous tension headaches, insomnia, neuralgia, and other ailments. The dried herbs are often stuffed (along with hops) in herbal sleep pillows. In aromatherapy, lavender oil with linalyl acetate and linalool is considered soothing and is often claimed to relieve headache.

....

LEMON BALM

(MELISSA OFFICINALIS)

Balm, Melissa

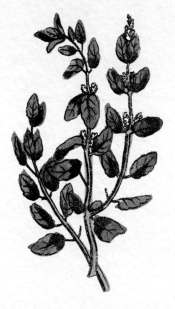

This herb is so well known to be an inhabitant almost in every garden. [Found throughout Europe and naturalized in North America as a wayside plant escaped from gardens.]

GOVERNMENT AND VIRTUES: It is an herb of Jupiter, and under Cancer, and strengthens nature much in all its actions. Let a syrup made with the juice of it and sugar be kept in every gentlewoman's house to relieve the weak stomachs and sick bodies of their poor sickly neighbors; as also the herb kept dry in the house, that so with other convenient simples, you may make it into an electuary with honey. The Arabian physicians have extolled the virtues thereof to the skies; although the Greeks thought it not worth mentioning. Seraphio says, it causes the mind and heart to become merry, and revives the heart, faintings and swoonings, especially of such who are overtaken in sleep, and drives away all troublesome cares and thoughts out of the mind, arising from. It is very good to help digestion, and open obstructions of the brain, and hath so much purging quality in it (saith Avicenna) as to expel those melancholy vapours from the spirits and blood which are in the heart and arteries, although it cannot do so in other parts of the body. Dioscorides says, that the leaves steeped in wine, and the wine drank, and the leaves externally applied, is a remedy against the stings of a scorpion, and the bitings of mad dogs; and commends the decoction thereof for women to bathe or sit in to procure their courses. It is good to wash aching teeth therewith, and profitable for those that have the bloody flux [dysentery]. The leaves also [as tea] helps the griping pains of the belly; and being made into an electuary, it is good for them that cannot fetch their breath. Used with salt, it takes away wens, kernels, or hard swelling in the flesh or throat; it cleanses foul sores, and eases pains of the gout. It is good for the liver and spleen. The herb bruised and boiled in a little wine and oil, and laid warm on a boil, will ripen it, and break it.

MODERN USES: Fresh lemon balm leaves have a pleasant citrus fragrance. The tea (up to 4.5 grams of the dried leaf per cup) is used as an herbal treatment for nervous sleeping disorders, nervousness due to stress, mild stomach upset (helping to relieve bloating and flatulence), and fevers. A 200:1 commercial extract (i.e., two hundred parts herb to one part extract) has shown clinical effectiveness in treating cold sores. Studied for use in relieving symptomatic complications of PMS. Culpeper was right; this herb should be kept in every gentlewoman's house.

....

LETTUCE

(LACTUCA SATIVA)

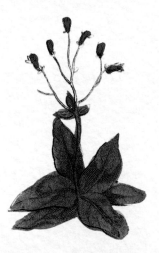

It is so well known, being generally used as a Salad-herb, that it is altogether needless to write any description thereof.

PLACE [Highly variable, cultivated in temperate climates as the familiar lettuce varieties of commerce.]

GOVERNMENT AND VIRTUES: The Moon owns them, and that is the reason they cool and moisten what heat and dryness Mars causeth. The juice of Lettuce mixed or boiled with Oil of Roses, applied to the forehead and temples procures sleep, and eases the headache proceeding of a hot cause: Being eaten boiled, it helps to loosen the belly. It helps digestion, quenches thirst, increases milk in nurses, eases griping pains in the stomach or bowels, that come of choler [bile]. Applied outwardly to the region of the heart, liver or kidneys, or by bathing the said places with the juice of distilled water, wherein some white Sanders, or red Roses are put; not only represses the heat and inflammations therein, but comforts and strengthens those parts, and also tempers the heat of urine. The seed and distilled water of Lettuce work the same effects in all things; but the use of Lettuce is chiefly forbidden to those that are short-winded, or have any imperfection in the lungs, or spit blood.

MODERN USES: The white latex in the leaves and stems of wild lettuce (the progenitor of garden lettuce) has long been used as a sedative. The condensed, concentrated bitter latex, known as *lactucarium* or *lettuce opium*, has been used to reduce anxiety and treat sleep disorders. Recent studies suggest the herb also has antioxidant, antimicrobial, anxiolytic, anti-inflammatory, digestive stimulant, and pain-relieving activity. In modern folk medicine, particularly in the Middle East, preparations are used for stomach problems such as indigestion and lack of appetite. **CAUTION:** May cause contact dermatitis in some individuals.

....

LICORICE

(GLYCYRRHIZA GLABRA)

Liquorice

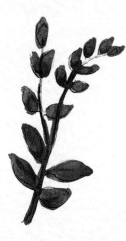

DESCRIPTION: Our English Liquorice rises up with woody stalks. This by many years continuance in a place, will bring forth flowers, of the form of [pale blue] pea blossoms. The roots run down deep into the ground, and shoot out suckers from the main roots.

PLACE: It is planted in fields and gardens, and [was commercially grown in England in Culpeper's time. Originating in much of Central and western Asia, it has been cultivated from southern Europe to England since ancient times; naturalized in the eastern Mediterranean and northern Africa].

GOVERNMENT AND VIRTUES: It is under the dominion of Mercury. Licorice boiled in fair water, with some Maidenhair and figs, makes a good drink for those that have a dry cough or hoarseness, wheezing or shortness of breath, and for all the griefs of the breast and lungs, phthisic [wasting] or consumptions caused by the distillation of salt humours on them. It is also good in all pains of the lower back, the strangury [painful, frequent urination], and heat of urine: The fine powder of Licorice blown through a quill into the eyes that have a pin and web (as they call it) or rheumatic distillations in them, doth cleanse and help them. The juice of Licorice is as effectual in all the diseases of the breast and lungs, the kidneys and bladder, as the decoction. The juice distilled in Rose-water, with some Gum Tragacanth, is a fine licking medicine for hoarseness, wheezing, etc.

MODERN USES: Dried licorice root and rhizome are used in tea to treat cough, sore throat, laryngitis, upper respiratory tract infections, urinary and intestinal irritations, and gastric and duodenal ulcers. Licorice and its extracts are also considered diuretic, demulcent, anti-inflammatory and antitussive, and mildly laxative. Up to 25 percent of the weight of the dried root is glycyrrhizic acid (glycyrrhizin), a glycoside that is fifty times sweeter than sugar. **CAUTION:** Licorice may cause hypertension and potassium loss and is contraindicated when diuretics or heart medications are prescribed. Use is limited to four to six weeks.

LILY OF THE VALLEY
(CONVALLARIA MAJALIS)

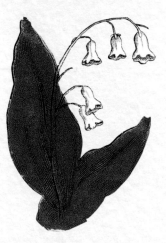

DESCRIPTION: The root is small, and creeps far in the ground. The leaves are many, a foot high, with many white flowers, like little bells.

PLACE: They grow plentifully [in shady, moist open woods; widely cultivated in gardens. Native to much of Europe and western and central Asia; naturalized in North America].

GOVERNMENT AND VIRTUES: It is under the dominion of Mercury, and therefore it strengthens the brain, recruits a weak memory, and makes it strong again: The distilled water dropped into the eyes, helps inflammations there; as also that infirmity which they call a pin and web. The spirit of the flowers distilled in wine, restores lost speech, helps the palsy, and is excellently good in the apoplexy, comforts the heart and vital spirits. Gerard saith, that the flowers being close stopped up in a glass, put into an ant-hill, and taken away again a month after, ye shall find a liquor in the glass, which, being outwardly applied, helps the gout.

MODERN USES: The root and other plant parts contain steroidal cardiac glycosides—called cardenolides (and derivative drugs such as convallotoxin)—which are used in highly controlled doses as a cardiotonic in the management and treatment of heart disease. **CAUTION:** This toxic plant is not appropriate for self-medication and is only used under the supervision of a qualified medical practitioner. Use of lily of the valley may cause cardiac arrhythmias and life-threatening interaction with prescription drugs containing cardiac digitalis glycosides or their chemical analogs. If ingested, it can be fatal to humans and pets.

··················

LIVERWORTS

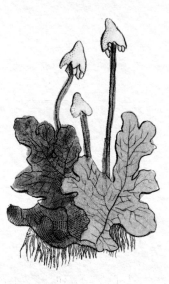

There are, according to some botanists, upwards of three hundred different kinds of Liverwort [a number that has grown to over nine thousand since Culpeper's time].

DESCRIPTION: Common Liverwort grows close, and spreads much upon the ground in moist and shady places, with many small green leaves, or rather (as it were) sticking flat to one another.

GOVERNMENT AND VIRTUES: It is under the dominion of Jupiter, and under the sign Cancer. It is a singularly good herb for all the diseases of the liver, both to cool and cleanse it, and helps the inflammations in any part, and the yellow jaundice likewise. Being bruised and boiled in small beer, and drank, it cools the heat of the liver and kidneys, and helps the running of the kidneys in men, and the whites [vaginal discharges] in women; it is a singular remedy to stay the spreading of tetters, ringworms, and other fretting and running sores and scabs, and is an excellent remedy for such whose livers are corrupted by surfeits, which cause their bodies to break out, for it fortifies the liver exceedingly, and makes it impregnable.

MODERN USES: Liverworts are little used today, but because of their superficial resemblance to the liver, they were traditionally used for the treatment of liver conditions.

··················

⇒⅄

LOOSESTRIFE

(LYTHRUM SALICARIA)

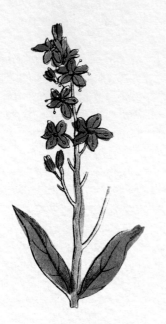

DESCRIPTION: This grows with many square stalks, about three feet high. The stalks are branched into many long stems of spiked [purple-blue] flowers half a foot long.

PLACE: It grows usually by rivers, and ditch-sides in wet ground. [Native to most of Europe, Asia, and North Africa. In North America it is a widespread, seriously invasive alien weed that displaces and overtakes native plant habitats.]

GOVERNMENT AND VIRTUES: It is an herb of the Moon, and under the sign Cancer; neither do I know a better preserver of the sight when it is well, nor a better cure for sore eyes than Eyebright, taken inwardly, and this used outwardly; it is cold in quality. This herb [loosestrife] is nothing inferior to the former [eyebright], it having not only all the virtues which the former hath, but more peculiar virtues of its own, found out by experience; as, namely, the distilled water is a present remedy for hurts and blows on the eyes, and for blindness, and this hath been sufficiently proved true by the experience of a man of judgment, who kept it long to himself as a great secret. It clears the eyes of dust, or anything gotten into them, and preserves the sight. It likewise cleanses and heals all foul ulcers, and sores whatsoever, and stays their inflammations by washing them with the water, and laying on them a green leaf or two in the Summer, or dry leaves in the Winter. This water gargled warm in the mouth, and sometimes drank also, doth cure the quinsy, or king's evil [unusual swelling of lymph nodes or scrofula] in the throat. The said water applied warm, takes away all spots, marks, and scabs in the skin; and a little of it drank, quenches thirst when it is extreme.

MODERN USES: The whole loosestrife plant, but especially the root, is used as a tea in folk medicine for the treatment of inflammatory conditions of the gastrointestinal system, especially diarrhea and dysentery. High in mucilage, it has also been used as a demulcent for bowel irritation. Modern research supports its traditional use as an antidiarrheal, anti-inflammatory, antimicrobial, and antioxidant. It may have antidiabetic effects.

....

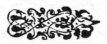

LOVAGE

(LEVISTICUM OFFICINALE)

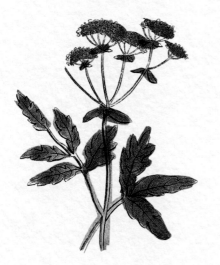

DESCRIPTION: It has many long and green stalks of large winged leaves, divided into many parts, every leaf being cut about the edges, broadest forward, and smallest at the stalk, from which rise up strong, hollow green stalks, five [to] eight feet high, bearing at their tops large umbels of yellow flowers, and after them flat brownish seed. The whole plant and every part of it smelling strong, and aromatically, and is of a hot, sharp, biting taste.

PLACE: It is usually planted in gardens, where, if it be suffered, it grows huge and great. [Found throughout much of Europe, though absent from the wild in the British Isles; naturalized in scattered parts of North America and temperate South America.]

GOVERNMENT AND VIRTUES: It is an herb of the Sun, under the sign Taurus. If Saturn offend the throat (as he always doth if he be occasioner of the malady, and in Taurus is the Genesis) this is your cure. It opens, cures and digests humours, and mightily provokes women's courses and urine.

Half a dram at a time of the dried root in powder taken in wine, doth wonderfully warm a cold stomach, helps digestion, and consumes all raw and superfluous moisture therein; eases all inward griping and pains, dissolves wind, and resists poison and infection. It is a known and much praised remedy to drink the decoction of the herb for any sort of ague, and to help the pains and torments of the body and bowels coming of cold. The seed is effectual to all the purposes aforesaid (except the last) and works more powerfully. The distilled water of the herb helps the quinsy in the throat [peritonsillar abscess], if the mouth and throat be gargled and washed therewith, and helps the pleurisy, being drank three or four times. It takes away spots or freckles in the face. The leaves bruised, and fried with a little hog's lard, and put hot to any blotch or boil, will quickly break it.

MODERN USES: Traditionally, lovage root is used for colic, flatulence, bladder ailments, cramps, stomachache, gout, insomnia, lumbago, and sciatica, among other ailments. Root extracts are strongly diuretic and have a mild sedative effect. Used as a diuretic in inflammatory conditions of the urinary tract and to prevent calculi in the kidneys. Also used for menstrual imbalances. In China, during the 1950s and 1960s, lovage root was used as a substitute for the famous Chinese herb dang-gui (*Angelica sinensis*) because of severe supply shortages of the latter. Lovage was called "European dang-gui." However, in 1984, the Chinese government banned it as a substitute. **CAUTION:** Lovage contains phototoxic compounds including bergapten and psoralens, which cause photodermatitis. Essential oil in the root can be irritating to mucous membranes.

. . . .

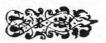

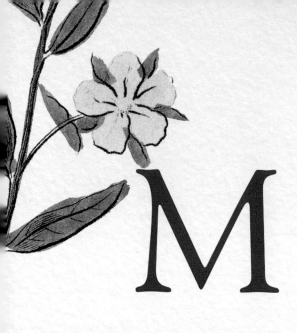

M

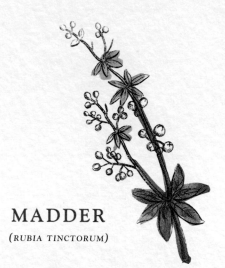

MADDER

(RUBIA TINCTORUM)

DESCRIPTION: Garden Madder shoots forth many very long, weak, four-square, reddish stalks, trailing on the ground a great way. At every one of these joints come forth diverse long and narrow leaves, standing like a star about the stalks, towards the tops whereof come forth many small pale-yellow flowers.

PLACE: Manured in gardens, or larger fields. [Originates in central and western Asia and the Mediterranean region of Europe. Cultivated and naturalized elsewhere in Europe and northern Africa.]

GOVERNMENT AND VIRTUES: It is an herb of Mars. It hath an opening quality, and afterwards to bind and strengthen. It is a sure remedy for the yellow jaundice, by opening the obstructions of the liver and gall, and cleansing those parts; it opens also the obstructions of the spleen, and diminishes the melancholy humour. It is available for the palsy and sciatica, and effectual for bruises inward and outward, and is therefore much used in vulnerary drinks. The root for all those aforesaid purposes, is to be boiled in wine or water, as the cause requires, and some honey and sugar put thereunto afterwards. The seed hereof taken in vinegar and honey, helps the swelling and hardness of the spleen. The leaves and roots beaten and applied to any part that is discoloured with freckles, morphew [skin blemishes], the white scurf, or any such deformity of the skin, cleanses thoroughly, and takes them away.

MODERN USES: Anthraquinones in the root and rhizome of madder are probably responsible for its anti-inflammatory, antibacterial, antidiarrheal, and antifungal activity as a folk medicine, especially for the treatment of bladder and kidney calculi. Components of the root have been studied for potential anti-cancer activity. Commercially, it is historically valued as a red and purple dye material.

....

PLACE: It grows upon old stone walls, and by springs, wells, and rocky moist and shady places, and is always green. [Found throughout temperate regions of the Northern and Southern Hemispheres.]

GOVERNMENT AND VIRTUES: [See White Maidenhair, below.]

MODERN USES: Little used today. Maidenhair fronds were once used as a tea substitute. The leaves were used as a folk medicine for the treatment of sore throat, bronchitis, and coughs. Antibacterial, anti-inflammatory, antioxidant, analgesic, and wound-healing activity are suggested by recent research. Used in various traditional cultures as a hair wash to prevent baldness and make dark hair shiny.

....

MAIDENHAIR
(ADIANTUM CAPILLUS-VENERIS)

Venus Maidenhair Fern

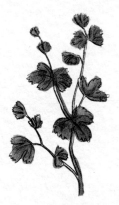

DESCRIPTION: Our common Maidenhair doth, from a number of hard black fibers, send forth a great many blackish shining brittle stalks, hardly a span long, in many not half so long, on each side set very thick with small, round, dark green leaves, and spitted on the back of them like a fern.

MAIDENHAIR, WHITE
(ASPLENIUM RUTA-MURARIA;
SYN. ADIANTUM RUTA-MURARIA)

Wall Rue

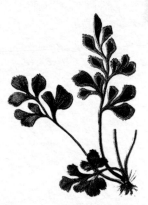

DESCRIPTION: This has very fine, pale green stalks, almost as fine as hairs, set confusedly with diverse pale green leaves on every short foot stalk.

PLACE: [A widespread fern on rocky outcrops. Native to East Asia, eastern North America, and much of Europe.]

GOVERNMENT AND VIRTUES: Both this and the former are under the dominion of Mercury, and so is that also which follows after, and the virtue of both are so near alike, that though I have described them and their places of growing severally, yet I shall in writing the virtues of them, join them both together as follows.

The decoction of the herb Maidenhair being drank, helps those that are troubled with the cough, shortness of breath, the yellow jaundice, diseases of the spleen, stopping of urine, and helps exceedingly to break the stone in the kidneys. It provokes women's courses, and stays both bleedings and fluxes of the stomach and belly, especially when the herb is dry; for being green, it loosens the belly, and voids choler [bile] and phlegm from the stomach and liver; it cleanses the lungs, and by rectifying the blood, causes a good colour to the whole body. The herb boiled in oil of Chamomile, dissolves knots, allays swellings, and dries up moist ulcers. The lye made thereof is singularly good to cleanse the head from scurf, and from dry and running sores, stays the falling or shedding of the hair, and causes it to grow thick, fair, and well coloured; for which purpose some boil it in wine, putting some Smallage seed thereto, and afterwards some oil. The Wall Rue is as effectual as Maidenhair, in all diseases of the head, or falling and recovering of the hair again, and generally for all the aforementioned diseases: And besides, the powder of it taken in drink for forty days together, helps the burstings in children.

MODERN USES: White maidenhair has fallen into obscurity and disuse.

·················

MALLOWS
(MALVA SPP.)

AND MARSHMALLOW
(ALTHAEA OFFICINALIS)

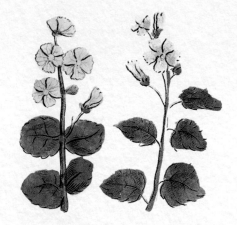

Common Mallows are generally so well known that they need no description.

Our common Marshmallows have diverse soft hairy white stalks, rising to be three or four feet high, spreading forth many branches, the leaves whereof are soft and hairy, somewhat less than the other Mallow leaves. The flowers are many, but smaller also than the other Mallows, and white, or tending to a bluish colour.

PLACE: The common Mallows grow [throughout Europe, Asia, and North America]. The common Marshmallows [grow] in most salt marshes [in Europe and eastern North America and are widely grown in herb gardens].

GOVERNMENT AND VIRTUES: Venus owns them both. The leaves of either of the sorts, both specified, and the roots also boiled in wine or water, or in broth with Parsley or Fennel roots, do help to open the body, and are very convenient in hot agues, or other distempers of the body, to apply the leaves so boiled warm to the belly. It not only voids hot, choleric, and other offensive humours, but eases the pains and torments of the belly coming thereby; and are therefore used in all clysters conducing to those purposes. The same used by nurses procures them store of milk. The decoction of the seed of any of the common Mallows made in milk or wine, doth marvelously help excoriations, the phthisic, pleurisy, and other diseases of the chest and lungs, that proceed of hot causes, if it be continued taking for some time together. The leaves and roots work the same effects. They help much also in the excoriations of the bowels, and hardness of the mother, and in all hot and sharp diseases thereof. Pliny saith, that whosoever takes a spoonful of any of the Mallows, shall that day be free from all diseases that may come unto him; and that it is especially good for the falling-sickness. The syrup also and conserve made of the flowers, are very effectual for the same diseases, and to open the body, being costive.

The leaves bruised, and laid to the eyes with a little honey, take away the imposthumations [inflammation] of them. The leaves bruised or rubbed upon any place stung with bees, wasps, or the like, presently take away the pain, redness, and swelling that rise thereupon. And Dioscorides saith, the decoction of the roots and leaves helps all sorts of poison, so as the poison be presently voided by vomit. A poultice made of the leaves boiled and bruised, with some bean or barley flower, and oil of Roses added, is an especial remedy against all hard tumours and inflammations, or imposthumes [abscesses], or swellings of the private parts, and other parts, and eases the pains of them; as also against the hardness of the liver or spleen, being applied to the places. The juice of Mallows boiled in old oil and applied, takes away all roughness of the skin, as also the scurf, dandruff, or dry scabs in the head, or other parts, if they be anointed there-

with, or washed with the decoction, and preserves the hair from falling off. It is also effectual against scaldings and burnings, St. Anthony's fire, and all other hot, red, and painful swellings in any part of the body. The flowers boiled in oil or water whereunto a little honey and alum is put, is an excellent gargle to wash, cleanse or heal any sore mouth or throat in a short space. If the feet be bathed or washed with the decoction of the leaves, roots, and flowers, it helps much the defluxions of rheum [watery discharge] from the head; if the head be washed therewith, it stays the falling and shedding of the hair. The green leaves (saith Pliny) beaten with nitre, and applied, draw out thorns or prickles in the flesh.

The Marshmallows are more effectual in all the diseases before mentioned.

You may remember that not long since there was a raging disease called the bloody-flux [dysentery with bleeding]; the college of physicians not knowing what to make of it, called it the inside plague, for their wits were at *Ne plus ultra* about it: My son was taken with the same disease, and the excoriation of his bowels was exceeding great; myself being in the country, was sent for, the only thing I gave him, was Mallows bruised and boiled both in milk and drink. In two days (the blessing of God being upon it) it cured him. And I here, to shew my thankfulness to God, in communicating it to his creatures, leave it to posterity.

MODERN USES: Mallow (*Malva* spp.) and marshmallow leaf and root are high in soothing mucilagin and continue to be used in modern phytomedicine. The leaf is used in tea to relieve dry, irritated coughs, and for inflammations of the mouth and throat. Marshmallow leaf tea soothes gastrointestinal mucous membrane inflammation. The root tea is used similarly and considered somewhat more effective than the leaf.

....

MARSH WOUNDWORT

(STACHYS PALUSTRIS)

Clown's Woundwort

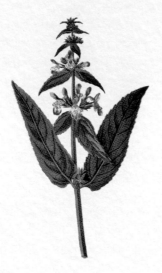

DESCRIPTION: It grows up sometimes to two or three feet high, with square green rough stalks, and two very long, somewhat narrow, leaves. The flowers stand towards the tops, end in a spiked top, having long and much gaping hoods of a purplish red colour, with whitish spots in them. This plant smells somewhat strong.

PLACE: It grows in [moist soils and ditches from Europe to Mongolia and the Western Himalayas. Naturalized in the northeastern United States, the northern Midwest, and adjacent provinces in Canada].

GOVERNMENT AND VIRTUES: It is under the dominion of the planet Saturn. It is singularly effectual in all fresh and green wounds, and therefore bears not this name for naught. And it is very available in staunching of blood and to dry up the fluxes of humours in old fretting ulcers, cankers, etc., that hinder the healing of them. A syrup made of the juice of it, is inferior to none for inward wounds, ruptures of veins, bloody flux [dysentery], vessels broken, spitting, urinating, or vomiting blood. Ruptures are excellent and speedily, ever to admiration, cured by taking now and then a little of the syrup, and applying an ointment or plaster of this herb to the place. Also, if any vein be swelled or muscle, apply a plaster of this herb to it, and if you add a little Comfrey to it, it will not be amiss. I assure thee the herb deserves commendation, though it has gotten such a clownish name; and whosoever reads this (if he try it, as I have done) will commend it; only take notice that it is of a dry earthy quality.

MODERN USES: Marsh woundwort is used traditionally for the external treatment of wounds. Its chemistry has been recently analyzed and shown to have biologically active compounds typical of its relatives in the mint family, with antioxidant, antispasmodic, antimicrobial, and possibly anti-inflammatory activity. With a slightly bitter-aromatic flavor (though unpleasant fragrance), the young leaves are used sparingly as a salad ingredient in eastern Europe. The roots are also considered edible along with the springtime shoots. It is surprisingly little researched.

....

MASTERWORT

(*PEUCEDANUM OSTRUTHIUM*; SYN.
IMPERATORIA OSTRUTHIUM)

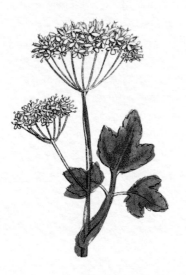

DESCRIPTION: Common Masterwort has diverse stalks of winged leaves divided, three for the most part standing together at a small foot-stalk; among which rise up two or three short stalks about two feet high, bearing umbels of white flowers, and after them thin, flat blackish seeds, bigger than Dill seeds.

PLACE: It is usually kept in gardens with us in England. [Native to most of western Europe. A garden plant that has escaped in Great Britain, Scandinavia, and eastern North America.]

GOVERNMENT AND VIRTUES: It is an herb of Mars. The root of Masterwort is hotter than pepper, and very available in cold griefs and diseases both of the stomach and body, dissolving very powerfully upwards and downwards. It is also used in a decoction with wine against all cold rheums, distillations upon the lungs, or shortness of breath, to be taken morning and evening. It also provokes urine, and helps to break the stone, and expel the gravel from the kidneys. It is effectual also against the dropsy, cramps, and falling sickness; for the decoction in wine being gargled in the mouth, draws down much water and phlegm, from the brain, purging and easing it of what oppresses it. It is of a rare quality against all sorts of cold poison, to be taken as there is cause; it provokes sweat. But lest the taste hereof, or of the seed (which works to the like effect, though not so powerfully) should be too offensive, the best way is to take the water distilled both from the herb and root. The juice hereof dropped, or tents dipped therein, and applied either to green wounds or filthy rotten ulcers, and those that come by envenomed weapons, doth soon cleanse and heal them. The same is also very good to help the gout coming of a cold cause.

MODERN USES: Masterwort is a famous folk medicine in Alpine areas of Western Europe. Traditionally, both the aboveground parts and the root were extracted in wine and used to treat joint pains. The plant was also soaked in schnapps, and this concoction was rubbed into painful limbs. Contains isoimperatorin and imperatorin, which are coumarins with pharmacological effects including analgesic, antiviral, anti-inflammatory, antibacterial, anti-hypertensive, and blood-thinning properties, plus experimental anticancer activity, among others. Plant preparations are used for gastrointestinal problems, cardiovascular conditions, inflammation of the upper respiratory tract, and tiredness. **CAUTION:** Furocoumarins, like those found in masterwort, can cause photodermatitis and, in some individuals, severe contact dermatitis. In so many words, Culpeper warns us that the root is acrid, bitter, and "hotter than pepper." Avoid products containing masterwort if you have been prescribed blood thinners.

. . . .

MAY LILY

(MAIANTHEMUM BIFOLIUM)

One-Blade, False Lily-of-the-Valley

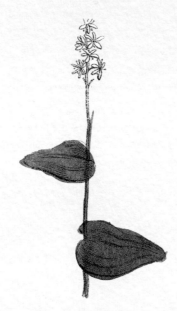

DESCRIPTION: This small plant never bears more than one leaf, but only when it rises up with his stalk, which thereon bears another, and seldom more, which are of a blueish green colour, pointed, with many ribs or veins therein [with] many small white flowers, star fashion.

PLACE: It grows in moist, shadowy and grassy places of woods. [Declined in England due to habitat loss; native to western Europe, and from Siberia to China and Japan.]

GOVERNMENT AND VIRTUES: It is a precious herb of the Sun. Half a dram, or a dram at most, in powder of the roots hereof taken in wine and vinegar, of each equal parts, and the party laid presently to sweat thereupon, is held to be a sovereign remedy for those that are infected with the plague, and have a sore upon them, by expelling the poison and infection, and defending the heart and spirits from danger. It is a singularly good wound herb, and is thereupon used with other the like effects in many compound balms for curing of wounds, be they fresh and green, or old and malignant, and especially if the sinews be burnt.

MODERN USES: May lily was once used topically as a folk remedy for wounds or sores. The fruits were harvested prior to the twentieth century and used for flavoring wine. The fruit contains anthocyanins, which may have antioxidant activity. Little used today.

....

MEADOWRUE

(THALICTRUM MINUS)

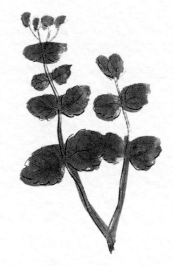

DESCRIPTION: Meadowrue rises up with a yellow stringy root, much spreading in the ground, shooting forth new sprouts round about, two feet high, and many large leaves on them, of a red green colour on the upper-side, and pale green underneath. The whole plant has a strong unpleasant scent.

PLACE: It grows in many places of this land, in the borders of moist meadows, and ditch-sides. [Occurs in most of Europe, Asia, and the Middle East.]

GOVERNMENT AND VIRTUES: Dioscorides saith, that this herb bruised and applied, perfectly heals old sores, and the distilled water of the herb and flowers doth the like. It is used by some among other pot-herbs to open the body, and make it soluble; but the roots washed clean, and boiled in ale and drank, provokes to stool more than the leaves, but yet very gently. The root boiled in water, and the places of the body most troubled with vermin and lice washed therewith while it is warm, destroys them utterly. In Italy it is good against the plague, and in Saxony against the jaundice, as Camerarius saith.

MODERN USES: Seldom used today. Meadow rue contains alkaloids (including berberine) that have antibacterial activity. Formerly used as a snake-bite remedy.

....

MEADOWSWEET
(*FILIPENDULA ULMARIA*)
Filipendula, Dropwort

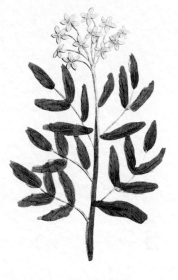

DESCRIPTION: This sends forth many leaves, some larger, some smaller, set on each side of a middle rib, and each of them dented about the edges; among which rise up one or more stalks, two or three feet high, spreading at the top into many white, sweet-smelling flowers.

PLACE: [It grows in fields and meadows throughout Europe and northern Asia; sporadically naturalized in North America.]

GOVERNMENT AND VIRTUES: It is under the dominion of Venus. It effectually opens the passages of the urine, helps the strangury; the stone in the kidneys or bladder, the gravel, and all other pains of the bladder and kidneys, by taking the roots in powder, or a decoction of them in white wine, with a little honey. The roots made into powder, and mixed with honey in the form of an electuary, doth much help them whose stomachs are swollen, dissolving and breaking the wind which was the cause thereof. It is also very effectual for all the diseases of the lungs, as shortness of breath, wheezing, hoarseness of the throat, and the cough; and to expectorate tough phlegm, or any other parts thereabout.

MODERN USES: Meadowsweet famously contains salicylates (the starting material of one of the first synthetic drugs, aspirin), which supports its traditional use as an antiseptic, fever reducer, and pain reliever for rheumatism and arthritis. It is also considered astringent, and a tea of the herb is used for dyspepsia with heartburn, diarrhea, and as a mild urinary antiseptic; also for supportive treatment of colds.

....

MEDLAR

(*CRATAEGUS GERMANICA;*
SYN. *MESPILUS GERMANICA*)

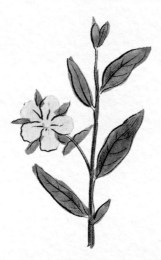

DESCRIPTION: The tree grows near the bigness of the Quince Tree, spreading branches reasonably large, with longer and narrower leaves. The fruit, of a brownish green colour, being ripe, bearing a crown as it were on the top. The fruit is very harsh before it is mellowed.

PLACE: [Cultivated and naturalized along fence rows and hedges in most of Western and central Europe. Native to Crimea, and from the Caucasus to Iran.]

GOVERNMENT AND VIRTUES: The fruit is old Saturn's, and sure a better medicine he hardly hath to strengthen the retentive faculty. They are powerful to stay any fluxes of blood or humours in men or women; the leaves also have this quality. The decoction of them is good to gargle and wash the mouth, throat and teeth, when there is any defluxions of blood to stay it, or of humours, which causes the pains and swellings. It is a good bath for women, that have their courses flow too abundant: or for the piles when they bleed too much. The dried leaves in powder strewed on fresh bleeding wounds restrains the blood, and heals up the wound quickly. The medlar-stones made into powder, and drank in wine, wherein some Parsley-roots have lain infused all night, or a little boiled, do break the stone in the kidneys, helping to expel it.

MODERN USES: Medlar is little used today; the fruit is hard, not tasty, and mostly inedible, but is considered styptic, astringent, and cooling. It was used as a folk medicine to treat diarrhea—and conversely, in preparations to treat constipation. Also used as a diuretic and treatment for kidney and bladder stones in southeastern Europe and western Asia. Leaf extracts have experimental antidiabetic activity.

....

MELANCHOLY THISTLE

(*CIRSIUM HETEROPHYLLUM;*
SYN. *CARDUUS HETEROPHYLLUS, CARDUUS HELENOIDES*)

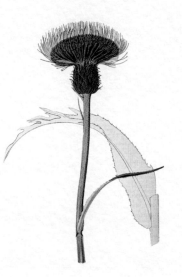

DESCRIPTION: It rises up with tender single hoary green stalks, bearing thereon four or five green leaves, dented about the edges; [not] prickly, and at the top usually but one head, scaly and prickly, with many reddish flowers in the middle, which being gathered fresh, will keep the colour a long time.

PLACE: They grow in many moist meadows, [grasslands, scrubs, and open woods in the British Isles and elsewhere in northern Europe and central Asia].

GOVERNMENT AND VIRTUES: It is under Capricorn, and therefore under both Saturn and Mars, one rids melancholy by sympathy, the other by antipathy. Their virtues are but few, but those not to be despised; for the decoction of the thistle in wine being drank, expels superfluous melancholy out of the body, and makes a man as merry as a cricket; superfluous melancholy causes care, fear, sadness, despair, envy, and many evils more besides; but religion teaches to wait upon God's providence, and cast our care upon him who cares for us. What a fine thing were it if men and women could live so? And yet seven years' care and fear makes a man never the wiser, nor a farthing richer. Dioscorides saith, the root borne about one doth the like, and removes all diseases of melancholy. Modern writers laugh at him; *Let them laugh that win*: my opinion is, that it is the best remedy against all melancholy diseases that grows; they that please may use it.

MODERN USES: No modern uses noted. Melancholy thistle was smoked instead of tobacco in Derbyshire, England, in the eighteenth century. It seems that modern societies, suffering from an epidemic of superfluous melancholy, should follow Culpeper's lead and research this herb.

....

MILK THISTLE

(*SILYBUM MARIANUM*)

Our Lady's Thistle

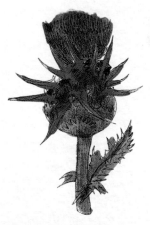

DESCRIPTION: Milk Thistle hath large and broad leaves, and as it were crumpled, of a white green shining colour, wherein are many lines and streaks of a milk white colour with many sharp and stiff prickles all about. At the end of every branch, is a great prickly Thistle-like head, strongly armed with prickles, and with bright purple [flowers]. The whole plant is bitter in taste.

PLACE: [Found in fields and wastelands throughout much of Europe; naturalized as a weed in California.]

GOVERNMENT AND VIRTUES: Milk Thistle is under Jupiter, and thought to be as effectual as *Carduus benedictus* for agues, and to prevent and cure the infection of the plague: as also to open the obstructions of the liver and spleen, and thereby is good against the jaundice. It provokes urine, breaks and expels the stone, and is good for the dropsy. It is effectual also for the pains in the sides, and many other inward pains and griping. The seed and distilled water is held powerful to all the purposes aforesaid, and besides, it is often applied both outwardly with cloths or sponges to the region of the liver, to cool the distemper thereof, and to the region of the heart, against swoonings and the passions of it. It cleanses the blood exceedingly: and in Spring, if you please to boil the tender plant (but cut off the prickles, unless you have a mind to choke yourself) it will change your blood as the season changes, and that is the way to be safe.

MODERN USES: Milk thistle is one of the best-studied and most widely used medicinal plants for the supportive treatment of chronic inflammatory liver disorders, including some forms of hepatitis, cirrhosis, and fatty infiltration of the liver by alcohol or other toxins. It is considered both a preventative and treatment for various liver conditions. A purified component from the seeds is used as an intravenous treatment for mushroom poisoning. The active constituents of the seed are a complex of components known as silymarin. Primarily used in products standardized to deliver 420 milligrams of silymarin per day, divided into three doses.

....

MINT
(*MENTHA SPICATA*)
Spearmint

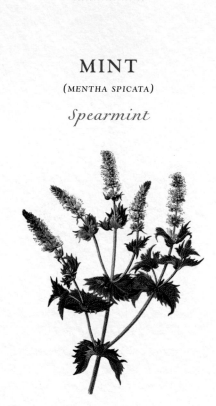

Of all the kinds of Mint, the Spear Mint, being most usual, I shall only describe as follows:

DESCRIPTION: Spear Mint has diverse round stalks, and long but narrowish leaves set thereon, of a dark green colour. The flowers stand in spiked heads at the tops of the branches, being of a pale blue colour.

PLACE: It is a usual inhabitant in gardens; and because it seldom gives any good seed, the seed is recompensed by the plentiful increase of the root, which being once planted in a garden, will hardly be rid out again.

GOVERNMENT AND VIRTUES: It is an herb of Venus. It stirs up venery, or bodily lust; two or three branches thereof taken in the juice of four pomegranates, stays the hiccough, vomiting, and allays the choler [bile]. It dissolves imposthumes [abscesses] being laid to with barley-meal. It is good to repress the milk in women's breasts, and for such as have swollen, flagging, or great breasts. Applied with salt, it helps the biting of a mad dog; with mead and honeyed water, it eases the pains of the ears, and takes away the roughness of the tongue, being rubbed thereupon. It suffers not milk to curdle in the stomach, if the leaves thereof be steeped or boiled in it before you drink it. Briefly it is very profitable to the stomach. The often use hereof is a very powerful medicine to stay women's courses and the whites [vaginal discharges]. Applied to the forehead and temples, it eases the pains in the head, and is good to wash the heads of young children therewith, against all manner of breakings-out, sores or scabs, therein. It is also profitable against the poison of venomous creatures. The distilled water of Mint is available to all the purposes aforesaid, yet more weakly. But if a spirit thereof be rightly and chemically drawn, it is much more powerful than the herb itself. Simeon Sethi saith, it helps a cold liver, strengthens the belly, causes digestion, stays vomits and hiccough. It is good against the gnawing of the heart, provokes appetite, takes away obstructions of the liver, and stirs up bodily lust; but therefore too much must not be taken, because it makes the blood thin and wheyish, and turns it into choler [bile], and therefore choleric persons must abstain from it. The powder of it being dried and taken after meat, helps digestion, and those that are splenetic. Taken with wine, it helps women in their sore travail in child-bearing. It is good against the gravel and stone in the kidneys, and the strangury [painful, frequent urination]. Being smelled unto, it is comfortable for the head and memory. The decoction hereof gargled in the mouth, cures the gums and mouth that are sore, and mends an ill-savored breath; as also the Rue and Coriander, causes the palate of the mouth to turn to its place, the decoction being gargled and held in the mouth.

MODERN USES: Spearmint was the most commonly used mint in Culpeper's day. Today's more widely used medicinal herb, peppermint (*Mentha* × *piperita*), a hybrid, was not known until decades after Culpeper's death. Both peppermint and spearmint leaf tea are used to soothe digestive problems, acting as carminatives, reducing nausea, and calming upset stomachs. The essential oil is also used to flavor chewing gum and dental products.

....

MISTLETOE

(*VISCUM ALBUM*)

Misselto, European Mistletoe

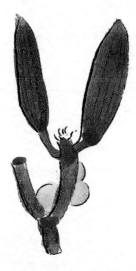

DESCRIPTION: This [parasitic shrub] rises up from the branch or arm of the tree whereon it grows, with a [green] woody stem. At the joints of the boughs and branches [are] small, round, white, transparent berries, three or four together, full of a glutinous moisture.

PLACE: It grows very rarely on oaks with us; plentifully in woody groves [throughout much of Europe; naturalized in California].

GOVERNMENT AND VIRTUES: This is under the dominion of the Sun, I do not question; and can also take for granted, that which grows upon oaks, participates something of the nature of Jupiter, because an oak is one of his trees; as also that which grows upon pear trees, and apple trees, participates something of his nature, because he rules the tree it grows upon, having no root of its own. But why that should have most virtues that grows upon oaks I know not, unless because it is rarest and hardest to come by; and our college's opinion is in this contrary to scripture, which saith, *God's tender mercies are over all his works*; and so it is, let the college of physicians walk as contrary to him as they please, and that is as contrary as the east to the west. Clusius affirms that which grows upon pear trees to be as prevalent, and gives order, that it should not touch the ground after it is gathered; and also saith, that, being hung about the neck, it remedies witchcraft. Both the leaves and berries of Mistletoe do heat and dry, and are of subtle parts. The Mistletoe itself of the oak (as the best) made into powder, and given in drink to those that have the falling sickness, does assuredly heal them, as Matthiolus saith: but it is fit to use it for forty days together. Some have so highly esteemed it for the virtues thereof, that they have called it *Lignum Sanctiæ Crucis*, Wood of the Holy Cross, believing it helps the falling sickness, apoplexy and palsy very speedily, not only to be inwardly taken, but to be hung at their neck.

MODERN USES: Controversially, extracts of mistletoe are used in injectable proprietary products in Europe for the supportive treatment of cancer, with a higher dose used for malignant tumors. In lower-dose intradermal injections, it has been used to treat joint inflammation. Obviously, these uses are not amenable to self-medication. As a tea, the herb is used as a folk medicine for mild hypertension. **CAUTION:** May cause allergies in some individuals. The translucent white berries have reportedly caused poisoning in children. Avoid ingestion.

....

MONEYWORT

(LYSIMACHIA NUMMULARIA)

Herb Twopence

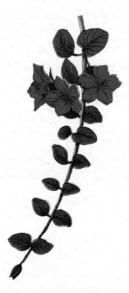

DESCRIPTION: The common Moneywort run[s] upon the ground two or three feet long or more, set with leaves two at a joint, which are almost round. At the joints with the leaves come forth one [or two] yellow flowers.

PLACE: It grows plentifully in moist [shaded grounds and fields throughout Europe; naturalized and weedy in North America].

GOVERNMENT AND VIRTUES: Venus owns it. Moneywort is singularly good to stay all fluxes in man or woman, whether they be lasks [diarrhea], bloody-fluxes [dysentery], bleeding inwardly or outwardly, or the weakness of the stomach that is given to casting. It is very good also for the ulcers or excoriations of the lungs, or other inward parts. It is exceedingly good for all wounds, either fresh or green, to heal them speedily, and for all old ulcers that are of spreading natures. For all which purposes the juice of the herb, or the powder drank in water wherein hot steel hath been often quenched; or the decoction of the green herb in wine or water drank, or used to the outward place, to wash or bathe them, or to have tents dipped therein and put into them, are effectual.

MODERN USES: Moneywort is a folk medicine used as an astringent for the treatment of diarrhea and dysentery. Also used topically for the treatment of wounds. Seldom used today.

....

MOONWORT
(BOTRYCHIUM LUNARIA)

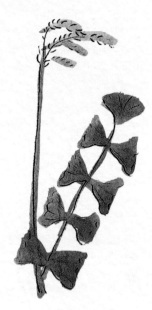

DESCRIPTION: [A small fern that] rises up usually but with one dark green, thick and flat leaf, with leaflets, resembling therein a half-moon.

PLACE: It grows on hills and heaths. [A widespread plant found in mountainous regions nearly worldwide; found in the Rocky Mountains and cooler regions of North America, Europe, Asia, and South America.]

GOVERNMENT AND VIRTUES: The Moon owns the herb. Moonwort is cold and drying more than Adder's Tongue, and is therefore held to be more available for all wounds both inward and outward. The leaves boiled in red wine, and drank, stay the immoderate flux of women's courses, and the whites. It also stays bleeding, vomiting, and other fluxes. It helps all blows and bruises, and to consolidate all fractures and dislocations. It is good for ruptures, but is chiefly used, by most with other herbs, to make oils or balsams to heal fresh or green wounds (as I said before) either inward or outward, for which it is excellently good.

Moonwort is an herb which (they say) will open locks, and unshod such horses as tread upon it: This some laugh to scorn, and those no small fools neither; but country people, that I know, call it Unshoe the Horse. Besides I have heard commanders say, that on White Down in Devonshire, there were found thirty horse shoes, pulled off from the feet of the Earl of Essex's horses, being there drawn up in a body, many of them being but newly shod, and no reason known. The herb described usually grows upon heaths.

MODERN USES: Moonwort is an obscure folk medicine, used internally much like Culpeper describes for the treatment of diarrhea, and externally for wounds or sores.

. . . .

MOTHERWORT

(*LEONURUS CARDIACA*)

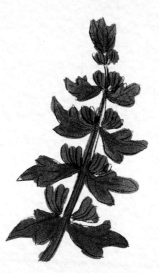

DESCRIPTION: This hath a hard, square, stalk, rising three or four feet high, whereon grow leaves on each side, as if it were rough or crumpled, and [toothed] deeply divided. The flowers are of a red or purple colour.

PLACE: It grows only in gardens in England. [Found in fields and wastelands throughout most of Europe and western Asia; naturalized throughout North America.]

GOVERNMENT AND VIRTUES: Venus owns the herb, and it is under Leo. There is no better herb to take melancholy vapours from the heart, to strengthen it, and make a merry, cheerful, blithe soul than this herb. It may be kept in a syrup or conserve; therefore the Latins called it Cardiaca. Besides, it makes women joyful mothers of children, and settles their wombs as they should be, therefore we call it Motherwort. It is held to be of much use for the trembling of the heart, and faintings and swoonings; from whence it took the name Cardiaca. The powder thereof, to the quantity of a spoonful, drank in wine, is a wonderful help to women in their sore travail, as also for the suffocating or risings of the mother, and for these effects, it is likely it took the name of Motherwort with us. It also provokes urine and women's courses, cleanses the chest of cold phlegm, oppressing it, kills worms in the belly. It is of good use to warm and dry up the cold humours, to digest and disperse them that are settled in the veins, joints, and sinews of the body, and to help cramps and convulsions.

MODERN USES: Traditionally, motherwort is used as a mild sedative, antispasmodic, cardiotonic, diuretic, hypotensive, and astringent. Used to treat menstrual irregularities, nervous heart complaints, and menopausal symptoms, among other ailments. Related species are commonly used in traditional Chinese medicine to regulate the menses, promote good blood circulation, and regulate the heart.

Motherwort is considered antioxidant, anti-inflammatory, immunomodulatory, and diuretic. European and Asian species share the alkaloids leonurine, stachydrine, and leonurinine.

....

MUGWORT

(ARTEMISIA VULGARIS)

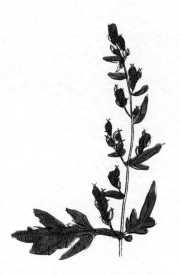

DESCRIPTION: Common Mugwort hath diverse leaves lying upon the ground, very much divided, or cut deeply in, of a dark green colour on the upper side, and very hoary white underneath. The stalks rise to be four or five feet high, with small, pale, flowers like buttons.

PLACE: It grows plentifully [in wastelands throughout Europe and Asia; weedy and widely naturalized in North America and elsewhere].

GOVERNMENT AND VIRTUES: This is an herb of Venus, therefore maintains the parts of the body she rules, remedies the diseases of the parts that are under her signs, Taurus and Libra. Mugwort is with good success put among other herbs that are boiled for women to apply the hot decoction to draw down their courses, to help the delivery of the birth, and expel the after-birth. As also for the obstructions and inflammations of the mother. It breaks the stone, and opens the urinary passages where they are stopped. The juice thereof made up with Myrrh, and put under as a pessary, works the same effects, and so does the root also. Being made up with hog's grease into an ointment, it takes away wens and hard knots and kernels that grow about the neck and throat, and eases the pains about the neck more effectually, if some Field Daisies be put with it. The herb itself being fresh, or the juice thereof taken, is a special remedy upon the overmuch taking of opium. Three drams of the powder of the dried leaves taken in wine, is a speedy and the best certain help for the sciatica. A decoction thereof made with Chamomile and Agrimony, and the place bathed therewith while it is warm, takes away the pains of the sinews, and the cramp.

MODERN USES: Like wormwood (*Artemisia absinthium*) mugwort has been used to expel roundworms and threadworms. Traditionally used for the treatment of nervous conditions, restlessness, anxiety, lack of sleep, and menstrual difficulties. Widely used in Asian traditional medicine systems as moxa (dried, compressed leaves burned on the skin to activate acupuncture points). The plant and its extracts have antioxidant, anti-bacterial, anti-inflammatory, anthelmintic, and mildly sedative effects. **CAUTION:** A source of airborne allergies; may cause contact dermatitis.

....

MULBERRY

(MORUS ALBA)

The Mulberry Tree

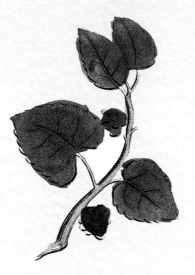

This is so well known where it grows, that it needs no description.

PLACE: [Native to Central Asia, mulberry has been cultivated since ancient times and occurs throughout Asia, much of Europe, temperate Africa, North America, and South America.]

GOVERNMENT AND VIRTUES: Mercury rules the tree, therefore are its effects variable as his are. The Mulberry is of different parts; the ripe berries, by reason of their sweetness and slippery moisture, opening the body, and the unripe binding it, especially when they are dried, and then they are good to stay fluxes, lasks [diarrhea], and the abundance of women's courses. The bark of the root kills the broad worms in the body. The juice, or the syrup made of the juice of the berries, helps all inflammations or sores in the mouth, or throat, and palate of the mouth when it is fallen down. The juice of the leaves is a remedy against the biting of serpents, and for those that have taken aconite. The leaves beaten with vinegar, are good to lay on any place that is burnt with fire. A decoction made of the bark and leaves is good to wash the mouth and teeth when they ache. If the root be a little slit or cut, and a small hole made in the ground next thereunto, in the Harvest-time, it will give out a certain juice, which being hardened the next day, is of good use to help the tooth-ache, to dissolve knots, and purge the belly. The leaves of Mulberries are said to stay bleeding at the mouth or nose, or the bleeding of the piles, or of a wound, being bound unto the places. A branch of the tree taken when the moon is at the full, and bound to the wrists of a woman's arm, whose courses come down too much, doth stay them in a short space.

MODERN USES: Mulberry leaf, mulberry root bark, mulberry twigs, and mulberry fruit, just as Culpeper enumerates from his era, are today all separate drugs in traditional Chinese medicine. The leaf is used in prescriptions for upper respiratory tract infections, dry coughs, headaches, and eye inflammations. Mulberry root bark is used to treat asthma and as a diuretic. The twigs are used for rheumatism and arthritis to help reduce aching and numbness of joints. The fruits are used to nourish the blood and to treat insomnia, diabetes, and thirst. Various pharmacological activities, including anti-inflammatory, antidiabetic, and antioxidant effects, are attributed to this plant.

....

MULLEIN

(VERBASCUM THAPSUS)

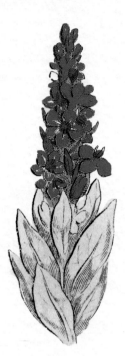

DESCRIPTION: Common Mullein has many fair, large, woolly white leaves, lying next the ground, somewhat longer than broad. The stalk rises up to be four or five feet high [the second year], set together in a long spike, [with yellow five-petaled flowers].

PLACE: It grows by way-sides and lanes, in many places [originating in the Balkans and southeast Europe, now found in wastelands, gravelly soils, and roadsides as a weed throughout most of the world].

GOVERNMENT AND VIRTUES: It is under the dominion of Saturn. A small quantity of the root given in wine, is commended by Dioscorides, against lasks [diarrhea] and fluxes of the belly. The decoction hereof drank, is profitable for those that are bursten, and for cramps and convulsions, and for those that are troubled with an old cough. The decoction thereof gargled, eases the pains of the toothache. And the oil made by the often infusion of the flowers, is of very good effect for the piles. The decoction of the root in red wine or in water, (if there be an ague) wherein red-hot steel hath been often quenched, doth stay the bloody-flux [dysentery]. The same also opens obstructions of the bladder and kidneys. A decoction of the leaves hereof, and of Sage, Marjoram, and Chamomile flowers, and the places bathed therewith, that have sinews stiff with cold or cramps, doth bring them much ease and comfort. Three ounces of the distilled water of the flowers drank morning and evening for some days together, is said to be the most excellent remedy for gout. The juice of the leaves and flowers being laid upon rough warts, as also the powder of the dried roots rubbed on, doth easily take them away, but doth no good to smooth warts. The powder of the dried flowers is an especial remedy for those that are troubled with the belly-ache, or the pains of the colic. The decoction of the root, and so likewise of the leaves, is of great effect to dissolve the tumours, swellings, or inflammations of the throat. The seed and leaves boiled in wine, and applied, draw forth speedily thorns or splinters gotten into the flesh, ease the pains, and heal them also. The seed bruised and boiled in wine, and laid on any member that has been out of joint, and newly set again, takes away all swelling and pain thereof.

MODERN USES: The flowers of mullein are used in tea as a soothing expectorant for congestion of the upper respiratory tract. When soaked in olive oil, the flowers are a popular herbal treatment for earache. The leaves are used in numerous cough and bronchial herbal preparations. Both the flowers and leaves contain soothing mucilage, along with various active constituents such as iridoids, saponins, and flavonoids. Mullein has anti-oxidant, antimicrobial, anti-inflammatory, and liver-protective activity.

·················

MUSTARD

(BRASSICA RAPA)

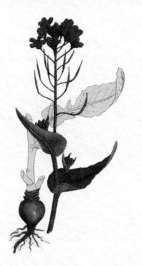

DESCRIPTION: Our common Mustard hath large and broad rough leaves, very much jagged with uneven and unorderly gashes, somewhat like turnip leaves, but less and rougher. The stalk rises to be more than a foot high [with] diverse yellow flowers one above another at the tops, after which come small rough pods [with] yellowish seed, sharp, hot, and biting upon the tongue.

PLACE: This grows with us in gardens only, and other manured places.

GOVERNMENT AND VIRTUES: It is an excellent sauce for such whose blood wants clarifying, and for weak stomachs, being an herb of Mars, but naught for choleric people, though as good for such as are aged, or troubled with cold diseases. Aries claims

something to do with it, therefore it strengthens the heart, and resists poison. Let such whose stomachs are so weak they cannot digest their meat, or appetite it, take of Mustard-seed a dram, Cinnamon as much, and having beaten them to powder, and half as much Mastic in powder, and with gum Arabic dissolved in rose-water, make it up into troches, of which they may take one of about half a dram weight an hour or two before meals; let old men and women make much of this medicine, and they will either give me thanks, or shew manifest ingratitude. Mustard seed hath the virtue of heat, discussing, ratifying, and drawing out splinters of bones, and other things of the flesh. It is of good effect to bring down women's courses, for the falling-sickness or lethargy, drowsy forgetful evil, to use it both inwardly and outwardly, to rub the nostrils, forehead and temples, to warm and quicken the spirits; for by the fierce sharpness it purges the brain by sneezing, and drawing down rheum [watery discharge] and other viscous humours, which by their distillations upon the lungs and chest, procure coughing, and therefore, with some, honey added thereto, doth much good therein. The seed taken either by itself, or with other things, either in an electuary or drink, doth mightily stir up bodily lust, and helps the spleen and pains in the sides, and gnawings in the bowels; and used as a gargle draws up the palate of the mouth, being fallen down; and also it dissolves the swellings about the throat, if it be outwardly applied. Being chewed in the mouth it oftentimes helps the toothache. The outward application hereof upon the pained place of the sciatica, eases the pains, as also gout, and other joint aches; and is much and often used to ease pains in the sides or loins, the shoulder, or other parts of the body. Upon the plying thereof to raise blisters, and cures the disease by drawing it to the outward parts of the body. It is also used to help the falling off of the hair. The seed bruised mixed with honey, and applied, or made up with wax, takes away the marks and black and blue spots of bruises, or the like, the roughness or scabbiness of the skin, as also the leprosy, and lousy evil. It helps also the crick in the neck. The distilled water of the herb, when it is in the flower, is much used to drink inwardly to help in any of the diseases aforesaid, or to wash the mouth when the palate is down, and for the disease of the throat to gargle, but outwardly also for scabs, itch, or other the like infirmities, and cleanses the face from morphew [blemishes], spots, freckles, and other deformities.

MODERN USES: Mustard seed is added to bathwater at about 1 percent by weight to stimulate circulation in arthritic hands or feet. The hot principles of mustard, known as glucosinolates, become pungent in the presence of the enzyme myrosinase. In mustards or mustard oil, these hot or pungent components can be irritating. Mustard and its preparations are used for rheumatism and arthritis, and in small quantities as an appetite and digestive stimulant. **CAUTION:** Prolonged exposure to mustard plaster or wraps can cause chemical burns and blistering.

....

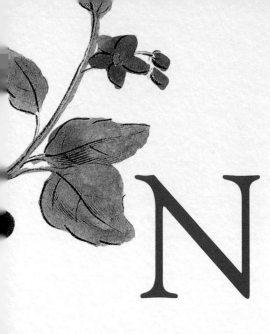

N

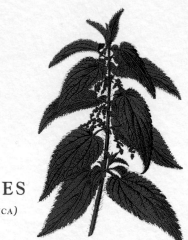

NETTLES
(URTICA DIOICA)

Nettles are so well known, that they need no description; they may be found by feeling, in the darkest night. [Native to Europe, North America, Asia, and elsewhere.]

GOVERNMENT AND VIRTUES: This is also an herb Mars claims dominion over. You know Mars is hot and dry, and you know as well that Winter is cold and moist; then you may know the reason as well why Nettle-tops eaten in the Spring consume the phlegmatic superfluities in the body of man, that the coldness and moistness of Winter hath left behind. The roots or leaves boiled, or the juice of either of them, or both made into an electuary with honey and sugar, is a safe and sure medicine to open the pipes and passages of the lungs, which is the cause of wheezing and shortness of breath, and helps to expectorate tough phlegm, as also to raise the imposthumed pleurisy; and spend it by spitting. The juice is also effectual to settle the palate of the mouth in its place, and to heal and temper the inflammations and soreness of the mouth and throat. The decoction of the leaves in wine, being drank, is singularly good to provoke women's courses. It is also applied outwardly with a little myrrh. The same also, or the seed provokes urine, and expels the gravel and stone in the kidneys or bladder, often proved to be effectual in many that have taken it. The same kills the worms in children, eases pains in the sides, and dissolves the windiness in the spleen, as also in the body, although others think it only powerful to provoke venery. The juice of the leaves taken two or three days together, stays bleeding at the mouth. The distilled water of the herb is also effectual (though not so powerful) for the diseases aforesaid; as for outward wounds and sores to wash them, and to cleanse the skin from morphew [blemishes], leprosy, and other discolourings thereof. The juice of the leaves, or the decoction of them, or of the root, is singularly good to wash either old, rotten, or stinking sores or fistulous, and gangrenes, and such as fretting, eating, or corroding scabs, manginess, and itch, in any part of the body, as also green wounds, by washing them therewith, or applying the green herb bruised thereunto, yea, although the flesh were separated from the bones. The same applied to our wearied members, refresh them, or to place those that have been out of joint, being first set up again, strengthens, dries, and comforts them, as also those places troubled with aches and gouts, and the defluxion of humours upon the joints or sinews; it eases the pains, and dries or dissolves the defluctions. An ointment made of the juice, oil, and a little wax, is singularly good to rub cold and benumbed members. A handful of the leaves of green Nettles, and another of Wallwort, or Deanwort, bruised and applied simply themselves to the gout, sciatica, or joint aches in any part, hath been found to be an admirable help thereunto.

MODERN USES: A tea of dried nettles is used as a diuretic, astringent, and blood builder to treat anemia due to its high iron content. A freeze-dried extract of nettle leaf is recommended for the treatment of allergies. Science confirms diuretic effects in patients with chronic venous insufficiency. Nettle root is used in preparations for the symptomatic relief of urinary difficulties associated with benign prostatic hyperplasia. **CAUTION:** Fresh nettle plants sting due to a combination of histamines, acetylcholine, and small amounts of formic acid in the hairs. Dried or cooked nettle does not have a stinging effect.

....

NIGHTSHADE, BLACK

(SOLANUM NIGRUM)

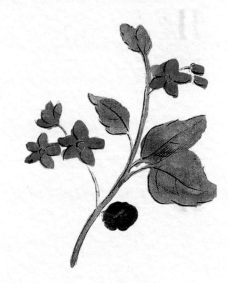

DESCRIPTION: Common Nightshade hath an upright stalk, about a foot or half a yard high, bushing forth, whereon grow many green leaves, somewhat broad, and pointed at the ends, soft and full of juice. At the tops of the stalks and branches come forth three or four more white flowers made of five small pointed [petals].

PLACE: It grows wild with us under our walls, and in rubbish, the common paths, and sides of hedges and fields, as also in our gardens, without any planting. [Native to southern Europe and western and central Asia; widely naturalized as a weed in East Asia, North America, and elsewhere.]

GOVERNMENT AND VIRTUES: It is a cold Saturnine plant. The common Nightshade is wholly used to cool hot inflammations either inwardly or outwardly, being no ways dangerous to any that use it, as most of the rest of the Nightshades are; yet it must be used moderately. The distilled water only of the whole herb is fittest and safest to be taken inwardly: The juice also clarified and taken, being mingled with a little vinegar, is good to wash the mouth and throat that is inflamed. It also doth much good for the shingles, ringworms, and in all running, fretting and corroding ulcers, applied thereunto. And Pliny saith, it is good for hot swellings under the throat. Have a care you mistake not the deadly Nightshade (*Atropa belladonna*) for this; if you know it not, you may let them both alone, and take no harm, having other medicines sufficient in the book.

MODERN USES: Little used due to toxicity. Contains solanine and other toxic alkaloids. Researched for antimicrobial, antiviral, and possible anti-cancer effects. The chemistry is highly variable, making toxicity unpredictable. **CAUTION:** All plant parts are poisonous. Do not follow Culpeper's recommendations, except for his warnings. Avoid.

....

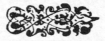

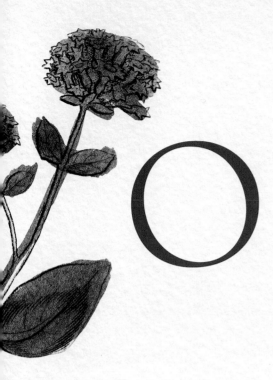

O

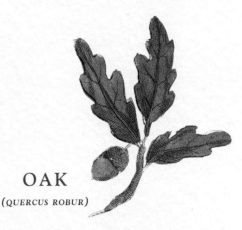

OAK
(QUERCUS ROBUR)

It is so well known (the timber thereof being the glory and safety of this nation by sea) that it needs no description. [Found throughout most of Europe; planted as a shade tree and occasionally naturalized elsewhere.]

GOVERNMENT AND VIRTUES: Jupiter owns the tree. The leaves and bark of the Oak, and the acorn cups, do bind and dry very much. The inner bark of the tree, and the thin skin that covers the acorn, are most used to stay the spitting of blood, and the bloody-flux [dysentery]. The decoction of that bark, and the powder of the cups, do stay vomiting, spitting of blood, bleeding at the mouth, or other fluxes of blood, in men or women; lasks [diarrhea] also, and the nocturnal involuntary flux of men. The acorn in powder taken in wine, provokes urine, and resists the poison of venomous creatures. The decoction of acorns and the bark made in milk and taken, resists the force of poisonous herbs and medicines. Galen applied them, being bruised, to cure green wounds. The distilled water of the Oaken bud, before they break out into leaves is good to be used either inwardly or outwardly, to assuage inflammations, and to stop all manner of fluxes in man or woman. The same is singularly good in pestilential and hot burning fevers; for it resists the force of the infection, and allays the heat: It cools the heat of the liver, breaking the stone in the kidneys, and stays women's courses. The decoction of the leaves works the same effects. The water that is found in the hollow places of old Oaks, is very effectual against any foul or spreading scabs. The distilled water (or concoction, which is better) of the leaves, is one of the best remedies that I know of for the whites [vaginal discharges] in women.

MODERN USES: During Culpeper's time, one or two oaks were recognized in England. Biological activity associated with oaks and their complex tannins includes antibacterial, antiviral, astringent, anti-inflammatory, and anticancer properties. Traditionally, the tea was used as a gargle for sore throat. Internally, a tea or decoction is used to allay diarrhea. Used as a wash for inflammatory skin diseases.

....

OATS
(AVENA SATIVA)

Are so well known that they need no description.

PLACE: [Cultivated since ancient times and thought to have originated in central Europe; sometimes found persisting in wastelands near where it may have once been cultivated.]

GOVERNMENT AND VIRTUES: Oats fried with bay salt, and applied to the sides, take away the pains of stitches and wind in the sides or the belly. A poultice made of meal of Oats, and some oil of Bays put thereunto, helps the itch and the leprosy, as also the fistulas of the fundament, and dissolves hard imposthumes [abscesses]. The meal of Oats boiled with vinegar, and applied, takes away freckles and spots in the face, and other parts of the body.

MODERN USES: Oatmeal itself is sometimes applied as a soothing poultice for inflammation. In modern phytomedicine, the primary use is that of oat straw in baths to treat inflammatory skin diseases with itching. Oat straw is also used in tea as a diuretic. The milky juice of fresh green tops of oats is considered a nerve tonic and antispasmodic for nervous disorders, exhaustion, and nervous debility.

....

ONIONS

(ALLIUM CEPA)

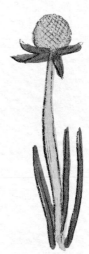

They are so well known, that I need not spend time about writing a description of them.

PLACE: [One of the oldest of cultivated vegetables, of unknown origin. Grown in home gardens.]

GOVERNMENT AND VIRTUES: Mars owns them, and they have gotten this quality, to draw any corruption to them, for if you peel one, and lay it upon a dunghill, you shall find it rotten in half a day, by drawing putrefaction to it; then, being bruised and applied to a plague sore, it is very probable it will do the like. Onions are flatulent, or windy; yet they do somewhat provoke appetite, increase thirst, ease the belly and bowels, provoke women's courses, help the biting of a mad dog, and of other venomous creatures, to be used with honey and rue, increase sperm, especially the seed of them. They also kill worms in children if they drink the water fasting wherein they have been steeped all night. Being roasted under the embers, and eaten with honey or sugar and oil, they much conduce to help an inveterate cough, and expectorate the cough phlegm. It hath been held by diverse country people a great preservative against infection, to eat Onions fasting with bread and salt: As also to make a great Onion hollow, filling the place with good treacle, and after to roast it well under the embers, which, after taking away the outermost skin thereof, being beaten together, is a sovereign salve for either plague or sore, or any other putrefied ulcer. The juice of Onions is good for either scalding or burning by fire, water, or gunpowder, and used with vinegar, takes away all blemishes, spots and marks in the skin. Applied also with figs beaten together, helps to ripen and break imposthumes [abscesses], and other sores.

Leeks are as like them in quality, as the pome-water is like an apple: They are a remedy against a surfeit of mushrooms, being baked under the embers and taken, and being boiled and applied very warm, help the piles. In other things they have the same property as the Onions, although not so effectual.

MODERN USES: Best known as a food rather than a medicinal herb, onion fits the adage that "your food should be your medicine." Onion bulbs are used for the prevention and treatment of age-dependent changes in the blood vessels (prevention of atherosclerosis), and as an appetite stimulant in cases of loss of appetite. In essence, the effects of onions are similar to those of garlic, though are considered somewhat weaker. Onions are antibacterial, blood thinning, and may help to lower blood pressure when consumed as a regular part of the diet.

....

ORCHIS

(ORCHIS SPP.)

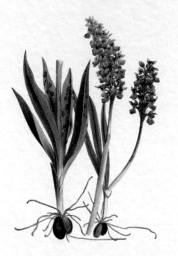

Not often used because of their rarity. All terrestrial orchids are restricted in international trade. Culpeper himself could not distinguish one from another. The most widely used medicinally was *Orchis mascula*—so named because the roots look like testicles. The roots have been shown to have antihypertensive activity. In India and Pakistan, this species has been used for sexual dysfunction, heart disease, and for the treatment of diarrhea, dysentery, and chronic inflammation. To quote William Curtis in *Flora Londinensis* (1772), "[We] readily subscribed to the opinion . . . in speaking of *Orchis* . . . that great names have introduced many absurd medicines."

....

DESCRIPTION: To describe all the several sorts of it were an endless piece of work; therefore I shall only describe the roots because they are to be used with some discretion. Now, it is that which is full which is to be used in medicines, the other being either of no use at all, or else, according to the humour of some, it destroys and disannuls the virtues of the other, quite undoing what that doth.

PLACE: [*Orchis* species are found in chalky grasslands and open woods; scattered throughout Europe and elsewhere.]

GOVERNMENT AND VIRTUES: They are hot and moist in operation, under the dominion of Dame Venus, and provoke lust exceedingly, which, they say, the dried and withered roots do restrain. They are held to kill worms in children; as also, being bruised and applied to the place, to heal the king's evil [unusual swelling of lymph nodes or scrofula].

MODERN USES: *Orchis* is a genus in the orchid family (Orchidaceae) with about three dozen species.

OREGANO

(ORIGANUM VULGARE)

Wild Marjoram, Wind Marjoram

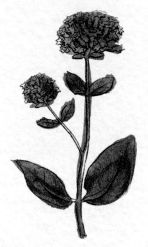

Called also Origanum, Eastward Marjoram; Wild Marjoram, and Grove Marjoram.

DESCRIPTION: Wild or field Marjoram send[s] up sundry brownish, square stalks, with small dark green leaves, very like those of Sweet Marjoram, at the top of the stalks stand tufts of flowers, of a deep purplish red colour.

PLACE: It grows plentifully in [fields throughout Europe and temperate Asia, and is naturalized in eastern North America].

GOVERNMENT AND VIRTUES: This is also under the dominion of Mercury. It strengthens the stomach and head much, there being scarce a better remedy growing for such as are troubled with a sour humour in the stomach; it restores the appetite being lost; helps the cough, and consumption of the lungs; it cleanses the body of choler [bile], expels poison, and remedies the infirmities of the spleen; helps the bitings of venomous beasts, and helps such as have poisoned themselves by eating Hemlock, Henbane, or Opium. It provokes urine and the terms in women, helps the dropsy, and the scurvy, scabs, itch, and yellow jaundice. The juice being dropped into the ears, helps deafness, pain and noise in the ears. And thus much for this herb, between which and adders, there is a deadly antipathy.

MODERN USES: Found wild throughout Europe, oregano has long been used as a folk medicine for indigestion, headaches, diarrhea, nervous tension, insect bites, toothache, earache, rheumatism, and coughs. Oregano has antitussive, carminative, diaphoretic, diuretic, and mild nervine properties. Oregano treats irritating coughs due to bronchitis (primarily due to its antispasmodic activity), urinary tract conditions, and painful menstruation. The essential oil contains carvacrol and thymol as the primary components and has confirmed antibacterial, antiviral, antispasmodic, and anti-inflammatory activity. **CAUTION:** All undiluted essential oils can be irritating.

....

ORPINE

(SEDUM TELEPHIUM; SYN. HELOTELEPHIUM TELEPHIUM)

Witch's Moneybags

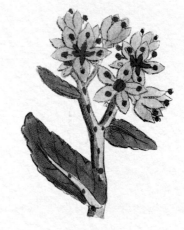

DESCRIPTION: Common Orpine rises up with diverse rough brittle stalks, thick set with fat and fleshy leaves, [with pinkish-white tufts of flowers].

PLACE: [Found throughout Europe and Asia; naturalized as a garden plant in the British Isles.]

GOVERNMENT AND VIRTUES: The Moon owns the herb, and he that knows but her exaltation, knows what I say is true. Orpine is seldom used in inward medicines with us, although Tragus saith from experience in Germany, that the distilled water thereof is profitable for gnawings or excoriations in the stomach or bowels, or for ulcers in the lungs, liver, or other inward parts, as also in the matrix, and helps all those diseases, being drank for certain days together. It stays the sharpness of humours in the bloody-flux [dysentery], and other fluxes in the body, or in wounds. The root thereof also performs the like effect. It is used outwardly to cool any heat or inflammation upon any hurt or wound, and eases the pains of them; as, also, to heal scaldings or burnings, the juice thereof being beaten with some green salad oil, and anointed. The leaf bruised, and laid to any green wound in the hand or legs, doth heal them quickly; and being bound to the throat, much helps the quinsy [peritonsillar abscess]; it helps also ruptures. If you please to make the juice thereof into a syrup with honey or sugar, you may safely take a spoonful or two at a time, (let my author say what he will) for a quinsy, and you shall find the medicine pleasant, and the cure speedy.

MODERN USES: Seldom used, orpine is an astringent. The tea is used as a folk medicine for the treatment of diarrhea. Like most fleshy-leaved sedums, the crushed leaves are considered cooling, anti-inflammatory, antioxidant, and were applied to wounds. Components of the plant may serve to simulate the immune system to enhance wound-healing.

....

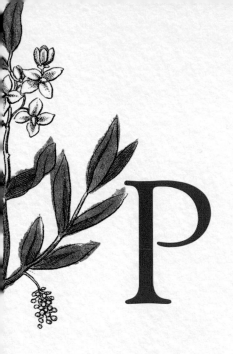

P

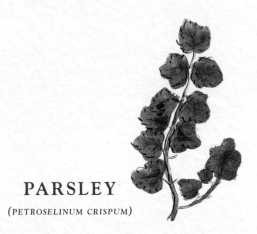

PARSLEY
(PETROSELINUM CRISPUM)

This is so well known, that it needs no description.

PLACE: [Originates in gravelly soils, near water seepage in southern Europe from Spain to Turkey. Cultivated in northern European monastary herb gardens during the Middle Ages. Introduced to English gardens in 1548 and commonly known in England by the 1640s.]

GOVERNMENT AND VIRTUES: It is under the dominion of Mercury; is very comfortable to the stomach; helps to provoke urine and women's courses, to break wind both in the stomach and bowels, and doth a little open the body, but the root much more. It opens obstructions both of liver and spleen, and is therefore accounted one of the five opening roots. Galen commended it against the falling sickness, and to provoke urine mightily; especially if the roots be boiled, and eaten like Parsnips. The seed is effectual to provoke urine and women's courses, to expel wind, to break the stone, and ease the pains and torments thereof. It is also effectual against the venom of any poisonous creature, and the danger that comes to them that have the lethargy, and is as good against the cough. The distilled water of Parsley is a familiar medicine with nurses to give their children when they are troubled with wind in the stomach or belly which they call the frets; and is also much available to them that are of great years. The leaves of Parsley laid to the eyes that are inflamed with heat, or swollen, doth much help them. If it be used with bread or meal; and being fried with butter, and applied to women's breasts that are hard through the curdling of their milk, it abates the hardness quickly; and also takes away black and blue marks coming of bruises or falls.

MODERN USES: Fresh parsley leaves are a well-known garnish for food, often included as a breath freshener at the end of a meal. The whole fresh herb or a tea of the dried herb is traditionally used as a diuretic and treatment for kidney stones or other urinary tract calculi. The root is considered a mild diuretic for flushing the urinary tract. Parsley is also used as a carminative for dyspepsia and an anti-inflammatory for urinary complaints. **CAUTION:** The seeds can be irritating to mucus membranes. Some individuals may have rare allergic reactions to parsley.

....

PARSNIPS
(*PASTINACA SATIVA*)

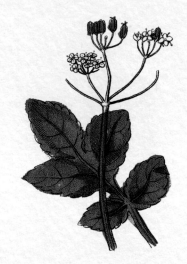

The garden kind thereof is so well known (the root being commonly eaten) that I shall not trouble you with any description of it. But the wild kind [is] of more physical use . . . and the root is shorter, woodier, and not so fit to be eaten, and therefore more medicinal.

PLACE: Wild parsnip grows in fields, and waste places. [Native to much of western Europe; naturalized in Scandinavia, Eastern Europe, North America, and temperate South America and South Africa.]

GOVERNMENT AND VIRTUES: The garden Parsnips are under Venus. The garden Parsnip nourishes much, and is good and wholesome nourishment, but a little windy, whereby it is thought to procure bodily lust; but it fastens the body much, if much need. It is conducive to the stomach and kidneys, and provokes urine. But the wild Parsnips hath a cutting, attenuating, cleansing, and opening quality therein. It resists and helps the bitings of serpents, eases the pains and stitches in the sides, and dissolves wind both in the stomach and bowels, which is the cholic, and provokes urine. The root is often used, but the seed much more. The wild being better than the tame, shews Dame Nature to be the best physician.

MODERN USES: The edible root of the garden parsnip is found at most supermarkets. It is considered sweet, aromatic, and diuretic; rather than treating flatulence, it may induce it. The root of the wild parsnip (even though it is the same plant species) is considered acrid and may induce vomiting. **CAUTION**: Wild parsnip is high in phototoxic compounds known as furanocoumarins. Ingesting or handling the plant can cause photodermatitis or contact dermatitis.

....

PEACH TREE

(PRUNUS PERSICA)

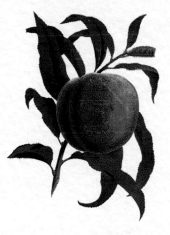

PLACE: [Peach trees have been cultivated since ancient times. The first known cultivated peaches date from China over eight thousand years ago.]

GOVERNMENT AND VIRTUES: Lady Venus owns this tree, and by it opposes the ill effects of Mars, and indeed for children and young people, nothing is better to purge choler [bile] and the jaundice, than the leaves or flowers of this tree being made into a syrup or conserve. Let such as delight to please their lust regard the fruit; but such as have lost their health, and their children's, let them regard what I say, they may safely give two spoonfuls of the syrup at a time; it is as gentle as Venus herself. The leaves bruised and laid on the belly, kill worms. The powder of them strewed upon fresh bleeding wounds stays their bleeding, and closes them up. The flowers steeped all night in a little wine standing warm, strained forth in the morning, and drank fasting, doth gently open the belly, and move it downward. The flowers made into a conserve, work the same effect. The liquor that dropped from the tree, being wounded, is given in the decoction of Coltsfoot, to those that are troubled with a cough or shortness of breath, by adding thereunto some sweet wine, and putting some saffron also therein. It is good for those that are hoarse, or have lost their voice; helps all defects of the lungs, and those that vomit and spit blood. The milk or cream of these kernels being drawn forth with some Vervain water and applied to the forehead and temples, doth much help to procure rest and sleep to sick persons wanting it. The oil drawn from the kernels, the temples being therewith anointed, doth the like. Being also anointed on the forehead and temples, it helps the migraine, and all other pains in the head. If the kernels be bruised and boiled in vinegar, until they become thick, and applied to the head, it marvelously procures the hair to grow again upon bald places, or where it is too thin.

MODERN USES: Peach pits and, more commonly, apricot pits, are famously the source of amygdalin and its analog, laetrile, developed in the 1920s and used controversially as an alternative cancer treatment. The flowers are a diuretic and used in traditional Chinese medicine as a purgative, increasing gastrointestinal motility; used also in cosmetics as an antioxidant to protect against skin damage. The leaves are considered to be demulcent, mildly sedative, diuretic, and expectorant, used as a folk medicine as Culpeper describes. Leaf extracts have been shown to have antidiabetic potential. However, most are content simply to eat the delicious fruit, which is high in antioxidant compounds and dietary fiber. **CAUTION:** The amygdalin in peach pits breaks down to hydrocyanic acid, which has the potential for cyanide-like toxicity.

....

PEAR TREE
(PYRUS COMMUNIS)

Pear Trees are so well known, that they need no description.

PLACE: [Pears are known to have occurred from Iran to the western coast of temperate Europe since prehistoric periods, and they have been cultivated since ancient times. Domestication occurred many centuries ago from China to the Middle East.]

GOVERNMENT AND VIRTUES: The Tree belongs to Venus, and so doth the Apple tree. For their physical use they are best discerned by their taste. All the sweet and luscious sorts, whether manured or wild, do help to move the belly downwards, more or less. Those that are hard and sour, do, on the contrary, bind the belly as much, and the leaves do so also: Those that are moist do in some sort cool, but harsh or wild sorts much more, and are very good in repelling medicines; and if the wild sort be boiled with mushrooms, it makes them less dangerous. The said Pears boiled with a little honey, help much the oppressed stomach, as all sorts of them do, some more, some less: but the harsher sorts do cooler and bind, serving well to be bound to green wounds, to cool and stay the blood, and heal up the green wound without farther trouble, or inflammation, as Galen saith he hath found by experience. The wild Pears do sooner close up the lips of green wounds than others.

Schola Selerni advises to drink much wine after Pears, or else (say they) they are as bad as poison; nay, and they curse the tree for it too; but if a poor man find his stomach oppressed by eating Pears, it is but working hard, and it will do as well as drinking wine.

MODERN USES: Pears are enjoyed as a fruit. Aside from their food value, they are little used medicinally, though pear syrup has been used as a component in cough syrup.

....

PELLITORY-
OF-THE-WALL

(*PARIETARIA OFFICINALIS*)

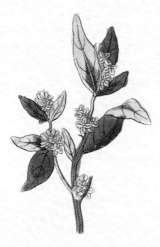

DESCRIPTION: It rises with brownish, red, tender, weak, clear, and almost transparent stalks, about two feet high, at the joints with the leaves from the middle of the stalk upwards, stand many small, pale, purplish flowers in hairy, rough husks.

PLACE: It grows wild, about the borders of fields, and by the sides of walls, and in waste places. [Native to much of western Europe and a weed in Great Britain; sometimes naturalized in North America and South America.]

GOVERNMENT AND VIRTUES: It is under the dominion of Mercury. The dried herb Pellitory made up into an electuary with honey, or the juices of the herb, or the decoction thereof made up with sugar or honey, is a singular remedy for an old or dry cough, the shortness of breath, and wheezing in the throat. Three ounces of the juice thereof taken at a time, doth wonderfully help stopping of the urine, and to expel the stone or gravel in the kidneys or bladder, and is therefore usually put among other herbs used in clysters to miti-

gate pains in the back, sides, or bowels, proceeding of wind, stopping of urine, the gravel or stone, as aforesaid. If the bruised herb, sprinkled with some Muskadel, be warmed upon a tile, or in a dish upon a few quick coals in a chafing-dish, and applied to the belly, it works the same effect. The decoction of the herb being drank, eases pains of the mother, and brings down women's courses: It also eases those griefs that arise from obstructions of the liver, spleen, and kidneys. The same decoction, with a little honey added thereto, is good to gargle a sore throat. The juice held a while in the mouth, eases pains in the teeth. The distilled water of the herb drank with some sugar, works the same effects, and cleanses the skin from spots, freckles, purples, wheals, sun-burn, morphew [blemishes], etc. The juice, or the distilled water, assuages hot and swelling imposthumes [abscesses], burnings and scaldings by fire or water; as also all other hot tumours and inflammations, or breakings-out, of heat, being bathed often with wet cloths dipped therein: The said juice made into a liniment with ceruss, and oil of roses, and anointed therewith, cleanses foul rotten ulcers, and stays spreading or creeping ulcers, and running scabs or sores in children's heads; and helps to stay the hair from falling off the head. The said ointment, or the herb opens the piles, and eases their pains; and being mixed with goats' tallow, helps the gout. The juice is very effectual to cleanse fistulas, and to heal them up safely; or the herb itself bruised and applied with a little salt. It is likewise also effectual to heal any green wound; if it be bruised and bound thereto for three days, you shall need no other medicine to heal it further. A poultice made hereof with Mallows, and boiled in wine and wheat bran and bean flour, and some oil put thereto, and applied warm to any bruised sinews, tendon, or muscle, doth in a very short time restore them to their strength, taking away the pains of the bruises, and dissolves the congealed blood coming of blows, or falls from high places.

The juice of Pellitory of the Wall clarified and boiled in a syrup with honey, and a spoonful of it drank every morning by such as are subject to the dropsy; if continuing that course, though but once a week, they ever have the dropsy, let them but come to me, and I will cure them *gratis*.

MODERN USES: Traditionally used as a diuretic and for coughs and cold, though seldom used today. Most of the modern scientific literature on pellitory-of-the-wall relates to the treatment of allergies and hay fever induced by the plant. **CAUTION:** A major hay allergy pollen source.

....

PENNYROYAL

(*MENTHA PULEGIUM*)

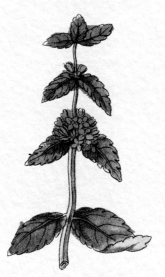

Pennyroyal is so well known unto all, I mean the common kind, that it needs no description.

PLACE: Common in gardens, grows in many moist places [in Europe. Naturalized in South America; escaped from cultivation in some locations in North America.]

GOVERNMENT AND VIRTUES: The herb is under Venus. Being boiled and drank, it and stays the disposition to vomit, being taken in water and vinegar mingled together. And being mingled with honey and salt, it voids phlegm out of the lungs, and purges melancholy by the stool. Drank with wine, it helps such as are bitten and stung with venomous beasts, and applied to the nostrils with vinegar, revives those that are fainting and swooning. Being dried and burnt, it strengthens the gums. It is helpful to those that are troubled with the gout, being applied of itself to the place until it was red; and applied in a plaster, it takes away spots or marks in the face; applied with salt, it profits those that are splenetic, or livergrown. The decoction doth help the itch, if washed therewith. The green herb bruised and put into vinegar, cleanses foul ulcers, and takes away the marks of bruises and blows about the eyes, and all discolourings of the face by fire, yea, and the leprosy, being drank and outwardly applied: Boiled in wine with honey and salt, it helps the toothache. It helps the cold griefs by the joints, taking away the pains, and warms the cold part, being fast bound to the place, after a bathing or sweating in a hot house.

MODERN USES: Aside from topical use to deter insects, pennyroyal is little used today except as a light tea to treat dyspepsia. Traditionally a menstruation-regulating herb, in classical antiquity it was employed by women of all social classes as an anti-fertility agent. Science confirms antimicrobial, insecticidal, and antioxidant activity. **CAUTION:** Ingestion of pennyroyal essential oil as an abortifacient has resulted in fatalities. Avoid.

....

PEONY

(PAEONIA OFFICINALIS AND PAEONIA LACTIFLORA)

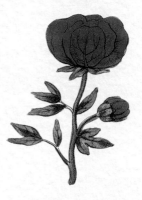

PAEONIA MAS

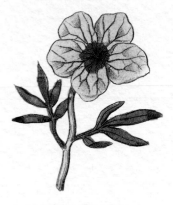

PAEONIA FEMINA

[In the West, the term *peony* almost always refers to one of the thousands of cultivated varieties of the Asia peony (*Paeonia lactiflora*) grown in China for at least three thousand years. These peonies have been grown in European horticulture since the 1550s, predating Culpeper's *English Physician* by a century. As many as eleven *Paeonia* species occur in Europe and twenty in the Mediterranean region, including *Paeonia officinalis*, once called *Paeonia femina* (the female peony of Culpeper), and *Paeonia mas* (the male peony of Culpeper), both of which are selected from the same highly variable species.]

PLACE: They grow in gardens. [Native to the Swiss mountains, southern Europe, and western Asia; cultivated in England since the early 1500s.]

GOVERNMENT AND VIRTUES: It is an herb of the Sun, and under the Lion. Physicians say, Male Peony roots are best; but Dr. Reason told me Male Peony was best for men, and Female Peony for women, and he desires to be judged by his brother Dr. Experience. The roots are held to be of more virtue than the seed; next the flowers; and, last of all, the leaves. The roots of the Male Peony, fresh gathered, having been found by experience to cure the falling sickness; but the surest way is, besides hanging it about the neck, by which children have been cured, to take the root of the Male Peony washed clean, and stamped somewhat small, and laid to infuse in sack for 24 hours at the least, afterwards strain it, and take it first and last, morning and evening, a good draught for sundry days together, before and after a full moon: and this will also cure old persons, if the disease be not grown too old, and past cure, especially if there be a due and orderly preparation of the body with posset-drink made of Betony, &c. The root is also effectual for women that are not sufficiently cleansed after child-birth, and such as are troubled with the mother; for which likewise the black seed beaten to powder, and given in wine, is also available. The black seed also taken before bed-time, and in the morning, is very effectual for such as in their sleep are troubled with the disease called Ephialtes, or Incubus, but we do commonly call it the Night-mare: a disease which melancholy persons are subject unto: It is also good against melancholy dreams. The distilled water or syrup made of the flowers, works the same effects that the root and seed do, although more weakly. The Female's is often used for the purpose aforesaid, by reason the Male is so scarce a plant, that it is possessed by few, and those great lovers of rarities in this kind.

MODERN USES: The root of Chinese peony and European peony are traditionally used similarly. Chinese peony is used in prescriptions for hypertensive headache, blood deficiencies, abdominal pains due to diarrhea or dysentery, appendicitis pain, abnormal or painful menstruation, fevers, and night sweats, among other uses. It is an official drug in pharmacies in the modern Chinese pharmacopeia. Experimentally, it lowers blood pressure and is anticonvulsive, anti-inflammatory, antispasmodic, an emmenagogue, and an expectorant. Usually a practitioner-prescribed herbal drug.

....

PEPPERWORTS, DITTANDER, AND GARDEN CRESS

(*LEPIDIUM LATIFOLIA* AND *LEPIDIUM SATIVUM*)

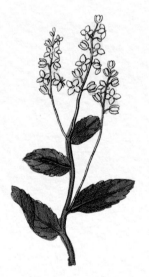

DESCRIPTION: Our common Pepperwort sends forth somewhat long and broad leaves, standing upon round hard stalks, three or four feet high, having many small white flowers at the tops of them. [Pepperwort grows in fields and wastelands; found throughout Europe and central Asia; naturalized elsewhere. *Lepidium sativum*, also known as garden cress, has a broader range, extending through most of Europe, northern Asia, India, and North Africa.]

GOVERNMENT AND VIRTUES: Here is another martial herb for you, make much of it. Pliny and Paulus Ægineta say, that Pepperwort is very successful for the sciatica, or any other gout or pain in the joints, or any other inveterate grief. The leaves hereof to be bruised, and mixed with old hog's grease, and applied to the place, and to continue thereon four hours in men, and two hours in women, the place being afterwards bathed with wine and oil mixed together, and then wrapped up with wool or skins, after they have sweat a little. It also amends the deformities or discolourings of the skin, and helps to take away marks, scars, and scabs, or the foul marks of burning with fire or iron. The juice hereof is by some used to be given in ale to drink, to women with child, to procure them a speedy delivery in travail.

MODERN USES: As mustard family members, pepperwort, dittander, and garden cress have peppery leaves and roots like those of many other *Lepidium* species. The leaves and seedpods are used in small amounts as a wild food flavoring. Garden cress seeds have been used as a folk medicine to mend broken bones and relieve joint pains. It is the most widely used *Lepidium* species worldwide, particularly in India, where it is used as a diuretic and appetite stimulant. Antidiabetic, antioxidant, antiasthmatic, antispasmodic, liver-protective, and anti-inflammatory activity are associated with garden cress and pepperwort.

....

PERIWINKLE

(VINCA MAJOR, VINCA MINOR)

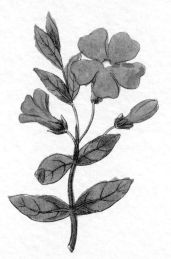

DESCRIPTION: The common sort hereof hath many branches trailing or running upon the ground. At the joints of these branches stand two small, dark-green, shining [evergreen] leaves with [blue-violet flowers].

PLACE: [Both greater periwinkle (*Vinca major*) and lesser periwinkle (*Vina minor*) were introduced into England in ancient times. They occur throughout Europe and are naturalized and weedy in North America and elsewhere.]

GOVERNMENT AND VIRTUES: Venus owns this herb, and saith, that the leaves eaten by man and wife together, cause love between them. The Periwinkle is a great binder, stays bleeding both at mouth and nose, if some of the leaves be chewed. The French used it to stay women's courses. Dioscorides, Galen, and Ægineta, commend it against the lasks and fluxes of the belly to be drank in wine.

MODERN USES: Seldom used, the leaves of greater and lesser periwinkle are astringent and were used to stop bleeding. Not to be confused with the tropical plant Madagascar periwinkle (*Catharanthus roseus*; syn. *Vinca rosea*), source of the toxic alkaloids vincristine and vinblastine and their analogs, which are widely used in chemotherapy, particularly for the treatment of childhood leukemias and Hodgkin's disease.

....

PLANTAIN

(PLANTAGO LANCEOLATA AND PLANTAGO MAJOR)

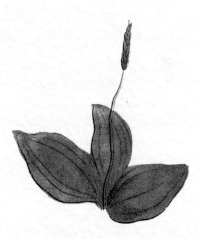

This grows usually in meadows and fields, and by path sides, and is so well known, that it needs no description.

PLACE: [Both English or lanceleaf plantain (*Plantago lanceolata*) and common or broad-leaved plantain (*Plantago major*) are ubiquitous weeds found in lawns, roadsides, fields, sidewalk cracks, and wastelands wherever Europeans have settled. In many places, both are considered noxious weeds.]

GOVERNMENT AND VIRTUES: It is true, Misaldus and others, yea, almost all astrology-physicians, hold this to be an herb of Mars, because it cures the diseases of the head and private parts, which are under the houses of Mars, Aries, and Scorpio: The truth is, it is under the command of Venus, and cures the head by antipathy to Mars, and the privities by sympathy to Venus; neither is there hardly a martial disease, but it cures.

The juice of Plantain clarified and drank for diverse days together, either of itself, or in other drink, prevails wonderfully against all torments or excoriations in the intestines or bowels, helps the distillations of rheum [watery discharge] from the head, and stays all manner of fluxes, even women's courses, when they flow too abundantly. It is good to stay spitting of blood and other bleedings at the mouth, or the making of foul and bloody water, by reason of any ulcer in the kidneys or bladder, and also stays the too free bleeding of wounds. It is held an especial remedy for those that are troubled with the phthisic [tuberculosis], or consumption of the lungs, or ulcers of the lungs, or coughs that come of heat. The herb (but especially the seed) is held to be profitable against the dropsy, the falling-sickness, the yellow jaundice, and stoppings of the liver and kidneys. The roots of Plantain, and Pellitory of Spain, beaten into powder, and put into the hollow teeth, takes away the pains of them. The clarified juice, or distilled water, dropped into the eyes, cools the inflammations in them, and takes away the pin and web; and dropped into the ears, eases the pains in them, and heals and removes the heat. The same also with the juice of Houseleek is profitable against all inflammations and breakings out of the skin, and against burnings and scaldings by fire and water. The juice or decoction made either of itself, or other things of the like nature, is of much use and good effect for old and hollow ulcers that are hard to be cured, and for cankers and sores in the mouth or private parts of man or woman; and helps also the pains of the piles.

The juice mixed with oil of roses, and the temples and forehead anointed therewith, eases the pains of the head proceeding from heat, and helps lunatic and frantic persons very much; as also the biting of serpents, or a mad dog. The same also is profitably applied to all hot gouts in the feet or hands, especially in the beginning. It is also good to be applied where any bone is out of joint, to hinder inflammations, swellings, and pains that presently rise thereupon. The powder of the dried leaves taken in drink, kills worms of the belly. One part of Plantain water, and two parts of the brine of powdered beef, boiled together and clarified, is a most sure remedy to heal all spreading scabs or itch in the head and body, all manner of tetters, ringworms, the shingles, and all other running and fretting sores. Briefly, the Plantains are singularly good wound herbs, to heal fresh or old wounds or sores, either inward or outward.

MODERN USES: Broad-leaved common plantain (*Plantago major*) and English or lanceleaf plantain (*Plantago lanceolata*) are among the most widely used herbs in folk medicine worldwide. Numerous studies have shown wound-healing, mild antibiotic, and anti-inflammatory activity. Preparations are used for astringent and soothing action for inflamed mucous membranes of the upper respiratory tract. The fresh or dried leaves are used externally for wounds, insect bites, and stings. The seed and seed husks of various *Plantago* species are the source of the psyllium seed, used as a fiber laxative.

....

PLUMS

(PRUNUS DOMESTICA)

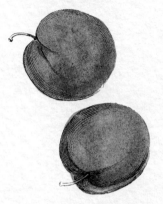

Are so well known that they need no description.

PLACE: [Originated in southwest Asia and the Caucasus; domesticated centuries ago. Naturalized in hedgerows, open woods, and wastelands throughout England and much of Europe, central Asia, and eastern and western North America.]

GOVERNMENT AND VIRTUES: All Plums are under Venus, and are like women, some better, and some worse. As there is great diversity of kinds, so there is in the operation of Plums, for some that are sweet moisten the stomach, and make the belly soluble; those that are sour quench thirst more, and bind the belly; the moist and waterish do sooner corrupt in the stomach, but the firm do nourish more, and offend less. The dried fruit sold by the grocers under the names of Damask Prunes, do somewhat loosen the belly, and being stewed, are often used, both in health and sickness, to relish the mouth and stomach, to procure appetite, and a little to open the body, allay choler [bile], and cool the stomach. Plum-tree leaves boiled in wine, are good to wash and gargle the mouth and throat, to dry the flux of rheum [watery discharge] coming to the palate [or] gums. The gum of the tree is good to break the stone. The gum or leaves boiled in vinegar, and applied, kills tetters and ringworms.

MODERN USES: Dried plums (prunes) and prune juice are well known as laxatives. Though not scientifically proven, such effects are easily observed by anyone who drinks a quantity of prune juice. Prune juice, rich in dietary fiber, is used to help restore normal bowel function in cases of constipation.

....

POLYPODY OF THE OAK

(POLYPODIUM VULGARE)

DESCRIPTION: [A small evergreen fern that often grows on the horizontal branches of oak trees.] The root is smaller than one's little finger, brownish on the outside and greenish within, of a sweetish harshness in taste, having also much mossiness or yellow hairiness upon it.

PLACE: It grows [also] on old rotten stumps, or trunks of trees, as oak, beech, hazel, willow, or others. [Found in northern Europe and Asia.]

GOVERNMENT AND VIRTUES: Polypodium of the Oak, that which grows upon the earth is best; it is an herb of Saturn, to purge melancholy; if the humour be otherwise, choose your Polypodium accordingly. Meuse (who is called the Physician's Evangelist for the certainty of his medicines, and the truth of his opinion) saith, that it dries up thin humours, digests thick and tough, and purges burnt choler [bile], and especially tough and thick phlegm, and thin phlegm also, even from the joints, and therefore good for those that are troubled with melancholy, or quartan agues [intermittent fevers such as malaria], especially if it be taken in whey or honied water, or in barley-water, or the broth of a chicken with Dodder, or with Beets and Mallows. It is good for the hardness of the spleen, and for pricking or stitches in the sides, as also for the cholic: Some use to put to it some Fennel seeds, or Anise seeds, or Ginger, to correct that loathing it brings to the stomach, which is more than needs, it being a safe and gentle medicine, fit for all persons, which daily experience confirms; and an ounce of it may be given at a time in a decoction, if there be not Senna, or some other strong purge put with it. A dram or two of the powder of the dried roots, taken fasting in a cup of honied water, works gently, and for the purposes aforesaid. The distilled water both of roots and leaves, is much commended for the quartan ague, to be taken for many days together, as also against melancholy, or fearful and troublesome sleeps or dreams; and with some sugar-candy dissolved therein, is good against the cough, shortness of breath, and wheezing, and those distillations of thin rheum [watery discharge] upon the lungs, which cause phthisis, and oftentimes consumptions. The fresh roots beaten small, or the powder of the dried roots mixed with honey, and applied to the member that is out of joint, doth much help it; and applied also to the nose, cures the disease called Polypus, which is a piece of flesh growing therein, which in time stops the passage of breath through that nostril; and it helps those clefts or chops that come between the fingers or toes.

MODERN USES: Traditionally used for upper respiratory tract infections and for relieving cough. The root (rhizome) of polypody of the oak has a bittersweet flavor and is considered laxative. A compound called osladin, which is up to five hundred times sweeter than sugar, was identified in the root. The root also contains steroid-like compounds that probably protect it from insects. Seldom used and not found in commercial trade. **CAUTION:** Extracts of the plant are known to interact with prescription drugs (increasing their effective dose), leading to potentially toxic effects.

....

POPLAR TREE

(POPULUS SPP.)

Black Poplar, White Poplar

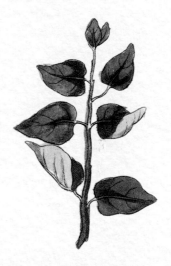

There are two sorts of Poplars, which are most familiar with us, *viz.* the Black [*Populus nigra*] and White [*Populus alba*], both which I shall here describe unto you.

DESCRIPTION: The White Poplar [is] reasonably high, covered with thick, smooth, white bark, especially the branches. The Black Poplar grows higher and straighter than the White, with a greyish bark, bearing broad green leaves, somewhat like ivy leaves, not cut in on the edges like the White, but whole and dented, ending in a point, and not white underneath, hanging by slender long foot stalks, which with the air are continually shaken, like as the Aspen leaves are. On both these trees [especially on leaf hairs, a deterrent to beetles] grows a sweet kind of musk, which in former times was used to put into sweet ointments.

PLACE: [White poplar was introduced into England in ancient times and occurs throughout most of Europe, East Asia, North Africa, eastern North America, and temperate South America. Black poplar has a similar range, though occurs less frequently.] They grow in moist woods, and by water-sides in sundry places of this land; yet the White is not so frequent as the other.

GOVERNMENT AND VIRTUES: Saturn hath dominion over both. White Poplar, saith Galen, is of a cleansing property: the weight of an ounce in powder, of the bark thereof, being drank, saith Dioscorides, is a remedy for those that are troubled with the sciatica, or the strangury. The juice of the leaves dropped warm into the ears, eases the pains in them. The young clammy buds or eyes, before they break out into leaves, bruised, and a little honey put to them, is a good medicine for a dull sight. The Black Poplar is held to be more cooling than the White, and therefore the leaves bruised with vinegar and applied, help the gout. The seed drank in vinegar, is held good against the falling-sickness. The water that drops from the hollow places of this tree, takes away warts, pushes, wheals, and other the like breakings-out

of the body. The young Black Poplar buds, saith Matthiolus, are much used by women to beautify their hair, bruising them with fresh butter, straining them after they have been kept for some time in the sun. The ointment called Populneon, which is made of this Poplar, is singularly good for all heat and inflammations in any part of the body, and tempers the heat of wounds. It is much used to dry up the milk of women's breasts when they have weaned their children.

MODERN USES: The unopened leaf buds of various poplars (especially Black Poplar) are sticky with resin, and the barks and buds contain components such as populin and salicin (the precursor to aspirin). They are used as an expectorant, antiseptic, and anti-inflammatory for acute or chronic upper respiratory tract infections, as well as a gargle to treat laryngitis. Used topically (especially in ointments) for treating skin ailments such as cuts and superficial wounds, hemorrhoids, frostbite, and sunburn. Studies have shown moderate antioxidant, anti-inflammatory, and liver-protective effects.

....

POPPIES

(PAPAVER SOMNIFERUM, PAPAVER HYBRIDUM,
AND PAPAVER RHOEAS)

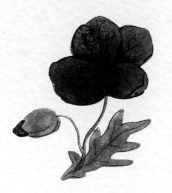

Of this I shall describe three kinds, *viz.* the White and Black of the Garden, and the erratic Wild Poppy.

DESCRIPTION: The White Poppy [opium poppy (*Papaver somniferum*)], hath at first four or five whitish green leaves lying upon the ground, which rise with the stalk. The flowers [have] four very large, white, [pink, red, or purple] round [petals], with many whitish round threads in the middle, set about a round, green head, having a crown, or star-like cover, which growing ripe, contains a great number of small round seeds. The whole plant, leaves, stalks, and heads, while they are fresh, young, and green, yield a milk when they are broken, of an unpleasant bitter taste, of a strong heady smell, which being condensed, is called Opium.

The Black Poppy [*Papaver hybridum*] little differs from the former, until it bears its flower, which is somewhat less, and of a black purplish colour, but without any purple spots in the bottom of the leaf. The head of the seed is much less than the former.

The wild Poppy, or Corn Rose [*Papaver rhoeas*], hath long and narrow leaves, very much cut in on the edges into many divisions, of a light green colour, sometimes hairy. The stalk is blackish and hairy also, but not so tall as the garden kind. The flower is of a fair yellowish red or crimson colour. A small green head, which when it is ripe, is not bigger than one's little finger's end, wherein is contained much black seeds smaller than that of the garden.

PLACE: The garden kinds do not naturally grow wild in any place, but all are sown in gardens where they grow.

The Wild Poppy or Corn Rose, is plentifully enough, and many times too much so in the corn fields [considered weedy in much of Europe].

GOVERNMENT AND VIRTUES: The herb is Lunar, and of the juice of it is made opium; only for lucre of money they cheat you, and tell you it is a kind of tear, or some such like thing, that drops from Poppies when they weep, and that is somewhere beyond the seas, I know not where beyond the Moon. The garden Poppy heads with seeds made into a syrup, is frequently, and to good effect used to procure rest, and sleep, in the sick and weak, and to stay catarrhs and defluxions [watery discharge] of thin rheums from the head into the stomach and lungs, causing a continual cough, the fore-runner of a consumption; it helps also hoarseness of the throat, and when one have lost their voice, which the oil of the seed doth likewise. The black seed boiled in wine, and drank, is said also to dry the flux of the belly, and women's courses. The empty shells, or poppy heads, are usually boiled in water, and given to procure rest and sleep. So doth the leaves in the same manner; as also if the head and temples be bathed with the decoction warm, or with the oil of Poppies, the green leaves or the heads bruised and applied with a little vinegar, or made into a poultice with barley-meal or hog's grease, cools and tempers all inflammations, as also the disease called St. Anthony's fire. It is generally used in treacle and mithridate, and in all other medicines that are made to procure rest and sleep, and to ease pains in the head as well as in other parts. It is also used to cool inflammations, agues, or frenzies, or to stay defluxions which cause a cough, or consumptions, and also other fluxes of the belly or women's courses; it is also put into hollow teeth, to ease the pain, and hath been found by experience to ease the pains of the gout.

The Wild Poppy, or Corn Rose (as Matthiolus saith) is good to prevent the falling-sickness. The syrup made with the flower, is with good effect given to those that have the pleurisy; and the dried flowers also, either boiled in water, or made into powder and drank, either in the distilled water of them, or some other drink, works the like effect. The distilled water of the flowers is held to be of much good use against surfeits, being drank evening and morning; It is also more cooling than any of the other Poppies, and therefore cannot but be as effectual in hot agues, frenzies, and other inflammations either inward or outward. Galen saith, the seed is dangerous to be used inwardly.

MODERN USES: Used since ancient times as a famous pain-killer and sedative, the white latex in poppy capsules contains more than two dozen alkaloids, including morphine and codeine, associated with pain relief. Today, semisynthetic and synthetic forms have largely replaced morphine and codeine extracted from the plant, and are used in virtually every hospital. Heroin is a purified form of the alkaloid morphine and is widely abused. **CAUTION:** Crude opium, morphine, and heroin are among the dangerous addictive drugs from opium poppies and are responsible for destroying countless lives. They are controlled narcotics worldwide.

....

PRIVET
(LIGUSTRUM VULGARE)

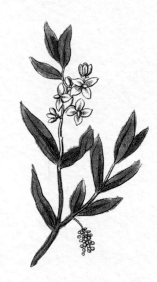

DESCRIPTION: Our common Privet is carried up with many slender branches to cover arbors, bowers and banqueting houses, and brought, wrought, and cut into so many forms, of men, horses, birds, etc. which though at first supported, grows afterwards strong of itself. It bears long and narrow green leaves by the couples, and sweet-smelling white flowers in tufts at the end of the branches, which turn into small black berries.

PLACE: [It grows throughout Europe; naturalized in North America.]

GOVERNMENT AND VIRTUES: The Moon is lady of this. It is little used in physic with us in these times, more than in lotions, to wash sores and sore mouths, and to cool inflammations, and dry up fluxes. Yet Matthiolus saith, it serves all the uses for which Cypress, or the East Privet, is appointed by Dioscorides and Galen. He further saith, that the oil that is made of the flowers of Privet infused therein, and set in the Sun, is singularly good for the inflammations of wounds, and for the headache, coming of a hot cause. There is a sweet water also distilled from the flowers, that is good for all those diseases that need cooling and drying, and therefore helps all fluxes of the belly or stomach, bloody-fluxes [dysentery], and women's courses, being either drank or applied; as all those that void blood at the mouth, or any other place, and for distillations of rheum [watery discharge] in the eyes, especially if it be used with them.

MODERN USES: The bitter, astringent leaves, as well as the flowers of privet, have been used in tea to treat sore throat and canker sores. The bitter black berries are purgative and turn the urine brown. Various species of *Ligustrum* have been used to prevent hypertension, inflammation, and diabetes, and are considered antioxidant, anti-inflammatory, immunomodulatory, and anti-diabetic. Related species are used in traditional Chinese medicine. **CAUTION:** The flowers are responsible for allergies and the fruits are considered potentially toxic.

....

PURSLANE

(*PORTULACA OLERACEA*)

Purslain

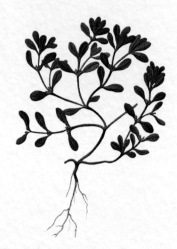

Garden Purslane (being used as a salad herb) is so well known that it needs no description; I shall therefore only speak of its virtues as follows.

PLACE: [Purslane is thought to originate in the Mediterranean region and is now considered weedy worldwide; recorded as a weed in in China by the tenth century and known in North and South America in Culpeper's lifetime.]

GOVERNMENT AND VIRTUES: 'Tis an herb of the Moon. It is good to cool any heat in the liver, blood, kidneys, and stomach, and in hot agues nothing better. It stays hot and choleric fluxes of the belly, women's courses, the whites, and gonorrhea, or running of the kidneys, the distillation from the head, and pains therein proceeding from heat, want of sleep, or the frenzy. The seed is more effectual than the herb, and is of singular good use to cool the heat and sharpness of urine, venereous dreams, and the like; insomuch that the over frequent use hereof extinguishes the heat and virtue of natural procreation. The seed bruised and boiled in wine, and given to children, expels the worms. The juice of the herb is held as effectual to all the purposes aforesaid; as also to stay vomiting, and taken with some sugar or honey, helps an old and dry cough, shortness of breath, and the phthisic, and stays immoderate thirst. The distilled water of the herb is used by many (as the more pleasing) with a little sugar to work the same effects. The juice also is singularly good in the inflammations and ulcers in the secret parts of man or woman, as also the bowels and hemorrhoids, when they are ulcerous. The herb bruised and applied to the forehead and temples, allays excessive heat therein, that hinders rest and sleep; and applied to the eyes, takes away the redness and inflammation in them, and those other parts where pushes, wheals, pimples, St. Anthony's fire and the like, break forth; if a little vinegar be put to it, and laid to the neck, with as much of galls and linseed together, it takes away the pains therein, and the crick in the neck. The juice is used with oil of roses for the same causes, or for blasting by lightning, and burnings by gunpowder, or for women's sore breasts, and to allay the heat in all other sores or hurts. Applied also to the navels of children that stick forth, it helps them; it is also good for sore mouths and gums that are swollen, and to fasten loose teeth. Camerarius saith, the distilled water used by some, took away the pain of their teeth, when all other remedies failed, and the thickened juice made into pills with the powder of gum Tragacanth and Arabic, being taken, prevails much to help those that make bloody water. Applied to the gout it eases pains thereof, and helps the hardness of the sinews, if it come not of the cramp, or a cold cause.

MODERN USES: The edible fresh succulent leaves of purslane are considered a cooling astringent, mostly applied externally to reduce inflammation. Used internally as a diuretic for painful urination. The seed oil contains omega-3 fatty acids and the neurohormone norepinephrine, which may reduce bleeding. First recorded in China in the year 934, the dried herb is used in traditional Chinese medicine (as *ma-chi-xian*) to stop bleeding and reduce heat for dysentery with bloody stools, hemorrhoids, and excessive uterine bleeding; externally the fresh herb is poulticed for boils, bug bites, and stings. The World Health Organization lists it among the most used medicinal plants in the world.

....

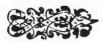

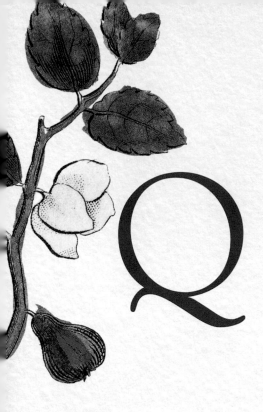

Q

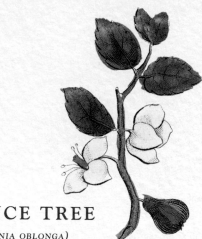

QUINCE TREE
(CYDONIA OBLONGA)

DESCRIPTION: The ordinary Quince Tree grows often to the height and bigness of a reasonable apple tree, but more usually lower and crooked. The flowers are large and white, sometimes dashed over with a blush. The fruit that follows is yellow, being near ripe, of a strong heady scent, and not durable to keep, and is sour, harsh, and of an unpleasant taste to eat fresh; but being scalded, roasted, baked, or preserved, becomes more pleasant.

PLACE: It best likes to grow near ponds and water sides. [Native to the Middle East and central Asia; naturalized through most of Europe (except Scandinavia), North Africa, and northeastern North America.]

GOVERNMENT AND VIRTUES: Old Saturn owns the Tree. Quinces, when they are green, help all sorts of fluxes in men or women, and choleric lasks, casting, and whatever needs astriction, more than any way prepared by fire. If a little vinegar be added [to the juice of conserve of the fruit], it stirs up the languishing appetite; some spices being added, comforts and strengthens the decaying and fainting spirits, and helps the liver oppressed, that it cannot perfect the digestion, or corrects choler [bile] and phlegm. If you would have them purging, put honey to them instead of sugar. To take the crude juice of Quinces, is held a preservative against the force of deadly poison; for it hath been found most certainly true, that the very smell of a Quince hath taken away all the strength of the poison of white Hellebore. If there be need of any outwardly binding and cooling of hot fluxes, the oil of Quinces, or other medicines that may be made thereof, are very available to anoint the belly or other parts therewith; it likewise strengthens the stomach and belly, and the sinews that are loosened by sharp humours falling on them, and restrains immoderate sweating. The mucilage taken from the seeds of Quinces, and boiled in a little water, is very good to cool the heat and heal the sore breasts of women. The same, with a little sugar, is good to lenify the harshness and hoarseness of the throat, and roughness of the tongue. The cotton or down of Quinces boiled and applied to plague sores, heals them up: and laid as a plaster, made up with wax, it brings hair to them that are bald, and keeps it from falling, if it be ready to shed.

MODERN USES: Quince fruit extract is considered antioxidant and was traditionally used as a digestive tonic, antidiarrheal, anti-inflammatory, a treatment for gastric ulcers, and to reduce bleeding internally and externally. The seeds have an antacid mucilage, used traditionally to treat skin conditions and historically to treat eye inflammation. The seed mucilage was also used as a hair dressing.

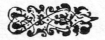

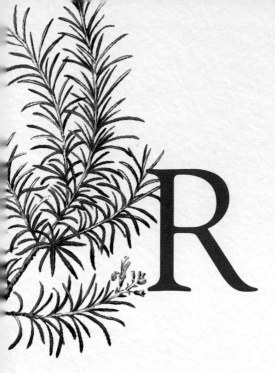

R

RAGWORT

(*SENECIO JACOBAEA, JACOBAEA VULGARIS*)

Tansy Ragwort

DESCRIPTION: The greater common Ragwort hath many large and long, dark green leaves, rent and torn on the sides, from among which rise up sometimes but one, sometimes two or three stalks, three or four feet high, bearing diverse yellow flowers.

PLACE: [Grows wild in cultivated fields, pastures, and wastelands; a weed of Eurasian origin, but widely naturalized as an invasive alien elsewhere.]

GOVERNMENT AND VIRTUES: Ragwort is under the command of Dame Venus, and cleanses, digests, and discusses. The decoction of the herb is good to wash the mouth or throat that hath ulcers or sores therein, and for swellings, hardness, or imposthumes [abscesses], for it thoroughly cleanses and heals them; as also the quinsy, and the king's evil. It helps to stay catarrhs, thin rheums [watery discharge], and defluxions from the head into the eyes, nose, or lungs. The juice is found by experience to be singularly good to heal green wounds, and to cleanse and heal all old and filthy ulcers in the private parts, and in other parts of the body, as also inward wounds and ulcers; stays the malignity of fretting and running cankers, and hollow fistulas. It is also much commended to help aches and pains either in the fleshy part, or in the nerves and sinews, as also the sciatica, or pain of the hips or knuckle-bone, to bathe the places with the decoction of the herb.

MODERN USES: Ragwort is of historical interest only. **CAUTION:** The primary modern concern with ragwort is eliminating it from pastures; it contains liver-toxic pyrrolizidine alkaloids, which accumulate in the liver, and in this case, are responsible for numerous livestock fatalities. Starting in the 1930s, Irish farmers were fined if they did not remove the plant from their fields.

....

PLACE: They grow in meadows [throughout Europe, in subarctic regions of North America, and East Asia].

GOVERNMENT AND VIRTUES: [Yellow Rattle] is under the dominion of the Moon. The yellow Rattle is held to be good for those that are troubled with a cough, or dimness of sight, if the herb, being boiled with beans, and some honey put thereto, be drank or dropped into the eyes.

MODERN USES: Yellow rattle is a minor folk medicine that has fallen into disuse. In his 1777 *Flora Londinensis*, William Curtis remarks, "Agriculturally considered, we may rank it with the useless plants."

....

RATTLE GRASS
(RHINANTHUS MINOR)

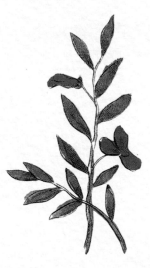

DESCRIPTION: The common Yellow Rattle hath, leaves set at a joint, deeply cut in on the edges, resembling the comb of a cock. The flowers [are] hooded, of a fair yellow colour. The seed is contained in large husks, and being ripe, will rattle.

RED CLOVER
(TRIFOLIUM PRATENSE);

WHITE CLOVER
(TRIFOLIUM REPENS)

Meadow Trefoil

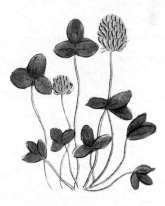

It is so well known, especially by the name of Honeysuckles, white [white clover (*Trifolium repens*)] and red [red clover (*Trifolium pratense*)], that

I need not describe them. [Not to be confused with honeysuckle, shrubs and vines in the genus *Lonicera*.]

PLACE: They grow [in almost every field, lawn, grassland, and roadside worldwide].

GOVERNMENT AND VIRTUES: Mercury hath dominion over the common sort. Dodoens saith, the leaves and flowers are good to ease the griping pains of the gout, the herb being boiled and used in a clyster. If the herb be made into a poultice, and applied to inflammations, it will ease them. The juice dropped in the eyes, is a familiar medicine, with many country people, to take away the pin and web (as they call it) in the eyes; it also allays the heat and blood shooting of them. Country people do also in many places drink the juice thereof against the biting of an adder; and having boiled the herb in water, they first wash the place with the decoction, and then lay some of the herb also to the hurt place. The herb also boiled in swine's grease, and so made into an ointment, is good to apply to the biting of any venomous creature. The herb also bruised and heated between tiles, and applied hot to the share, causes them to make water who had it stopped before. It is held likewise to be good for wounds, and to take away seed. The decoction of the herb and flowers, with the seed and root, taken for some time, helps women that are troubled with the whites. The seed and flowers boiled in water, and afterwards made into a poultice with some oil, and applied, helps hard swellings and imposthumes [abscesses].

MODERN USES: Culpeper describes traditional uses of astringent red clover for the treatment of wounds, inflammation, and skin conditions such as eczema and psoriasis. It has phytoestrogenic compounds, which has led to the development of products for reducing symptoms associated with menopause, such as hot flashes. Several clinical studies suggest safety and efficacy. White clover is seldom used as a folk medicine today. **CAUTION:** The herb's estrogenic-like components suggest that it should not be used during pregnancy and lactation.

....

RESTHARROW

(ONONIS SPINOSA)

Cammock

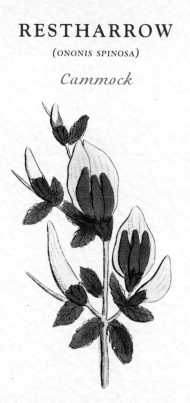

DESCRIPTION: Common Rest Harrow rises up with rough woody twigs half a yard, with short and sharp thorns. The flowers fashioned like peas blossoms, but lesser, flatter, and somewhat closer, [are] of a faint purplish colour.

PLACE: It grows in many places of this land, as well in the arable as waste ground. [Found throughout Europe.]

GOVERNMENT AND VIRTUES: It is under the dominion of Mars. It is singularly good to provoke urine when it is stopped, and to break and drive forth the stone, which the powder of the bark of the root taken in wine performs effectually. The decoction thereof made with some vinegar, gargled in the mouth, eases the toothache, especially when it comes of rheum [watery discharge]; and the said decoction is very powerful to open obstructions of the liver and spleen, and other parts. The powder of the said root made into an electuary, or lozenges, with sugar, as also the bark of the fresh roots boiled tender, and afterwards beaten to a conserve with sugar, works the like effect. The powder of the roots strewed upon the brims of ulcers, or mixed with any other convenient thing, and applied, consumes the hardness, and causes them to heal the better.

MODERN USES: The root and rhizome of restharrow are used as a diuretic for supportive treatment of inflammatory infections of the lower urinary tract and to prevent and treat kidney gravel. Isoflavones are thought to be responsible for the mild diuretic activity.

....

RHUBARB
(RHEUM RHAPONTICUM)
Rephontic

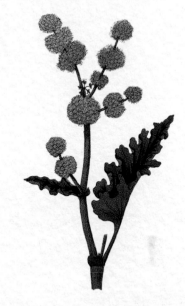

Do not start, and say, this grows you know not how far off: and then ask me, how it comes to pass that I bring it among our English simples? For though the name may speak it foreign, yet it grows with us in England, and that frequent enough in our gardens; and when you have thoroughly pursued its virtues, you will conclude it nothing inferior to that which is brought out of China, and by that time this hath been as much used as that hath been, the name which the other hath gotten will be eclipsed by the fame of this; take therefore a description at large of it as follows:

DESCRIPTION: At the first appearing out of the ground, which opens itself into sundry leaves one after another, very much crumpled or folded together at the first, but afterwards it spreads itself, and becomes smooth, very large and almost round, the leaf itself, being also two feet, the breadth thereof from edge to edge, in the broadest place, of a fine tart or sourish taste, much more pleasant than the garden or wood sorrel. The roots that are to be dried and kept all the year following, are not to be taken up before the stalk and leaves be quite turned red and gone, and that is not until the middle or end of October, and if they be taken a little before the leaves do spring, or when they are sprung up, the roots will not have half so good a colour in them.

PLACE: It grows in gardens, and flowers about the beginning and middle of June, and the seed is ripe in July.

MODERN USES: Rhubarb is best known today for the sour but edible leaf stalks that are consumed in the spring. Not used medicinally. Instead, Asian species such as *Rheum palmatum* and *Rheum officinale*, originating from northwest China and cultivated elsewhere, are used. These have large roots, which when dried and aged for a year contain strongly laxative components that are used as a stimulant laxative to induce propulsive contractions in the colon. **CAUTION:** Contraindicated in intestinal inflammation, Crohn's disease, colitis, appendicitis, and whenever medical advice suggests refraining from the use of stimulant laxatives. May cause electrolyte imbalances. Fresh leaves of cultivated rhubarb are considered toxic and should be avoided.

....

ROCKET, ARUGULA

(ERUCA VESICARIA; SYN. ERUCA SATIVA)

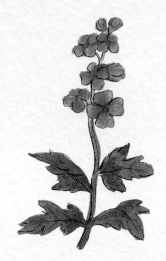

DESCRIPTION: The common wild Rocket has long and narrow leaves, much divided into slender cuts and jags, which rise up diverse stalks two or three feet high, bearing sundry yellow flowers on them [with] small reddish seed, in small long pods, more bitter and hot biting taste than the garden kinds.

PLACE: It is found wild in diverse places of this land. [Scattered throughout Europe in wastelands, mostly as a waif; primarily cultivated in vegetable gardens.]

GOVERNMENT AND VIRTUES: The wild Rockets are forbidden to be used alone, in regard their sharpness fumes into the head, causing aches and pains therein, and are less hurtful to hot and choleric persons, for fear of inflaming their blood, and therefore for such we may say a little doth but a little harm, for angry Mars rules them, and he sometimes will be restive when he meets with fools. The wild Rocket is stronger and more effectual to increase sperm and venerous qualities, whereunto all the seed is more effectual than the garden kind. It serves also to help digestion, and provokes urine exceedingly. The seed is used to cure the biting of serpents, the scorpion, and the shrew mouse, and other poisons, and expels worms, and other noisome creatures that breed in the belly. The herb boiled or stewed, and some sugar put thereto, helps the cough in children, being taken often. The seed also taken in drink, takes away the ill scent of the arm-pits, increases milk in nurses, and wastes the spleen. The seed mixed with honey, and used on the face, cleanses the skin from morphew [blemishes], and used with vinegar, takes away freckles and redness in the face, or other parts; and with the gall of an ox, it mends foul scars, black and blue spots, and the marks of the small-pox.

MODERN USES: Rocket (or arugula) is primarily used as a warming food in relatively small quantities as a bitter condiment, and more popularly as a salad green. Contains the pungent components of mustards (glucosinolates). Traditionally used as an antiphlogistic, diuretic, digestive, and as Culpeper suggests, an aphrodisiac, but then again, onions were also once considered an aphrodisiac. **CAUTION:** Has a strong mustard pungency, which can be irritating.

....

ROSE
(ROSA DAMASCENA, ROSA GALLICA, ROSA CANINA)

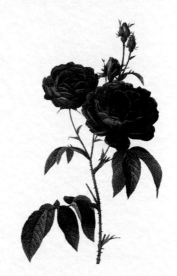

I hold it altogether needless to trouble the reader with a description of any of these, since both the garden Roses, and the Roses of the briars are well enough known.

PLACE: [With upwards of 150 species and thousands of varieties, roses are well-known in horticultural as well as in wild habitats throughout northern temperate regions in Europe, North America, and especially Asia, with ranges extending southward to tropical mountains in Mexico, the Philippines, and Ethopia.]

GOVERNMENT AND VIRTUES: What a pother [fuss] have authors made with Roses! What a racket have they kept? I shall add, red Roses are under Jupiter, Damask under Venus, White under the Moon, and Provence under the King of France. The white and red Roses are cooling and drying, and yet the white is taken to exceed the red in both the properties, but is seldom used inwardly in any medicine: The bitterness in the Roses when they are fresh, especially the juice, purges choler [bile], and watery humours; but being dried, and that heat which caused the bitterness being consumed, they have then a binding and astringent quality: Those also that are not full [in full bloom], do both cool and bind more than those that are in full [bloom], and the white Rose more than the Red. The decoction of red Roses made with wine and used, is very good for the headache, and pains in the eyes, ears, throat, and gums; as also for, the lower part of the belly and the matrix, being bathed or put into them. The same decoction with the Roses remaining in it, is profitably applied to the region of the heart to ease the inflammation therein; as also St. Anthony's fire, and other diseases of the stomach. Being dried and beaten to powder, and taken in steeled wine or water, it helps to stay women's courses. The yellow threads in the middle of the Roses (which are erroneously called the Rose Seed) being powdered and drank in the distilled water of Quinces, stays the overflowing of women's courses, and doth wonderfully stay the defluctions of rheum [watery discharge] upon the gums and teeth, preserving them from corruption, and fastening them if they be loose, being washed and gargled therewith, and some vinegar of Squills added thereto. The heads with the seed being used in powder, or in a decoction, stays the lask [diarrhea] and spitting of blood. Red Roses do strengthen the heart, the stomach and the liver, and the retentive faculty. They mitigate the pains that arise from heat, assuage inflammations, procure rest and sleep, stay both whites and reds in women, the gonorrhea, or running of the kidneys, and fluxes of the belly: the juice of them doth purge and cleanse the body from choler [bile] and phlegm. The husks of the Roses [rosehips], with the beards and nails of the Roses, are binding and cooling, and the distilled water of either of them is good for the heat and redness in the eyes, and to stay and dry up the rheums and watering of them.

Of the Red Roses are usually made many compositions, all serving to sundry good uses, *viz.*

Electuary of Roses, Conserve, both moist and dry, which is more usually called Sugar of roses, Syrup of dry Roses, and Honey of Roses. The cordial powder called *Diarrhoden Abbatis*, and *Aromatica Rosarum*. The distilled Water of Roses, Vinegar of Roses, Ointment, and Oil of Roses, and the Rose leaves dried, are of great use and effect. To write at large of every one of these, would make my book smell too big, it being sufficient for a volume of itself, to speak fully of them.

The simple water of Damask Roses is chiefly used for fumes to sweeten things, as the dried leaves thereof to make sweet powders, and fill sweet bags; and little use they are put to in physic, although they have some purging quality; the wild Roses also are few or none of them used in physic, but are generally held to come near the nature of the manured Roses. The fruit of the wild briar, which are called Hips, being thoroughly ripe, and made into a conserve with sugar, besides the pleasantness of the taste, doth gently bind the belly, and stay defluctions from the head upon the stomach, drying up the moisture thereof, and helps digestion. The pulp of the hips dried into a hard consistence, like to the juice of the licorice, or so dried that it may be made into powder and taken into drink, stays speedily the whites in women. The briar ball is often used, being made into powder and drank, to break the stone, to provoke urine when it is stopped, and to ease and help the cholic; some appoint it to be burnt, and then taken for the same purpose. In the middle of the balls are often found certain white worms, which being dried and made into powder, and some of it drank, is found by experience of many to kill and drive forth the worms of the belly.

MODERN USES: Damask rose, source of the expensive oil of roses, is used in aromatherapy to treat asthma, nausea, impotence, and female disorders.

In cosmetics, it is an important fragrance ingredient thought to rejuvenate the skin. Preparations of the flowers are used in tea or as an astringent gargle for mild inflammation of the throat and oral mucosa. Rose hips (mostly from the dog rose, *Rosa canina*) are used as a diuretic for urinary tract inflammation, as well as an anti-inflammatory for rheumatism, gout, sciatica, and other ailments.

....

ROSEMARY

(*ROSMARINUS OFFICINALIS*;
SYN. *SALVIA ROSMARINUS*)

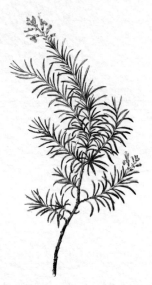

Our garden Rosemary is so well known, that I need not describe it.

PLACE: [Native to the Mediterranean coasts of France, Portugal, Spain, and Morocco. Cultivated elsewhere in Europe since ancient times.]

GOVERNMENT AND VIRTUES: The Sun claims privilege in it, and it is under the celestial Ram. It is an herb of as great use with us in these days as any whatsoever, not only for physical but civil purposes. The physical use of it (being my present task) is very much used both for inward and outward diseases, for by the warming and comforting heat thereof it helps all cold diseases, both of the head, stomach, liver, and belly. The decoction thereof in wine, helps the cold distillations of rheum [watery discharge] into the eyes, and all other cold diseases of the head and brain, as the giddiness or swimmings therein, drowsiness or dullness of the mind and senses like a stupidness, the dumb palsy, or loss of speech, the lethargy, and fallen-sickness, to be both drank, and the temples bathed therewith. It helps the pains in the gums and teeth, by rheum falling into them, not by putrefaction, causing an evil smell from them, or a stinking breath. It helps a weak memory, and quickens the senses. It is very comfortable to the stomach in all the cold griefs thereof, helps both retention of meat, and digestion, the decoction or powder being taken in wine. It is a remedy for the windiness in the stomach, bowels, and spleen, and expels it powerfully. It helps those that are liver-grown, by opening the obstructions thereof. It helps dim eyes, and procures a clear sight, the flowers thereof being taken all the while it is flowering every morning fasting, with bread and salt. Both Dioscorides and Galen say, that if a decoction be made thereof with water, and they that have the yellow jaundice exercise their bodies directly after the taking thereof, it will certainly cure them. The flowers and conserve made of them, are singularly good to comfort the heart, and to expel the contagion of the pestilence; to burn the herb in houses and chambers, corrects the air in them. Both the flowers and leaves are very profitable for women that are troubled with the whites, if they be daily taken. The dried leaves shred small, and taken in a pipe, as tobacco is taken, helps those that have any cough, phthisic, or consumption, by warming and drying the thin distillations which cause those diseases. The leaves are very much used in bathings; and made into ointments or oil, are singularly good to help cold benumbed joints, sinews, or members. The essential oil drawn from the leaves and flowers, is a sovereign help for all the diseases aforesaid, to touch the temples and nostrils with two or three drops for all the diseases of the head and brain spoken of before; as also to take one drop, two, or three, as the case requires, for the inward griefs: Yet must it be done with discretion, for it is very quick and piercing, and therefore but a little must be taken at a time. There is also another oil made by insolation in this manner: Take what quantity you will of the flowers, and put them into a strong glass close stopped, tie a fine linen cloth over the mouth, and turn the mouth down into another strong glass, which being set in the sun, an oil will distil down into the lower glass, to be preserved as precious for diverse uses, both inward and outward, as a sovereign balm to heal the disease before-mentioned, to clear dim sights, and to take away spots, marks, and scars in the skin.

MODERN USES: Rosemary leaf and its preparations, such as tea, are primarily used today to treat mild dyspeptic problems, such as an upset stomach. Applied externally as a stimulant rubefacient wash to treat circulatory disorders and rheumatic complaints. "It helps a weak memory and quickens the senses," as Culpeper reminds us, of its long-standing use to improve memory. Indeed, as shown in a clinical study, rosemary has components that might help improve brain function, reduce anxiety and depression, and increase memory performance. It also has liver-protective, anti-inflammatory, analgesic, and other activities.

....

ROUND-LEAVED DOCK
(RUMEX ALPINUS)
Bastard Rhubarb

MONK'S RHUBARB
(RUMEX PATIENTIA)
Patient Dock, Garden Patience

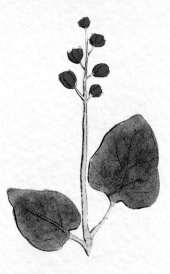

DESCRIPTION: Round-leaved Dock [*Rumex alpinus*] has large, round, thin yellowish green leaves rising from the root, a little waved about the edges, from among which rises up a pretty big stalk, about two feet high, with a long spike [of] many small brownish flowers, which turn into a hard three square shining brown seed. Monk's Rhubarb [*Rumex patientia*] is a Dock bearing the name of Rhubarb for some purging quality therein, and grows up with large tall stalks, set with somewhat broad and long, fair, green leaves; the stalks being divided into many small branches, bear reddish or purplish flowers, and three-square seed.

PLACE: These grow in gardens. [Round-leaved dock is native to wet fields in much of Europe, except Scandinavia. Monk's rhubarb is native to southeastern Europe and naturalized elsewhere in Europe, eastern North America, and the mountainous regions of western South America.]

GOVERNMENT AND VIRTUES: Mars claims predominance over all these wholesome herbs: You cry out upon him for an unfortunate, when God created him for your good (only he is angry with fools.) What dishonor is this, not to Mars, but to God himself? A dram of the dried root of Monk's Rhubarb, with a scruple of Ginger made into powder, and taken fasting in a draught or mess of warm broth, purges choler [bile] and phlegm downwards very gently and safely without danger. The seed thereof contrary doth bind the belly, and helps to stay any sort of lasks [diarrhea] or bloody-flux [dysentery]. The distilled water thereof is very profitably used to heal scabs; also foul ulcerous sores, and to allay the inflammation of them; the juice of the leaves or roots or the decoction of them in vinegar, is used as the most effectual remedy to heal scabs and running sores.

The Bastard Rhubarb hath all the properties of the Monk's Rhubarb, but more effectual for both inward and outward diseases. The decoction thereof without vinegar dropped into the ears, takes away the pains; gargled in the mouth, takes away the toothache; and being drank, heals the jaundice. The seed thereof taken, eases the gnawing and griping pains of the stomach, and takes away the loathing thereof unto meat. The root thereof helps the ruggedness of the nails, and being boiled in wine helps the swelling of the throat, commonly called the king's evil [unusual swelling of lymph nodes or scrofula], as also the swellings of the kernels of the ears. It helps them that are troubled with the stone, provokes urine, and helps the dimness of the sight. The roots of this Bastard Rhubarb are used in opening and purging diet-drinks, with other things, to open the liver, and to cleanse and cool the blood.

MODERN USES: Culpeper writes of "Bastard Rhubarb" (*Rumex alpinus*) and what he called "Patience," or Monk's Rhubarb (*Rumex patientia*), the dried roots of which were used as laxatives and the dried tops to reduce bleeding or act as an astringent on the bowels. The leaves of both are used as wild edibles and are seldom used today except as folk medicines for the same uses that Culpeper describes. **CAUTION:** May cause nausea, diarrhea (if not properly cured), and gastric upset.

....

ROYAL FERN
(OSMUNDA REGALIS)

Osmond Royal, Water Fern

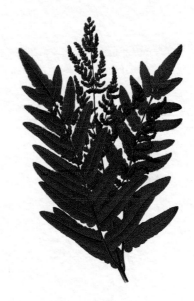

DESCRIPTION: This shoots forth in Spring time (for in the Winter the leaves perish) diverse rough hard stalks, half round, and yellowish, or flat on the other side, two feet high, having diverse branches of winged yellowish green leaves on all sides, set one against another, long and narrow.

PLACE: It grows on moors, bogs, and watery places, in many parts of [northern Europe and eastern North America. As one of the largest temperate-climate ferns, it is commonly grown as an ornamental in suitable moist, acidic soils].

GOVERNMENT AND VIRTUES: Saturn owns the plant. This has all the virtues mentioned in the former Ferns, and is much more effectual than they, both for inward and outward griefs, and is accounted singularly good in wounds, bruises, or the like. The decoction to be drank, or boiled into an ointment of oil, as a balsam or balm, and so it is singularly good against bruises, and bones broken, or out of joint, and gives much ease to the cholic and splenetic diseases: as also for ruptures or burstings. The decoction of the root in white wine, provokes urine exceedingly, and cleanses the bladder and passages of urine.

MODERN USES: Seldom used today, the royal fern has a large root, which, when soaked in water, produces a highly mucilaginous mass that was formerly used in the treatment of coughs, diarrhea, dysentery, and other ailments. Also considered styptic. Used as an external folk remedy for the treatment of lower back pain and rickets (caused by vitamin D deficiency). In the Cantabria region of Spain, it has a little studied folk-medicine use for treating bone fracture, joint disorders, rheumatic pain, and arthritis.

....

RUE

(RUTA GRAVEOLENS)

Garden-Rue

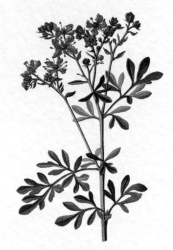

Garden-rue is so well known by this name, and the name Herb of Grace. [Originating in the Balkans, rue is found throughout much of Europe, North Africa, and South Africa. Commonly grown in herb gardens and as an ornamental for its wispy, gray-green leaves.]

GOVERNMENT AND VIRTUES: It is an herb of the Sun, and under Leo. It provokes urine and women's courses, being taken either in meat or drink. The leaves taken either by themselves, or with figs and walnuts, is called Mithridate's counter-poison against the plague, and causes all venomous things to become harmless; being often taken in meat and drink, it abates venery. Being boiled or infused in oil, it is good to help the wind cholic, the hardness and windiness of the mother. It kills and drives forth the worms of the belly, if it be drank after it is boiled in wine to the half, with a little honey; it helps the gout or pains in the joints, hands, feet or knees, applied thereunto; and with figs it helps the dropsy, being bathed therewith. Being bruised and put into the nostrils, it stays the bleeding thereof. It takes away wheals and pimples, if being bruised with a few myrtle leaves, it be made up with wax, and applied. It cures the morphew [skin blemishes]. An ointment made of the juice thereof with oil of roses, ceruse, and a little vinegar, and anointed, cures St. Anthony's fire, and all running sores in the head, and the stinking ulcers of the nose, or other parts. What a sot is he that knows not if he had accustomed his body to cold poisons, but poisons would have dispatched him? On the contrary, if not, corrosions would have done it.

MODERN USES: Rue has traditionally been used for menstrual disorders, uterine stimulation, nervous conditions, and in small amounts (nibbling an edge of the very bitter leaf) to stimulate digestion in cases of loss of appetite. Externally, it has been used for sprains, arthritic conditions, rheumatism, and a long list of other uses, as described by Culpeper. It is seldom used in modern herbal medicine because of toxicity concerns. **CAUTION:** Causes phototoxicity due to the furanocoumarins found in the leaf. Commonly causes contact dermatitis. Tragic cases of pregnant women attempting to use the herb for abortion have resulted in fatalities. Rue can also cause liver and kidney failure and other systemic toxicity. The fresh leaves are irritating. Avoid.

....

RUPTUREWORT

(*HERNIARIA GLABRA*)

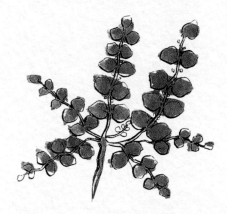

DESCRIPTION: This spreads very many thready branches round about upon the ground, about a span long, divided into many other smaller parts full of small joints set very thick together, whereat come forth two very small leaves, also a number of exceedingly small yellowish flowers. This has neither smell nor taste at first, but afterwards has a little astringent taste, without any manifest heat; yet a little bitter and sharp withal.

PLACE: It grows in dry, sandy, and rocky places. [Found through Europe, much of northern Asia, North Africa, and the Canadian Maritime Provinces.]

GOVERNMENT AND VIRTUES: They say Saturn causes ruptures; if he do, he does no more than he can cure; if you want wit, he will teach you, though to your cost. This herb is Saturn's own, and is a noble antivenereal. Rupture-wort hath not its name in vain: for it is found by experience to cure the rupture, not only in children but also in elder persons, if the disease be not too inveterate, by taking a dram of the powder of the dried herb every day in wine, or a decoction made and drank for certain days together. The juice or distilled water of the green herb, taken in the same manner, helps all other fluxes either of man or woman; vomiting also, and the gonorrhea, being taken any of the ways aforesaid. It doth also most assuredly help those that have the strangury, or are troubled with the stone or gravel in the kidneys or bladder. The same also helps stitches in the sides, griping pains of the stomach or belly, the obstructions of the liver, and cures the yellow jaundice; likewise it kills also the worms in children. Being outwardly applied, it conglutinates wounds notably, and helps much to stay defluctions of rheum [watery discharge] from the head to the eyes, nose, and teeth, being bruised green and bound thereto; or the forehead, temples, or the nape of the neck behind, bathed with the decoction of the dried herb. It also dries up the moisture of fistulous ulcers, or any other that are foul and spreading.

MODERN USES: Rupturewort is a traditional remedy for disorders of the kidney and urinary tract, inflammation of the upper respiratory tract, arthritis, and rheumatism. Also used as a "blood purifier." The plant is mildly diuretic, antihypertensive, and antispasmodic. Little used and little researched today.

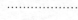

RUSTYBACK, SCALE FERN

(CETERACH OFFICINARUM; SYN. ASPLENIUM CETERACH)

Spleenwort, Ceterach, or Heart's Tongue

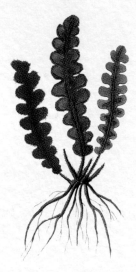

DESCRIPTION: [A small fern] sends forth many long single leaves, cut in on both sides each division being not always set opposite unto the other, cut between each, smooth, and of a light green on the upper side.

PLACE: It grows as well upon stone walls, as moist and shady places. [Native to the Mediterranean region and naturalized elsewhere.]

GOVERNMENT AND VIRTUES: Saturn owns it. It is generally used against infirmities of the Spleen: It helps the strangury, and wastes the stone in the bladder, and is good against the yellow jaundice and the hiccough; but the juice of it in women hinders conception. Matthiolus saith, that if a dram of the dust that is on the backside of the leaves be mixed with half a dram of amber in powder, and taken with the juice of purslane or plantain, it helps the gonorrhea speedily, and that the herb and root being boiled and taken, helps all melancholy diseases, and those especially that arise from the French diseases [syphilis]. Camerarius saith, That the distilled water thereof being drank, is very effectual against the stone in the kidneys and bladder; and that the lye that is made of the ashes thereof being drank for some time together, helps splenetic persons. It is used in outward remedies for the same purpose.

MODERN USES: Rustyback is little used today. A documented folk remedy for malaria with antibacterial activity.

....

RYE
(*SECALE CEREALE*)

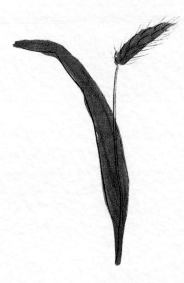

This is so well known in all the counties of this land, and especially to the country-people, who feed much thereon, that if I did describe it, they would presently say, I might as well have spared that labour. Its virtue follows.

PLACE: [Originating in southwest Asia and cultivated for two millenia; occasionally naturalized or a relic near cultivated fields.]

GOVERNMENT AND VIRTUES: Rye is more digesting than wheat; the bread and the leaven thereof ripens and breaks imposthumes [abscesses], boils, and other swellings: The meal of Rye put between a double cloth, and moistened with a little vinegar, and heated in a pewter dish, set over a chafing dish of coals, and bound fast to the head while it is hot, doth much ease the continual pains of the head. Matthiolus saith, that the ashes of Rye straw put into water, and steeped therein a day and a night, and the chops of the hands or feet washed therewith, doth heal them.

MODERN USES: Rye, of course, is a well-known grain, but little used medicinally.

....

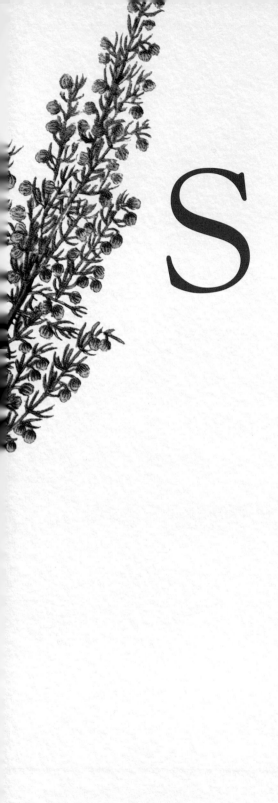

S

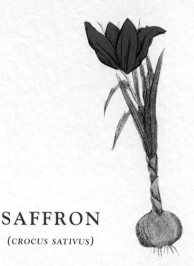

SAFFRON
(CROCUS SATIVUS)

The herb needs no description, it being known generally where it grows.

PLACE: [Native to Greece; naturalized in Turkey, Iran, Spain, and elsewhere.]

GOVERNMENT AND VIRTUES: It is an herb of the Sun, and under the Lion, and therefore you need not demand a reason why it strengthens the heart so exceedingly. Let not above ten grains be given at one time, for the Sun may dazzle the eyes, and make them blind; a cordial being taken in an immoderate quantity, hurts the heart instead of helping it. It quickens the brain, for the Sun is exalted in Aries, as he hath his house in Leo. It helps consumptions of the lungs, and difficulty of breathing. It is excellent in epidemical diseases, as pestilence, small-pox, and measles. It is a notable expulsive medicine, and a notable remedy for the yellow jaundice. My opinion is, (but I have no author for it) that hermodactyls [autumn crocus (*Colchicum autumnale*)] are nothing else but the roots of Saffron dried; and my reason is, that the roots of all crocus, both white and yellow, purge phlegm as hermodactyls do; and if you please to dry the roots of any crocus, neither your eyes nor your taste shall distinguish them from hermodactyls [Culpeper here reveals possible adulteration and confusion about the identity of the herb in the marketplace of his day].

MODERN USES: Saffron, one of the world most expensive spices, has a surprising array of health benefits. The hand-picked flower stigmas contain over 150 compounds with a range of effects including anti-inflammatory, antioxidant, and immunomodulatory activity. Saffron is used for neurodegenerative disorders, coronary artery disease, gastrointestinal conditions, and urinary disorders. Saffron extracts have been studied in clinical trials for treating anxiety, type 2 diabetes, and erectile dysfunction, as well as for their role in improving cognitive function in age-related dementia. **CAUTION:** Saffron's safety during pregnancy and lactation has not been established and may be associated with nausea and increased bleeding.

....

SAGE

(*SALVIA OFFICINALIS*)

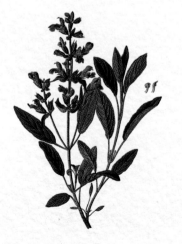

Our ordinary garden Sage needs no description.

PLACE: [Native to the Dalmatian coast; occurring in Croatia, Montenegro, and Albania, where wild-harvested sage accounts for about half of the world's supply; naturalized elsewhere in Europe and North America.]

GOVERNMENT AND VIRTUES: Jupiter claims it, and bids me tell you, it is good for the liver, and to breed blood. A decoction of the leaves and branches of Sage made and drank, saith Dioscorides, provokes urine, brings down women's courses, and causes the hair to become black. It stays the bleeding of wounds, and cleanses foul ulcers. Three spoonfuls of the juice of Sage taken fasting, with a little honey, doth presently stay the spitting or casting of blood of them that are in a consumption. Matthiolus saith, it is very profitable for all manner of pains in the head coming of cold and rheumatic humours: as also for all pains of the joints, whether inwardly or outwardly, and therefore helps the falling-sickness, the lethargy, such as are dull and heavy of spirit, the palsy; and is of much use in all defluctions of rheum [watery discharge] from the head, and for the diseases of the chest or breast. The leaves of Sage and nettles bruised together, and laid upon the imposthume [abscess] that rises behind the ears, doth assuage it much. The juice of Sage taken in warm water, helps a hoarseness and a cough. The leaves sodden in wine, and laid upon the place affected with the palsy, helps much, if the decoction be drank. Also Sage taken with wormwood is good for the bloody-flux [dysentery]. Pliny saith, it procures women's courses, and stays them coming down too fast: helps the stinging and biting of serpents. Sage is of excellent use to help the memory, warming and quickening the senses; and the conserve made of the flowers is used to the same purpose, and also for all the former recited diseases. The juice of Sage drank with vinegar, hath been of good use in time of the plague at all times. Gargles likewise are made with Sage, rosemary, honeysuckle, and plantain, boiled in wine or water, with some honey or alum put thereto, to wash sore mouths and throats, cankers, or the secret parts of man or woman, as need requires. And with other hot and comfortable herbs, Sage is boiled to bathe the body and the legs in the Summer time, especially to warm cold joints, or sinews, troubled with the palsy and cramp, and to comfort and strengthen the parts. It is much commended against the stitch, or pains in the side coming of wind, if the place be fomented warm with the decoction thereof in wine, and the herb also after boiling be laid warm thereunto.

MODERN USES: Common garden sage is best known as a culinary herb, but like rosemary, it is traditionally used to improve memory. A gargle of sage tea is used to treat mouth sores, canker sores, and sore throat. The fresh or dried leaves are used externally to treat rheumatic pain, sprains, and swelling. Sage is a folk remedy to reduce sweating and to dry up a mother's milk. Of research interest for possible antiobesity and antidiabetic activity. Confirmed pharmacological effects include anti-inflammatory, antioxidant, and antimicrobial activity, among others. Used to treat upset stomach and reduce night sweats. **CAUTION:** Avoid use during pregnancy or lactation.

....

ST.-JOHN'S-WORT

(HYPERICUM PERFORATUM)

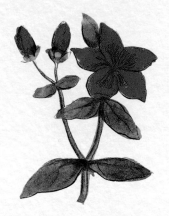

DESCRIPTION: Common St. John's Wort shoots forth, two feet high, with two small leaves set one against another at every place, and full of small holes in every leaf when they are held up to the light; at the tops of the stalks and branches stand yellow flowers of five [petals] a-piece, which being bruised do yield a reddish juice like blood.

PLACE: [Found in fields, roadsides, and open woods throughout Europe, Asia, North America, South America, and Australia—in short, a cosmopolitan weed in temperate climates worldwide.]

GOVERNMENT AND VIRTUES: It is under the celestial sign Leo, and the dominion of the Sun. It may be, if you meet a Papist, he will tell you, especially if he be a lawyer, that St. John made it over to him by a letter of attorney. It is a singular wound herb; boiled in wine and drank, it heals inward hurts or bruises; made into an ointment, it open obstructions, dissolves swellings, and closes up the lips of wounds. The decoction of the herb and flowers, especially of the seed, being drank in wine, with the juice of Knotgrass, helps all manner of vomiting and spitting of blood, is good for those that are bitten or stung by any venomous creature, and for those that cannot make water. Two drams of the seed of St. John's Wort made into powder, and drank in a little broth, doth gently expel choler [bile] or congealed blood in the stomach. The decoction of the leaves and seeds drank somewhat warm before the fits of agues, whether they be tertian or quartans [malaria] alters the fits, and, by often using, doth take them quite away. The seed is much commended, being drank for forty days together, to help the sciatica, the falling-sickness, and the palsy.

MODERN USES: One of the most thoroughly studied plants in modern times, St.-John's-wort is a widely used folk medicine for topical wound healing and lacerations involving nerve damage. It is also a diuretic, astringent, and mild sedative. The flowering tops soaked in olive oil are used to treat wounds, abrasions, and first-degree burns. St.-John's-wort extracts are widely used to treat symptoms of mild to moderate depression, anxiety, seasonal affective disorder, and other mild psychological disorders. **CAUTION**: Contraindicated for severe depression. Hypericin, a component in the flowering tops, may cause photodermatitis in lighted-skinned individuals. Like grapefruit, St.-John's-wort extract induces the cytochrome P450 enzyme system, which is involved in the intestinal uptake of conventional drugs, thereby interfering with the effective dose (by increasing it), making it one of the most significant herb-drug interactions. Best used under professional medical advice.

....

SAMPHIRE
(CRITHMUM MARITIMUM)

Sea Fennel

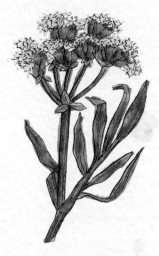

DESCRIPTION: Rock Samphire grows up with a tender green stalk about half a yard, branching forth with sundry thick and almost round (somewhat long) leaves, sappy, and of a pleasant, hot, and spicy taste. At the top of the stalks and branches stand umbels of white flowers.

PLACE: It grows on seaside rocks. [Grows in coastal regions at the demarcation of land and sea from the British Isles to Europe's Mediterranean region and North Africa.]

GOVERNMENT AND VIRTUES: It is an herb of Jupiter, and was in former times want to be used more than now it is; the more is the pity. It is well known almost to everybody, that ill digestions and obstructions are the cause of most of the diseases which the frail nature of man is subject to; both which might be remedied by a more frequent use of this herb. If people would have sauce to their meat, they may take some for profit as well as for pleasure. It is a safe herb, very pleasant both to taste and stomach, helps digestion, and in some sort opening obstructions of the liver and spleen: provokes urine, and helps thereby to wash away the gravel and stone engendered in the kidneys or bladder.

MODERN USES: More common as a wild edible or specialty vegetable than an herbal medicine, fresh samphire leaves are high in antioxidants including polyphenols, vitamin C, and vitamin E. Traditionally sold in local markets, the crisp, succulent, aromatic, and somewhat salty leaves were pickled and used in salads. Considered diuretic in effect.

....

SANICLE

(SANICULA EUROPAEA; SYN. SANICULA OFFICINALIS)

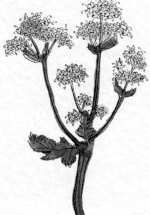

DESCRIPTION: Ordinary Sanicle [also called butterwort] sends forth many great round leaves, every one somewhat deeply cut or divided into five or six parts, and cut somewhat like the leaf of [buttercup], or Dovesfoot; it branches forth into flowers, which are small and white.

PLACE: It is found in many [shady, rich, deciduous] woods [in much of Europe].

GOVERNMENT AND VIRTUES: This is one of Venus's herbs, to cure the wounds or mischiefs Mars inflicts upon the body of man. It heals green wounds speedily, or any ulcers, imposthumes [abscesses], or bleedings inward, also tumours in any part of the body; for the decoction or powder in drink taken, and the juice used outwardly, dissipates the humours: and there is not found any herb that can give such present help either to man or beast, when the disease falleth upon the lungs or throat, and to heal up putrid malignant ulcers in the mouth, throat, by gargling or washing with the decoction of the leaves and roots made in water, and a little honey put thereto. It helps to stay women's courses, and all other fluxes of blood, either by the mouth, urine, or stool, and lasks of the belly; the ulcerations of the kidneys also, and the pains in the bowels, and gonorrhea, being boiled in wine or water, and drank. The same also is no less powerful to help any ruptures or burstings, used both inwardly and outwardly. And briefly, it is as effectual in binding, restraining, consolidating, heating, drying and healing, as Comfrey, Bugle, Self-heal, or any other of the vulnerary herbs.

MODERN USES: The dried sanicle leaves, somewhat bitter and mildly astringent, are used in teas for the treatment of mild catarrhs of the upper respiratory tract; nonspecific bleeding, including excessive menstrual bleeding; and as a treatment for hemorrhoids. Seldom used, except locally in parts of Europe as a folk medicine for the topical treatment of cuts and wounds. It is astringent, antiviral against influenza, and antioxidant due to the rosmarinic acid content.

....

SANTOLINA

(*SANTOLINA CHAMAECYPARISSUS*)

Lavender–Cotton

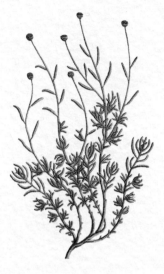

It being a common garden herb, I shall forbear the description. [Originating in dry soils of the Mediterranean region, gray santolina (*Santolina chamaecyparissus*) and green santolina (*Santolina virens*) are commonly grown in herb gardens.]

GOVERNMENT AND VIRTUES: It is under the dominion of Mercury. It resists poison, putrefaction, and heals the biting of venomous beasts: A dram of the powder of the dried leaves taken every morning fasting, stops the running of the kidneys in men, and whites in women. The seed beaten into powder, and taken as worm-seed, kills the worms, not only in children, but also in people of riper years; the like doth the herb itself, being steeped in milk, and the milk drank; the body bathed with the decoction of it, helps scabs and itch.

MODERN USES: Santolina was used as a folk medicine to expel worms; also used as a digestive stimulant and treatment for stomachache and leukorrhea. Antibacterial, analgesic, anti-inflammatory, anti-spasmodic, digestive, and immunostimulant activities have been described in recent scientific studies. **CAUTION:** Some individuals may have allergic reactions or experience contact dermatitis from santolina.

....

SARACEN'S CONFOUND, OR SARACEN'S WOUNDWORT

(*SENECIO OVATUS*; SYN. *SENECIO SARRACENICUS*)

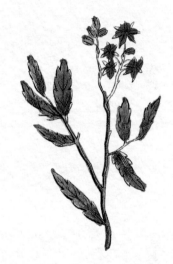

DESCRIPTION: This grows sometimes, to a man's height, having narrow green leaves snipped about the edges with many yellow star-like flowers. The taste hereof is strong and unpleasant; and so is the smell also.

PLACE: It grows in moist and wet grounds [in woods in Europe].

GOVERNMENT AND VIRTUES: Saturn owns the herb, and it is of a sober condition, like him. Among the Germans, this wound herb is preferred before all others of the same quality. Being boiled in wine, and drank, it helps the indisposition of the liver, and free[s] the gall from obstructions; whereby it is good for the yellow jaundice and for the dropsy in the beginning of it; for all inward ulcers of the kidneys, mouth or throat, and inward wounds and bruises, likewise for such sores as happen in the privy parts of men and women; being steeped in wine, and then distilled, the water thereof drank, is singularly good to ease all gnawings in the stomach, or other pains of the body, as also the pains of the mother: and being boiled in water, it helps continual agues; and the said water, or the simple water of the herb distilled, or the juice or decoction, are very effectual to heal any green wound, or old sore or ulcer whatsoever, cleansing them from corruption, and quickly healing them up: Briefly, whatsoever hath been said of Bugle or Sanicle, may be found herein.

MODERN USES: Saracen's confound is an obscure, little-used, little-researched medicinal plant once regarded as a folk remedy for the topical treatment of wounds. **CAUTION:** Contain liver-toxic pyrrolizidine alkaloids, which can cause veno-occlusive disease of the liver, a sometimes fatal, difficult-to-recognize condition. Contrary to what Culpeper suggests it is more likely to cause "indisposition of the liver" rather than help it.

....

SAVINE

(JUNIPERUS SABINA)

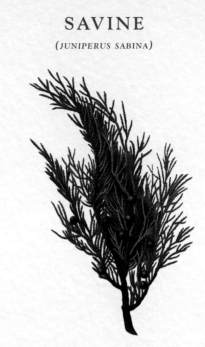

To describe a plant so well-known is needless, it being nursed up almost in every garden, and abides green all the Winter. [Occurs through southern and central Europe, continuously through East Asia.]

GOVERNMENT AND VIRTUES: It is under the dominion of Mars, being hot and dry in the third degree, and being of exceeding clean parts, is of a very digesting quality. If you dry the herb into powder, and mix it with honey, it is an excellent remedy to cleanse old filthy ulcers and fistulas; but it hinders them from healing. The same is excellently good to break carbuncles and plague-sores; also helps the king's evil [unusual swelling of lymph nodes or scrofula], being applied to the place. Being spread over a piece of leather, and applied to the navel, kills the worms in the belly, helps scabs and itch, running sores, cankers, tetters, and ring-worms; and being applied to the place, may haply cure venereal sores. This I thought good to speak of, as it may be safely used outwardly, for inwardly it cannot be taken without manifest danger.

MODERN USES: Savine is little used today either for the treatment of worms or plague-sores. Externally, it has a long history of folk use in China for treating rheumatoid arthritis. **CAUTION:** Savine is a poisonous plant that has highly irritating effects on the gastrointestinal system and kidneys and produces systemic toxicity. Topical use can cause chemical burns and blistering. Once used as a drastic worm treatment, it has fallen into disuse due to its high toxicity. Avoid.

....

SAVORY, WINTER AND SUMMER

(SATUREJA MONTANA AND SATUREJA HORTENSIS)

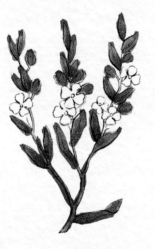

Both these are so well known (being entertained as constant inhabitants in our gardens) that they need no description. [From Europe, widely cultivated in herb gardens.]

GOVERNMENT AND VIRTUES: Mercury claims dominion over this herb, neither is there a better remedy against the colic and iliac passion, than this herb; keep it dry by you all the year, if you love yourself and your ease, and it is a hundred pounds to a penny if you do not; keep it dry, make conserves and syrups of it for your use, and withal, take notice that the Summer kind is the best. They are both of them hot and dry, especially the Summer kind, which is both sharp and quick in taste, expelling wind in the stomach and bowels, and is a present help for the rising of the mother procured by wind; provokes urine and women's courses, and is much commended for women with child to take inwardly, and to smell often unto. It cures tough phlegm in the chest and lungs, and helps to expectorate it the more easily; quickens the dull spirits in the lethargy, the juice thereof being snuffed up into the nostrils. The juice heated with the oil of Roses, and dropped into the ears, eases them of the noise and singing in them, and of deafness also. Outwardly applied with wheat flour, in manner of a poultice, it gives ease to the sciatica and palsied members, heating and warming them, and takes away their pains. It also takes away the pain that comes by stinging of bees, wasps, &c.

MODERN USES: Winter savory (*Satureja montana*), a woody perennial, and summer savory (*Satureja hortensis*), a garden annual, are traditionally used in tea as a digestive carminative, antispasmodic, and expectorant. Gargled for sore throat and sipped as tea for indigestion. A tea is also used as a treatment for diarrhea and acute enterocolitis. Fresh leaves are rubbed on insect stings. Considered antibacterial, antifungal, anti-inflammatory, and antioxidant, among other effects. **CAUTION:** Avoid use during pregnancy and lactation.

....

SCABIOUS, FIELD

(*KNAUTIA ARVENSIS, CENTAUREA SCABIOSA, SCABIOSA ATROPURPUREA*, AND OTHER SPECIES)

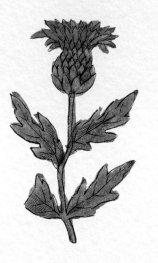

DESCRIPTION: Common field Scabious (*Knautia arvensis*) grows up with many hairy, soft, whitish green leaves, some whereof are very little, if at all jagged on the edges, others very much rent and torn on the sides, and have threads in them, which upon breaking may be plainly seen. At the tops thereof, stand round heads of flowers, of a pale blueish colour.

PLACE: Field Scabious grows more usually in meadows [throughout most of Europe].

There are many other sorts of Scabious, but I take these which I have here described to be most familiar with us. The virtues of both these and the rest, being much alike, take them as follows. [The common name "scabious" was applied to many plants in medieval England, a tea of which was given to treat scabies.]

GOVERNMENT AND VIRTUES: Mercury owns the plant. Scabious is very effectual for all sorts of coughs, shortness of breath, and all other diseases of the breast and lungs, ripening and digesting cold phlegm, and other tough humours, voids them forth by coughing and spitting. The green herb bruised and applied to any carbuncle or plague sore, is found by certain experience to dissolve and break it in three hours space. The same decoction also drank, helps the pains and stitches in the side. The juice or decoction drank, helps also scabs and breakings-out of the itch, and the like. The juice also made up into an ointment and used, is effectual for the same purpose. The same also heals all inward wounds by the drying, cleansing, and healing quality therein: And a syrup made of the juice and sugar, is very effectual to all the purposes aforesaid, and so is the distilled water of the herb and flowers made in due season, especially to be used when the green herb is not in force to be taken. The decoction of the herb and roots outwardly applied, doth wonderfully help all sorts of hard or cold swellings in any part of the body, is effectual for shrunk sinews or veins, and heals green wounds, old sores, and ulcers. The juice of Scabious, made up with the powder of Borax and Samphire, cleanses the skin of the face, or other parts of the body, not only from freckles and pimples, but also from morphew [blemishes] and leprosy; the head washed with the decoction, cleanses it from dandruff, scurf, sores, itch, and the like, used warm. The herb bruised and applied, doth in a short time loosen, and draw forth any splinter, broken bone, arrow head, or other such like thing lying in the flesh.

MODERN USES: The highly variable and ambiguous collection of plant species called "scabious" are seldom used today and of only historical interest.

....

SCARLET PIMPERNEL

(LYSIMACHIA ARVENSIS; SYN. ANAGALLIS ARVENSIS)

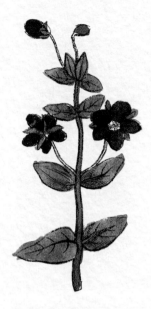

it very effectually cures in a short space. It is also effectual to ease the pains of the hemorrhoids or piles.

MODERN USES: Scarlet pimpernel is not used today, despite Culpeper's praise for its external effects on wounds. **CAUTION:** Usually considered a poisonous plant, it is associated with livestock toxicity and known to have caused the death of cattle and sheep in Australia and South America.

....

SCURVYGRASS

(COCHLEARIA OFFICINALIS)

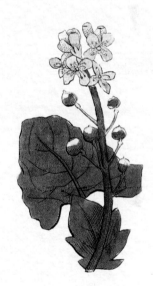

DESCRIPTION: Common Pimpernel hath diverse weak square stalks lying on the ground, beset all with two small and almost round leaves at every joint. The flowers stand singly [with] five small round-pointed [orange] petals.

PLACE: [A widespread weed in meadows and fields in most of Europe and North Africa; widely naturalized as a weed in North America, South America, and Asia.]

GOVERNMENT AND VIRTUES: It is a gallant solar herb, of a cleansing attractive quality, whereby it draws forth thorns or splinters, or other such like things gotten into the flesh; and put up into the nostrils, purges the head; and Galen saith also, they have a drying faculty, whereby they are good to solder the lips of wounds, and to cleanse foul ulcers. The decoction, or distilled water, is no less effectual to be applied to all wounds that are fresh and green, or old, filthy, fretting, and running ulcers, which

DESCRIPTION: The ordinary English Scurvygrass hath many thick flat leaves, more long than broad; sometimes also smooth on the edges, and sometimes a little waved. At the tops grow many whitish flowers.

PLACE: It grows all along [rivers and seashores in most of northern Europe].

GOVERNMENT AND VIRTUES: It is an herb of Jupiter. The English Scurvygrass is more used for the salt taste it bears, which doth somewhat open and cleanse; [it is] chiefly used (if it may be had) by those that have the scurvy, and is of singular good effect to cleanse the blood, liver, and spleen, taking the juice in the Spring every morning fasting in a cup of drink. The decoction is good for the same purpose, and opens obstructions, evacuating cold, clammy and phlegmatic humours both from the liver and the spleen, and bringing the body to a livelier colour. The juice also helps all foul ulcers and sores in the mouth, gargled therewith; and used outwardly, cleanses the skin from spots, marks, or scars that happen therein.

MODERN USES: A member of the mustard family, scurvygrass is a moderately succulent and pungent seaside green. Its juice and tea were used as a treatment for scurvy and as a diuretic. Eighteenth-century English authors recommended eating the pungent leaves between bread with butter. Until the mid-nineteenth century, scurvy (vitamin C deficiency) was a primarily a disease associated with months-long voyages at sea, but by the beginning of the seventeenth century, "land scurvy" was also recognized by non-seafaring peoples.

....

SELF-HEAL
(PRUNELLA VULGARIS)

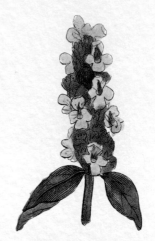

DESCRIPTION: The common Self-heal, which is called also Prunel, Carpenter's Herb, Hook-heal, and Sickle-wort, is a small, low, creeping herb, having many small, roundish pointed leaves, [from] which rise square hairy stalks, scarce a foot high, [with] flowers of a blueish purple.

PLACE: It is found in woods and fields everywhere. [Native to Europe, Asia, and North America; widely naturalized in South America.]

GOVERNMENT AND VIRTUES: Here is another herb of Venus, Self-heal, whereby when you are hurt you may heal yourself: It is a special herb for inward and outward wounds. Take it inwardly in syrups for inward wounds: outwardly in unguents, and plasters for outward, for inward wounds or ulcers whatsoever within the body, for bruises or falls, and such like hurts. Where there is cause to repress the heat and sharpness of humours flowing to any sore, ulcers, inflammations, swellings, or the like, or to stay the fluxes of blood in any wound or part, this is used with some good success; as also to cleanse the foulness of sores, and cause them more speedily to be healed. It is an especial remedy for all green wounds, to solder the lips of them, and to keep the place from any further inconveniencies. The juice hereof used with oil of roses to anoint the temples and forehead, is very effectual to remove headache, and the same mixed with honey of roses, cleanses and heals all ulcers, in the mouth, and throat, and those also in the secret parts. And the proverb of the Germans, French, and others, is verified in this, *that he needs neither physician nor surgeon that hath Self-heal and Sanicle to help himself.*

MODERN USES: Self-heal is a folk remedy used today in many cultures for the same or similar uses as Culpeper describes. Pharmacological studies confirm antiallergenic, antimicrobial, anti-inflammatory, anti-oxidant, immunostimulatory, pain-relieving, and potential anti-diabetic activity, among other effects. In traditional Chinese medicine, the dried flower heads are used to relieve pain and promote blood flow in the treatment of rheumatism, arthritis, sciatica, and traumatic injuries.

SERVICE TREE
(CORMUS DOMESTICA; SYN. SORBUS DOMESTICA)

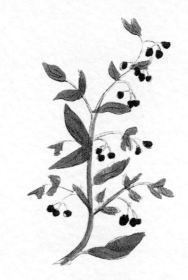

It is so well known in the place where it grows, that it needs no description.

PLACE: [Mostly cultivated, it is a small tree that grows along hedgerows, mountainsides, and roadsides; planted in yards throughout Europe.]

GOVERNMENT AND VIRTUES: Services, when they are mellow, are fit to be taken to stay fluxes, scouring, and casting, yet less than medlars. If they be dried before they be mellow, and kept all the year, they may be used in decoctions for the said purpose, either to drink, or to bathe the parts requiring it; and are profitably used in that manner to stay the bleeding of wounds, and of the mouth or nose, to be applied to the forehead and nape of the neck; and are under the dominion of Saturn.

MODERN USES: Considered inedible until completely ripe, the bitter fruits of the service tree have been traditionally used to stimulate digestion. Once used as a treatment for diarrhea and dysentery. Little used today.

SHEPHERD'S PURSE

(CAPSELLA BURSA-PASTORIS)

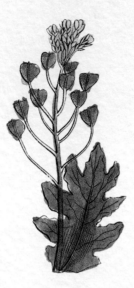

It is called Whoreman's Permacety, Shepherd's Scrip, Shepherd's Pounce, Toy-wort, Pickpurse, and Casewort.

DESCRIPTION: The leaves are small and long, of a pale green colour, and deeply cut in on both sides, among which spring up a stalk [with very small white flowers] after which come the little cases which hold the seed, which are flat [and heart-shaped].

PLACE: [A frequent roadside weed of farms and wastelands throughout Europe, Asia, North America, much of Africa, and South America.]

GOVERNMENT AND VIRTUES: It is under the dominion of Saturn, and of a cold, dry, and binding nature, like to him. It helps all fluxes of blood, either caused by inward or outward wounds; as also flux of the belly, and bloody flux [dysentery], spitting blood, and bloody urine, stops the terms in women; being bound to the wrists of the hands, and the soles of the feet, it helps the yellow jaundice. The herb being made into a poultice, helps inflammations and St. Anthony's fire. The juice being dropped into the ears, heals the pains, noise, and mutterings thereof. A good ointment may be made of it for all wounds, especially wounds in the head.

MODERN USES: Shepherd's purse is one of the best-known herbal hemostatics to stop bleeding both internally and externally. Used for the supportive treatment of excessive menstrual bleeding; applied topically to treat varicose veins; used to stop nosebleeds, staunch wounds, and resolve bruising. Also used in the treatment of edema and hypertension. Has confirmed styptic, antioxidant, anti-inflammatory, and antimicrobial, and effects. **CAUTION:** Avoid use in cases of kidney stones.

....

SILVERWEED

(AGERTINA ANSERINA; SYN. POTENTILLA ANSERINA)

Wild Tansy

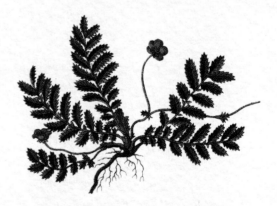

This is also so well-known, that it needs no description. [It has a distinctive silver-green sheen on the underside of finely divided leaves and yellow five-petaled flowers.]

PLACE: It grows in every place [throughout Europe, Asia, and much of northeastern and western North America].

GOVERNMENT AND VIRTUES: Now Dame Venus hath fitted women with two herbs of one name, the one to help conception, and the other to maintain beauty, and what more can be expected of her? What now remains for you, but to love your husbands, and not to be wanting to your poor neighbors? [Silverweed] stays the lask [diarrhea], and all the fluxes of blood in men and women, which some say it will do, if the green herb be worn in the shoes, so it be next the skin; and it is true enough, that it will stop the terms, if worn so, and the whites [vaginal discharges] too, for ought I know. It stays also spitting or vomiting of blood. The powder of the herb taken in some of the distilled water, helps the whites in women, but more especially if a little coral and ivory in powder be put to it. It is also recommended to help children that are bursten, and have a rupture, being boiled in water and salt. Being boiled in water and drank, it eases the griping pains of the bowels, and is good for the sciatica and joint-aches. The same boiled in vinegar, with honey and alum, and gargled in the mouth, eases the pains of the toothache, fastens loose teeth, helps the gums that are sore, and settles the palate of the mouth in its place, when it is fallen down. It cleanses and heals ulcers in the mouth, or secret parts, and is very good for inward wounds, and to close the lips of green wounds, and to heal old, moist, and corrupt running sores in the legs or elsewhere. Being bruised and applied to the soles of the feet and hand wrists, it wonderfully cools the hot fits of agues, be they never so violent. The distilled water cleanses the skin of all discolourings therein, as morphew [blemishes], sun-burnings, etc., as also pimples, freckles, and the like.

MODERN USES: Botanist William Curtis wrote in *Flora Londinensis* in 1777 that silverweed's "Medicinal virtues are wholly out of repute." He did suggest the roots could be a potential hog food. However, the herb has made a comeback in Europe and is a traditional medicine to treat inflammation, wounds, bacterial infections, mild acute diarrhea, and particularly premenstrual syndrome, for which it functions as a calming antispasmodic. **CAUTION:** May increase gastrointestinal irritation.

....

SLOE-BUSH

(*PRUNUS SPINOSA*)

Black Thorn

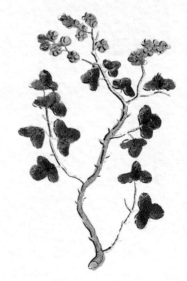

It is so well known, that it needs no description.

PLACE: [A common thorny shrub or small tree found in hedges and borders of fields throughout Europe and western Asia; naturalized in Canada.]

GOVERNMENT AND VIRTUES: All the parts of the Sloe-Bush are binding, cooling, and dry, and all effectual to stay bleeding at the nose and mouth, or any other place; the lask of the belly or stomach, or the bloody flux [dysentery], the too much abounding of women's courses, and helps to ease the pains of the sides, and bowels, that come by overmuch scouring, to drink the decoction of the bark of the roots, or more usually the decoction of the berries, either fresh or dried. The conserve also is of very much use, and more familiarly taken for the purposes aforesaid. The leaves also are good to make lotions to gargle and wash the mouth and throat, wherein are swellings, sores, or kernels; and to stay the defluctions of rheum [watery discharge] to the eyes, or other parts; as also to cool the heat and inflammations of them, and ease hot pains of the head, to bathe the forehead and temples therewith. The simple distilled water of the flowers is very effectual for the said purposes, and the condensate juice of the Sloes. The distilled water of the green berries is used also for the said effects.

MODERN USES: In European phytomedicine, dried sloe-bush flowers are used as an ingredient in preparations for colds, upper respiratory tract infections, gastric disorders (both prevention and treatment), and bladder and kidney spasms. Also used as a diuretic and "blood purifier." Both the fruits and leaves are used as a gargle for sore throat. The fruits are used as a diuretic and a laxative, as well as for convalescing patients with weak stomachs. There is little scientific validation of the claimed uses, though the flowers and fruits of sloe-bush contain antioxidant phenolic compounds. **CAUTION:** May contain hydrogen cyanide, a serious toxin.

....

SOAPWORT

(SAPONARIA OFFICINALIS)

Sopewort, Bruisewort

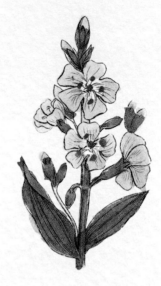

DESCRIPTION: The roots creep underground, shooting forth in diverse places weak round stalks, set with two leaves, set with flowers at the top, made of five [petals] a-piece, round at the ends, and dented in the middle, of a rose colour, almost white, sometimes deeper, sometimes paler; of a reasonable scent.

PLACE: It grows wild in low and wet grounds [throughout most of Europe. Naturalized in Asia, North America, and temperate South America].

GOVERNMENT AND VIRTUES: Venus owns it. The country people in diverse places do use to bruise the leaves of Soapwort, and lay it to their fingers, hands or legs, when they are cut, to heal them up again. Some make great boast thereof, that it is diuretic to provoke urine, and thereby to expel gravel and the stone in the lower back or kidneys, and do also account it singularly good to void hydropical waters: and they no less extol it to perform an absolute cure in the French pox [syphilis], more than either sarsaparilla, guaiacum, or China can do; which, how true it is, I leave others to judge.

MODERN USES: Soapwort contains high levels (up to 8 percent by weight) of saponins in the root, which if agitated in water, create suds, hence the name soapwort. A folk medicine for the treatment of upper respiratory tract infections such as bronchitis. Seldom used in modern herbal medicine, but of research interest for the emulsifying and surfactant properties of the roots, which may have industrial applications in bioremediation of environmental toxins such as diesel fuel.

....

SOLOMON'S SEAL

(POLYGONATUM MULTIFLORUM, POLYGONATUM BIFLORUM)

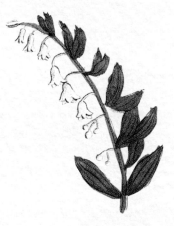

DESCRIPTION: The common Solomon's Seal rises up with a round stalk half a yard high, bowing or bending down to the ground, set with single leaves one above another. At the foot of every leaf, come forth small, long, white and hollow pendulous flowers. The root is of the thickness of one's finger or thumb, white and knotted in some places, a flat round circle representing a Seal, whereof it took the name.

PLACE: [Found in moist, rich, shaded situations, with a native range in most of Europe, eastward to the Caucasus, and the Himalayas. Naturalized in eastern North America or used interchangeably with the North American *Polygonatum biflorum*.]

GOVERNMENT AND VIRTUES: Saturn owns the plant, for he loves his bones well. The root of Solomon's Seal is found by experience to be available in wounds, hurts, and outward sores, to heal and close up the lips of those that are green, and to dry up and restrain the flux of humours to those that are old. It is singularly good to stay vomiting and bleeding wheresoever, as also all fluxes in man or woman; also, to knit any joint, which by weakness uses to be often out of place, or will not stay in long when it is set; also to knit and join broken bones in any part of the body, the roots being bruised and applied to the places; yea, it hath been found by experience, and the decoction of the root in wine, or the bruised root put into wine or other drink, and after a night's infusion, strained forth hard and drank, hath helped both man and beast, whose bones hath been broken by any occasion, which is the most assured refuge of help to people of diverse counties of the land that they can have. It is no less effectual to help ruptures and burstings, the decoction in wine, or the powder in broth or drink, being inwardly taken, and outwardly applied to the place. The same is also available for inward or outward bruises, falls or blows, both to dispel the congealed blood, and to take away both the pains and the black and blue marks that abide after the hurt. The same also, or the distilled water of the whole plant, used to the face, or other parts of the skin, cleanses it from morphew [skin blemishes], freckles, spots, or marks whatsoever, leaving the place fresh, fair, and lovely; for which purpose it is much used by the Italian Dames.

MODERN USES: The root (rhizome) of related species of Solomon's seal are used in traditional Chinese medicine to resolve phlegm due to dry cough, as a blood tonic (strengthener), and to treat diabetes. Traditionally considered astringent, demulcent, and tonic; used for gout and rheumatism. Applied externally to treat wounds. The rhizome is also nibbled on during hikes as a wild edible. **CAUTION:** Do not confuse with lily of the valley, which has cardioactive and potentially dangerous constituents.

....

SORREL

(RUMEX ACETOSA)

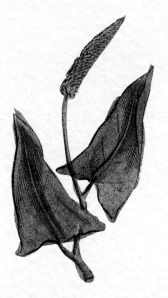

Our ordinary Sorrel, which grows in gardens, and also wild in the fields, is so well known, that it needs no description. [Through centuries of cultivation, sorrel is well-established throughout Europe and temperate Asia; naturalized in most of Canada and the northern United States.]

GOVERNMENT AND VIRTUES: It is under the dominion of Venus. Sorrel is prevalent in all hot diseases, to cool any inflammation and heat of blood in agues pestilential or choleric, or sickness and fainting, arising from heat, and to refresh the overspent spirits with the violence of furious or fiery fits of agues; to quench thirst, and procure an appetite in fainting or decaying stomachs. It resists the putrefaction of the blood, kills worms, and is a cordial to the heart, which the seed doth more effectually, being more drying and binding, and thereby stays the hot fluxes of women's courses, or of humours in the bloody flux [dysentery], or flux of the stomach. The root also in a decoction, or in powder, is effectual for all the said purposes. Both roots and seeds, as well as the herb, are held powerful to resist the poison of the scorpion. The decoction of the roots is taken to help the jaundice, and to expel the gravel and the stone in the kidneys. The decoction of the flowers made with wine and drank, helps the black jaundice, as also the inward ulcers of the body and bowels. A syrup made with the juice of Sorrel and fumitory, is a sovereign help to kill those sharp humours that cause the itch. The juice thereof, with a little vinegar, serves well to be used outwardly for the same cause, and is also profitable for tetters, ringworms, etc. The leaves wrapped in a colewort leaf and roasted in the embers, and applied to a hard imposthume [abscess], boils, or plague sore, doth both ripen and break it. The distilled water of the herb is of much good use for all the purposes aforesaid.

MODERN USES: Sorrel extracts are of research interest for antibacterial activity (for the prevention of periodontitis and inhibition of the influenza virus) and antioxidant activity of proanthocyanidins in the leaves. Mostly used in small amounts as a specialty vegetable. The bitter-sour flavor of the leaves is due to high oxalic acid content. Not widely used today.

....

SOUTHERNWOOD

(ARTEMISIA ABROTANUM)

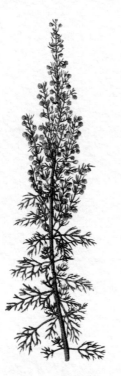

Southern Wood is so well known to be an ordinary inhabitant in our gardens, that I shall not need to trouble you with any description thereof. [Cultivated in herb gardens for many centuries; origin unknown.]

GOVERNMENT AND VIRTUES: It is a gallant mercurial plant, worthy of more esteem than it hath. The oil thereof anointed on the back-bone before the fits of agues come, takes them away. Boiled with barley-meal it takes away pimples, pushes or wheals that arise in the face, or other parts of the body. The herb bruised and laid to, helps to draw forth splinters and thorns out of the flesh. The ashes thereof dries up and heals old ulcers, that are without inflammation, although by the sharpness thereof it bites sore, and puts them to sore pains; as also the sores in the private parts of man or woman. The ashes mingled with old salad oil, helps those that have hair fallen, and are bald, causing the hair to grow again either on the head or beard. Daranters saith, That the oil made of Southernwood, and put among the ointments that are used against the French disease [syphilis], is very effectual, and likewise kills lice in the head. The distilled water of the herb is said to help them much that are troubled with the stone, as also for the diseases of the spleen and mother. The Germans commend it for a singular wound herb, and therefore call it Stabwort. It is held by all writers, ancient and modern, to be more offensive to the stomach than Wormwood.

MODERN USES: A pleasantly aromatic *Artemisia*, southernwood is seldom used except in small amounts as an aromatic bitter. Once used to flavor beers. Bundles of the dried herb are sometimes used as an insect repellant in clothing dressers. Contains antioxidant polyphenols and components with strong antifungal and antispasmodic activity, among other effects. A nasal spray for the treatment of allergic rhinitis has been developed from southernwood extracts. Traditionally used as a folk medicine for the treatment of worms and fevers. **CAUTION:** May cause allergic reactions or contact dermatitis in some individuals.

....

SOW THISTLES

(SONCHUS ASPER, SONCHUS OLERACEUS)

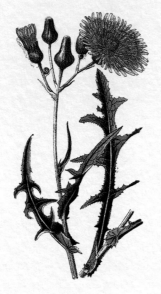

Sow Thistles are generally so well known, that they need no description.

PLACE: They grow near gardens [and in fields. Originating in Eurasia, the sow thistles (*Sonchus* spp.) are among the most successful weeds worldwide.]

GOVERNMENT AND VIRTUES: This is under the influence of Venus. Sow Thistles are cooling, and somewhat binding, and are very fit to cool a hot stomach, and ease the pains thereof. The herb boiled in wine, is very helpful to stay the dissolution of the stomach, and the milk that is taken from the stalks when they are broken, given in drink, is beneficial to those that are short winded, and have wheezing. Pliny saith, that it caused the gravel and stone to be voided by urine, and that the eating thereof helps a stinking breath. The decoction of the leaves and stalks causes abundance of milk in nurses, and their children to be well coloured. The juice or distilled water is good for all hot inflammations, wheals, and eruptions or heat in the skin, itching of the hemorrhoids. It is wonderful good for women to wash their faces with, to clear the skin, and give it a lustre.

MODERN USES: Leaves of various sow thistles are used topically as cooling, anti-inflammatory poultices for wounds and sores. *Sochus arvensis* has been studied for antioxidant, antibacterial, and liver-protective effects. Used as a folk medicine for liver and kidney disorders, asthma, and oxidative stress to the liver. Seldom used.

....

SPIGNEL

(MEUM ATHAMANTICUM)

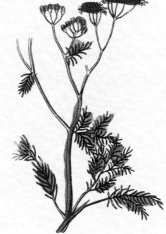

DESCRIPTION: The roots of common Spignel do spread much and deep in the ground, from whence rise long stalks of most fine cut leaves like hair, smaller than dill, set thick on both sides of the stalks, and of a good scent. Among these leaves rise up round stiff stalks, with a few joints and leaves on them, and at the tops an umbel of pure white flowers.

PLACE: It grows wild and is also planted in gardens. [Originating in Western and central Europe and Morocco.]

GOVERNMENT AND VIRTUES: It is an herb of Venus. Galen saith, the roots of Spignel are available to provoke urine, and women's courses; but if too much thereof be taken, it causes head-ache. The roots boiled in wine or water, and drank, helps the strangury and stoppings of the urine, the wind, swellings and pains in the stomach, pains of the mother, and all joint-aches. If the powder of the root be mixed with honey, and the same taken as a licking medicine, it breaks tough phlegm, and dries up the rheum [watery discharge] that falls on the lungs. The roots are accounted very effectual against the stinging or biting of any venomous creature.

MODERN USES: A little used or researched aromatic member of the carrot family, spignel is a folk medicine for rheumatism. **CAUTION:** May cause photodermatitis or contact dermatitis in some individuals.

....

STAR THISTLE
(CENTAUREA CALCITRAPA)

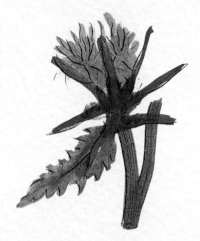

DESCRIPTION: Star Thistle has narrow leaves lying next the ground, cut on the edges somewhat deeply into many parts [with] small whitish green heads, set with sharp white pricks [with many small purple flowers in heads].

PLACE: It grows wild in the fields. [A weedy thistle found throughout Europe and the Middle East; naturalized in North America, arriving in ballast from sailing ships.]

GOVERNMENT AND VIRTUES: This, as almost all Thistles are, is under Mars. The seed of this Star Thistle made into powder, and drank in wine, provokes urine, and helps to break the stone, and drives it forth. The root in powder, and given in wine and drank, is good against the plague and pestilence; and drank in the morning fasting for some time together, it is very profitable for fistulas in any part of the body. Baptista Sardas doth much commend the distilled water thereof, being drank, to help the French disease [syphilis], to open the obstructions of the liver, and cleanse the blood from corrupted humours, and is profitable against the quotidian or tertian ague [malaria].

MODERN USES: Star thistle has historically been used as a balsamic tonic for intermittent fevers. Still found in local markets in Sicily, the young leaves are eaten as a wild food, boiled then eaten with olive oil. An enzyme from the plant is suggested as a possible vegetarian alternative to rennet to produce high-quality cheeses.

....

STONECROP

(SEDUM ACRE)

Prick–Madam, Small–Houseleek, Wall Pepper

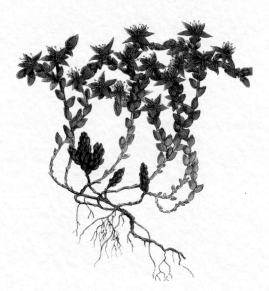

DESCRIPTION: It grows with trailing branches, set with many thick, flat, roundish, leaves with [yellow, star-shaped] flowers.

PLACE: It grows upon the stone walls and mud walls, and in gravelly places. [Found throughout Europe and North Africa; naturalized in North America and South America. A common garden succulent.]

GOVERNMENT AND VIRTUES: It is under the dominion of the Moon, cold in quality, and binding, and therefore very good to stay defluctions, especially such as fall upon the eyes. It stops bleeding, both inward and outward, helps cankers, and all fretting sores and ulcers; it abates the heat of choler [bile]. It expels poison much, resists pestilential fevers, being exceeding good also for tertian agues [intermittent fevers; malaria]: You may drink the decoction of it, if you please, for all the foregoing infirmities. It is so harmless an herb, you can scarce use it amiss [but Culpeper misses the fact that it is irritating and acrid]: Being bruised and applied to the place, it helps the king's evil, and any other knots or kernels in the flesh; as also the piles.

MODERN USES: At first has a bland taste but beomes acrid due to piperidine alkaloids, hence the name "wall pepper." Once used as an emetic and purgative. Fresh leaves were formerly applied to cancerous sores and warts. Seldom used today. **CAUTION:** Topical application may cause irritation and blistering. May irritate the gastrointestinal tract.

....

STRAWBERRIES

(FRAGARIA VESCA)

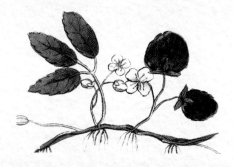

These are so well known through this land, that they need no description.

PLACE: [Found in field edges and open woods throughout Europe, much of Asia, and eastern North America.]

GOVERNMENT AND VIRTUES: Venus owns the herb. Strawberries, when they are green, are cool and dry; but when they are ripe, they are cool and moist: The berries are excellently good to cool the liver, the blood, and the spleen, or an hot choleric stomach; to refresh and comfort the fainting spirits, and quench thirst. They are good also for other inflammations. The leaves and roots boiled in wine and water, and drank, do likewise cool the liver and blood, and assuage all inflammations in the kidneys and bladder, provoke urine, and allay the heat and sharpness thereof. The same also being drank stays the bloody flux [dysentery] and women's courses, and helps the swelling of the spleen. The water of the berries carefully distilled, is a sovereign remedy and cordial in the panting and beating of the heart, and is good for the yellow jaundice. The juice dropped into foul ulcers, or they washed therewith, or the decoction of the herb and root, doth wonderfully cleanse and help to cure them. Lotions and gargles for sore mouths, or ulcers therein, or in the private parts or elsewhere, are made with the leaves and roots thereof; which is also good to fasten loose teeth, and to heal spongy foul gums. It helps also to stay catarrhs, or defluctions of rheum [watery discharge] in the mouth, throat, teeth, or eyes. It is also of excellent property for all pushes, wheals and other breakings forth of hot and sharp humours in the face and hands, and other parts of the body, to bathe them therewith, and to take away any redness in the face, or spots, or other deformities in the skin, and to make it clear and smooth.

MODERN USES: Wild strawberries are collected in various parts of eastern Europe. The European wild strawberry crosses the line between food and medicine. Traditionally, the astringent leaves have been used for diarrhea, dysentery, and to stop bleeding. The fruits are antioxidant, antiscorbutic, diuretic, and considered a digestive tonic. A folk medicine eaten as a preventative for gout.

....

SUNDEW
(DROSERA ROTUNDIFOLIA)

Rosa Solis, Sun Dew

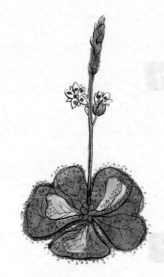

It is likewise called Red-rot, and Youth-wort.

DESCRIPTION: It hath, diverse small, round leaves, full of certain red hairs. The leaves are continually moist in the hottest day, yea, the hotter the sun shines on them, the moister they are, with a sliminess that will rope (as we say,) the small hairs always holding the moisture.

PLACE: It grows usually in bogs and wet places, and sometimes in moist woods [throughout the Northern Hemisphere].

GOVERNMENT AND VIRTUES: The Sun rules it, and it is under the sign Cancer. Sundew is accounted good to help those that have a salt rheum [watery discharge] distilling on their lungs, which breeds a consumption, and therefore the distilled water thereof in wine is held fit and profitable for such to drink, which water will be of a good yellow colour. The same water is held to be good for all other diseases of the lungs, as phthisic [tuberculosis], wheezing, shortness of breath, or the cough; as also to heal the ulcers that happen in the lungs; and it comforts the heart and fainting spirits. The leaves, outwardly applied to the skin will raise blisters, which has caused some to think it dangerous to be taken inwardly.

MODERN USES: A tiny, insectivorous plant, sundew is seldom used because of conservation concerns over sustainable sources. Considered antitussive and antispasmodic with antibacterial, antifungal, and antiviral activity. Used in preparations for excessive coughing and dry cough.

....

SWEET CICELY

(*MYRRHIS ODORATA*)

Sweet Chervil

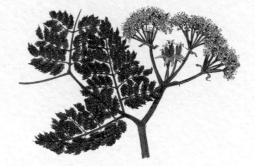

DESCRIPTION: This grows very like the great hemlock, having large spread leaves cut into diverse parts, but of a fresher green colour than the Hemlock, tasting as sweet as the Aniseed. At the tops of the branched stalks [are] umbels of white flowers; after which comes long crested black shining seed, sweet and pleasant.

PLACE: [Native to meadows and field edges in the Alps, Pyrenees, and the Apennine Mountains, extending to the Balkan peninsula. Widely naturalized elsewhere in western Europe, where it has been grown in gardens for centuries.]

GOVERNMENT AND VIRTUES: These are all three of them of the nature of Jupiter, and under his dominion. This whole plant, besides its pleasantness in salads, has its physical virtue. The root boiled, and eaten with oil and vinegar, (or without oil) do much please and warm old and cold stomachs oppressed with wind or phlegm, or those that have the phthisic or consumption of the lungs. The same drank with wine is a preservation from the plague. It provokes women's courses, procures an appetite to meat, and expels wind. The juice is good to heal the ulcers of the head and face; the candied root hereof are held as effectual as Angelica, to preserve from infection in the time of a plague, and to warm and comfort a cold weak stomach.

MODERN USES: A common plant in herb gardens, sweet cicely has a pleasant flavor and fragrance due to the anethole content of the essential oil, which gives it the scent and taste we have come to associate with "licorice flavor." The leaves and seeds (fruits) are traditionally used for their mild expectorant, carminative, stomachic, and diuretic qualities. A tea of the roots is used to allay coughs and as a diuretic. **CAUTION:** Do not confuse with poison hemlock.

....

SWEET MARJORAM

(ORIGANUM MAJORANA)

Pot Marjoram

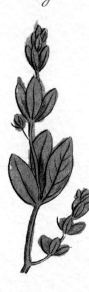

Sweet Marjoram is so well known, being an inhabitant in every garden, that it is needless to write any description thereof, neither of the Winter Sweet Marjoram, or Pot Marjoram.

PLACE: They grow commonly in gardens; some sorts grow wild in the borders of corn fields and pastures, in sundry places of this land; but it is not my purpose to insist upon them. The garden kinds being most used and useful.

GOVERNMENT AND VIRTUES: It is an herb of Mercury, and under Aries, and therefore is an excellent remedy for the brain and other parts of the body and mind, under the dominion of the same planet. Our common Sweet Marjoram is warming and comfortable in cold diseases of the head, stomach, sinews, and other parts, taken inwardly, or outwardly applied. The decoction thereof being drank, helps all diseases of the chest which hinder the freeness of breathing, and is also profitable for the obstructions of the liver and spleen. It helps the cold griefs of the womb, and the windiness thereof, and the loss of speech, by resolution of the tongue. Being made into powder, and mixed with honey, it takes away the black marks of blows, and bruises, being thereunto applied. It is profitably put into those ointments and salves that are warm, and comfort the outward parts, as the joints and sinews; for swellings also, and places out of joint. The powder thereof chewed in the mouth, draws forth much phlegm. The oil made thereof, is very warm and comfortable to the joints that are stiff, and the sinews that are hard, to mollify and supple them. Marjoram is much used in all odoriferous water, powders, &c. that are for ornament or delight.

MODERN USES: Used similarly to oregano (pages 172–73).

....

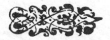

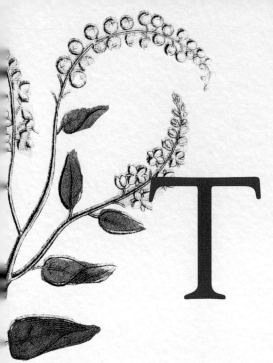

T

TAMARISK
(TAMARIX GALLICA, TAMARIX AFRICANA)

It is so well known in the place where it grows, that it needs no description.

PLACE: [Introduced in England at an early date, both species are from sandy soils near coastal areas in the Mediterranean region.]

GOVERNMENT AND VIRTUES: A gallant Saturnine herb it is. The root, leaves, young branches, or bark boiled in wine, and drank, stays the bleeding of the hemorrhoidal veins, the spitting of blood, the too abounding of women's courses, the jaundice, the cholic, and the biting of all venomous serpents, except the asp [Egyptian cobra]; and outwardly applied, is very powerful against the hardness of the spleen, and toothache, pains in the ears, red and watering eyes. The decoction, with some honey put thereto, is good to stay gangrenes and fretting ulcers, and to wash those that are subject to nits and lice. Alpinus and Veslingius affirm, That the Egyptians do with good success use the wood of it to cure the French disease [syphilis], and give it also to those who have the leprosy, scabs, ulcers, or the like. Its ashes doth quickly heal blisters raised by burnings or scaldings. It helps the dropsy, arising from the hardness of the spleen, and therefore to drink out of cups made of the wood is good for splenetic persons. It is also helpful for melancholy, and the black jaundice that arise thereof.

MODERN USES: Growing in marginal sandy soils, tamarisk is traditionally used for liver disorders and marketed widely in the Middle East. Science confirms strong antioxidant activity, and antioxidant flavonoids from the plant have been of research interest to inhibit amyloid cell aggregation (associated with the development of Alzheimer's disease). Also of research interest in type 2 diabetes. A folk cancer remedy of research interest in potential inhibition of cancer cell growth.

....

TANSY

(*TANACETUM VULGARE*;
SYN. *CHRYSANTHEMUM VULGARE*)

Garden Tansy

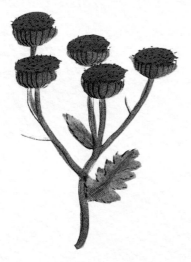

Garden Tansy is so well known, that it needs no description. [Commonly grown in herb gardens; found in fields through Europe, Asia, and in cooler parts of North America.]

GOVERNMENT AND VIRTUES: Dame Venus was minded to pleasure women with child by this herb, for there grows not an herb, fitter for their use than this is; it is just as though it were cut out for the purpose. This herb bruised and applied to the navel, stays miscarriages; I know no herb like it for that use: Boiled in ordinary beer, and the decoction drank, doth the like; and if her womb be not as she would have it, this decoction will make it so. Let those women that desire children love this herb, it is their best companion, their husbands excepted. Also it consumes the phlegmatic humours, the cold and moist constitution of Winter most usually affects the body of man with, and that was the first reason of eating tansies in the Spring. The decoction of the common Tansy, or the juice drank in wine, is a singular remedy for all the griefs that come by slopping of the urine, helps the strangury and those that have weak kidneys. It is also very profitable to dissolve and expel wind in the stomach, belly, or bowels, to procure women's courses, and expel windiness in the matrix, if it be bruised and often smelled unto, as also applied to the lower part of the belly. It is used also against the stone in the kidneys, especially to men. The herb fried with eggs (as it is the custom in the Spring-time) which is called a Tansy, helps to digest and carry downward those bad humours that trouble the stomach. The seed is very profitably given to children for the worms, and the juice in drink is as effectual. Being boiled in oil, it is good for the sinews shrunk by cramps, or pained with colds, if thereto applied.

MODERN USES: Tansy was once widely used for various menstrual problems and as a worm expellant, carminative, and antispasmodic. Used sparingly to treat roundworm or threadworm in children.

A weak tea has been used to increase appetite and digestion. Pharmacological activities include anti-inflammatory, immunostimulatory, and antibacterial effects, among others. Various chemotypes with different chemical compositions in the essential oil thwart proper dosage. **CAUTION:** The essential oil is considered toxic (fatalities have been reported) and is prohibited from food use. Tansy can cause contact dermatitis. Contraindicated during pregnancy and lactation due to toxicity, despite Culpeper's musings to the contrary.

....

TEASEL

(DIPSACUS FULLONUM, DIPSACUS SATIVUS)

Fuller's Thistle, or Teasel

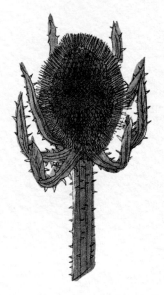

[Garden Teasel (*Dipsacus sativus*)] is so well known, that it needs no description. [The seed heads are] used by clothworkers. The wild Teasel (*Dipsacus fullonum*) is in all things like the former, but that the prickles are small, soft, and upright,

not hooked or stiff, and the flowers are of a fine blueish, or pale carnation colour.

PLACE: The Garden Teasel grows, in gardens or fields for the use of clothworkers: The other [grows wild near ditches. Teasels are of Eurasian origin and are widespread weeds elsewhere.]

GOVERNMENT AND VIRTUES: It is an herb of Venus. Dioscorides saith, That the root bruised and boiled in wine, till it be thick, and kept in a brazen vessel, and after spread as a salve, and applied to the fundament, doth heal the cleft thereof, cankers and fistulas therein, also takes away warts and wens. The juice of the leaves dropped into the ears, kills worms in them. The distilled water of the leaves is often used by women to preserve their beauty, and to take away redness and inflammations, and all other heat or discolourings.

MODERN USES: Teasel has traditionally been used as a diuretic and as an astringent for the treatment of diarrhea. The root is used as a digestive stimulant. Seldom used today. The dried seed heads were historically used for dressing or finishing of cloth. The genus name *Dipsacus* means "beautifying," which relates to the use of the seed heads in raising the nap or "fulling" (cleaning) of woven cloth, especially wool. The process is also called *teaseling*.

....

THYME

(THYMUS VULGARIS)

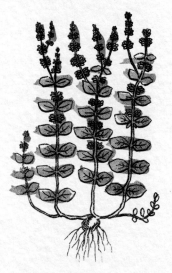

It is in vain to describe an herb so commonly known. [Native to gravelly soils in France, Spain, and Italy; widely planted and naturalized elsewhere.]

GOVERNMENT AND VIRTUES: It is a noble strengthener of the lungs, as notable a one as grows; neither is there scarce a better remedy growing for that disease in children which they commonly call the Chin-cough, than it is. It purges the body of phlegm, and is an excellent remedy for shortness of breath. It kills worms in the belly, and being a notable herb of Venus, provokes the terms. An ointment made of it takes away hot swellings and warts, helps the sciatica and dullness of sight, and takes away pains and hardness of the spleen. 'Tis excellent for those that are troubled with the gout. It eases pains in the loins and hips. The herb taken any way inwardly, comforts the stomach much, and expels wind.

MODERN USES: As in Culpeper's day, thyme is associated with treatments for lung conditions. It is used for bronchitis, whooping cough (pertussis), and general catarrhs of the upper respiratory tract. A tea of the herb is also used as a digestive carminative. Also used as a folk remedy to regulate the menses. Pharmacologically, it acts as an antispasmodic on the bronchial passages and is expectorant, antibacterial, antioxidant, and antitussive. **CAUTION:** Contraindicated during pregnancy.

....

THYME, WILD

(THYMUS SERPYLLUM)

Mother of Thyme

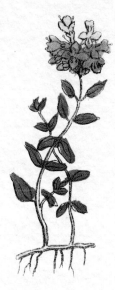

Wild Thyme also is so well known, that it needs no description.

PLACE: It may be found commonly [in fields and rocky areas throughout temperate Europe and cooler regions of Asia. Dozens of species of wild thyme are collectively used in a similar manner to *Thymus serpyllum*, many now aggregated under *Thymus pulegioides* or *Thymus polytrichus*.]

GOVERNMENT AND VIRTUES: It is under the dominion of Venus, and under the sign Aries, and therefore chiefly appropriated to the head. It provokes urine and the terms, and eases the griping pain of the belly, cramps, ruptures, and inflammation of the liver. If you make a vinegar of the herb, as vinegar of roses is made (you may find out the way in my translation of the London Dispensatory) and anoint the head with it, it presently stops the pains thereof. It is excellently good to be given either in phrenzy or lethargy, although they are two contrary diseases: It helps spitting and voiding of blood, coughing, and vomiting; it comforts and strengthens the head, stomach, kidneys, and womb, expels wind, and breaks the stone.

MODERN USES: Used similarly to thyme, but considered weaker. Traditionally used as a stomachic, expectorant, antitussive, antioxidant, antibacterial, and a mild diuretic. Used externally for bruises, sprains, and rheumatic complaints. Mostly used as a calming digestive tea to relieve flatulence or bloating. Sometimes an ingredient in cough drops or cough syrups.

....

TOADFLAX

(*LINARIA VULGARIS*)

Butter–and–Eggs, Flaxweed

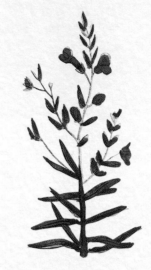

DESCRIPTION: Our common [toadflax] has diverse stalks full fraught with long and narrow ash-coloured leaves, and from the middle of them almost upward, a number of pale-yellow flowers, of a strong unpleasant scent.

PLACE: Grows throughout [Europe in meadows and fields; widely naturalized in eastern North America].

GOVERNMENT AND VIRTUES: Mars owns the herb: In Sussex we call it Gallwort, and lay it in our chicken's water to cure them of the gall; it relieves them when they are drooping. This is frequently used to spend the abundance of those watery humours by urine which cause the dropsy. The decoction of the herb, both leaves and flowers, in wine, taken and drank, doth somewhat move the belly downwards, opens obstructions of the liver, and helps the yellow jaundice; expels poison. The distilled water of the herb and flowers is effectual for all the same purposes; being drank with a dram of the powder of the seeds of bark or the roots of

Wallwort, and a little Cinnamon, it is held a singular remedy for the dropsy. The juice or water put into foul ulcers, whether they be cancerous or fistulous, with tents rolled therein, or parts washed and injected therewith, cleanses them thoroughly from the bottom, and heals them up safely. The same juice or water also cleanses the skin of all sorts of deformity, as leprosy, morphew [skin blemishes], scurf, wheals, pimples, or spots, applied of itself, or used with some powder of Lupines.

MODERN USES: Toadflax leaf tea was formerly used as a folk medicine for its laxative and diuretic effect. A flower ointment was used externally for hemorrhoids and skin blemishes. Allergy-preventative, antioxidant, and fever-reducing effects are also reported. **CAUTION:** Contains potentially toxic components.

....

TOBACCO
(NICOTIANA RUSTICA)

English Tobacco

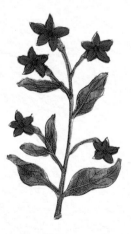

DESCRIPTION: This rises up with a round thick stalk, about two feet high, whereon do grow thick, flat green leaves, nothing so large as the other Indian kind [*Nicotiana tabacum*]. The stalk branches forth, and bear at the tops flowers of a greenish yellow colour.

PLACE: [Widely diffused throughout the Americas before the arrival of Europeans, tobacco may have originated in Peru. Cultivated in Mexico before the Spanish conquest. *Nicotiana rustica* is the tobacco species first seen by English colonists in Virginia. To quote Culpeper's contemporary William Coles, from his book *Adam in Eden* (1657), "English tobacco, which is so called (not for that it is natural in England, but) because it is more common with us growing in every country Garden almost, and endureth better here than the other."]

GOVERNMENT AND VIRTUES: It is a martial plant. It is found by good experience to be available to expectorate tough phlegm from the stomach, chest, and lungs. The juice thereof made into a syrup, or the distilled water of the herb drank with some sugar, or without, if you will, or the smoke taken by a pipe, as is usual, but fainting, helps to expel worms in the stomach and belly, and to ease the pains in the head, or megrim [depression], and the griping pains in the bowels. It is profitable for those that are troubled with the stone in the kidneys, both to ease the pains by provoking urine, and also to expel gravel and the stone engendered therein, and hath been found very effectual to expel windiness, and other humours, which cause the strangling of the mother. The seed hereof is very effectual to expel the toothache, and the ashes of the burnt herb to cleanse the gums, and make the teeth white. The herb bruised and applied to the place grieved with the king's evil [unusual swelling of lymph nodes or scrofula], helps it in nine or ten days effectually. Monardes saith, it is a counter poison against the biting of any venomous creature, the herb also being outwardly applied to the hurt place. The distilled water is often given with some sugar before the fit of an ague [malaria], to lessen it, and take it away in three or four times using. The juice is also good to kill lice in children's heads. The green herb bruised and applied to any green wounds, cures any fresh wound or cut whatsoever: and the juice put into old sores, both cleanses and heals them. There is also made hereof a singularly good salve to help imposthumes [abscesses], hard tumours, and other swellings by blows and falls.

MODERN USES: The plant Culpeper calls "English Tobacco" is the small, yellow-flowered *Nicotiana rustica*, rather than the familiar, six-foot tall, pink-flowered "Indian tobacco" (*Nicotiana tabacum*), the commercial source of tobacco. Culpeper is perhaps the only author to claim that the ashes of tobacco can "make the teeth white." Do not expect to see it as an ingredient in teeth-whitening products anytime soon! The former is considered milder than common tobacco, though it is acrid and contains nicotine and related alkaloids. **CAUTION:** The dangers of tobacco use in any form are well-known worldwide.

. . . .

TORMENTIL

(*POTENTILLA ERECTA; SYN. TOMATILLO ERECTA*)

Septfoil

DESCRIPTION: This hath reddish, slender, weak branches rising from the root, lying on the ground, whereof [the leaves] are like cinquefoil, but somewhat long, [divided into five to seven leaflets]. At the tops of the branches stand diverse small five-petalled yellow flowers.

PLACE: It grows as well in woods and shady places [in most of Europe and western Asia].

GOVERNMENT AND VIRTUES: This is a gallant herb of the Sun. Tormentil is most excellent to stay all kind of fluxes of blood or humours in man or woman, whether at nose, mouth, or belly. The root taken inwardly is most effectual to help any flux of the belly, stomach, spleen, or blood; and the juice wonderfully opens obstructions of the liver and lungs, and thereby helps the yellow jaundice. The powder or decoction drank, or to sit thereon as a bath, is an assured remedy against abortion, if it proceed from the over flexibility or weakness of the inward retentive faculty; as also a plaster made therewith, and vinegar applied to the lower back, doth much help not only this, but also those that cannot hold their water, the powder being taken in the juice of plantain, and is also commended against the worms in children. It is very powerful in ruptures and burstings, as also for bruises and falls, to be used as well outwardly as inwardly. Tormentil is no less effectual and powerful a remedy against outward wounds, sores and hurts, than for inward, and is therefore a special ingredient to be used in wound drinks, lotions and injections, for foul corrupt rotten sores and ulcers of the mouth, secrets, or other parts of the body. The juice or powder of the root put in ointments, plasters, and such things that are to be applied to wounds or sores, is very effectual, as the juice of the leaves and the root bruised and applied to the throat or jaws, heals the king's evil [unusual swelling of lymph nodes or scrofula], and eases the pain of the sciatica. The same used with a little vinegar, is a special remedy against the running sores of the head or other parts; scabs also, and the itch or any such eruptions in the skin, proceeding of salt and sharp humours. The same is also effectual for the piles or hemorrhoids, if they be washed or bathed therewith, or with the distilled water of the herb and roots. It is found also helpful to dry up any sharp rheum [watery discharge] that distills from the head into the eyes, causing redness, pain, waterings, itching, or the like, if a little prepared tutia, or white amber, be used with the distilled water thereof. And here is enough, only remember the Sun challenges this herb.

MODERN USES: Dried tormentil root is used to check bleeding internally and externally, and because it is very astringent (containing about 7 percent tannins and flavonoids), it is used to treat acute diarrhea or dysentery. A tea is used as a gargle or wash for inflammation of the mouth, gums,

or sore throat. Used exernally for slow-to-heal wounds and hemorrhoids. Pharmacologically, it has antiviral, antimicrobial, anti-inflammatory, immunostimulant, and antioxidant effects.

....

TURNSOLE, OR HELIOTROPIUM

(HELIOTROPIUM EUROPAEUM; SYN. HELIOTROPIUM MAJUS)

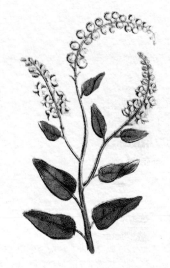

DESCRIPTION: The greater Turnsole rises with one upright stalk, about a foot high, [with] diverse small branches, of a hoary colour; [with] small broad [hoary white] leaves. At the tops [are] small white flowers, set in order one above another, upon a small crooked spike, which turns inwards like a bowed finger.

PLACE: It grows in gardens [native to disturbed ground in southern Europe and through central Asia, India, and North Africa].

GOVERNMENT AND VIRTUES: It is an herb of the Sun,

and a good one too. Dioscorides saith, that a good handful of this, which is called the Great Turnsole, boiled in water, and drank, purges both choler [bile] and phlegm; and boiled with cumin, helps the stone in the kidneys, or bladder, provokes urine and women's courses. The leaves bruised and applied to places pained with the gout, or that have been out of joint and newly set, and full of pain, do give much ease; the seed and juice of the leaves also being rubbed with a little salt upon warts and wens, and other kernels in the face, eye-lids, or any other part of the body, will, by often using, take them away.

MODERN USES: Not used today. **CAUTION:** In 1974, an epidemic outbreak of veno-occlusive liver disease occurred in Afghanistan, affecting over 7,800 people and resulting in 1,600 deaths because a wheat bread was contaminated with heliotrope seeds (*Heliotropium gillianum*). After this tragic outbreak, scientists looked at the pyrrolizidine alkaloids in other members of the borage family, such as comfrey, leading to the current toxicological science warning against consuming plants that contain these insidious liver toxins (found in 3 percent of flowering plants, or about six thousand plant species).

....

TUSTAN

(*HYPERICUM ANDROSAEMUM*)

Park Leaves

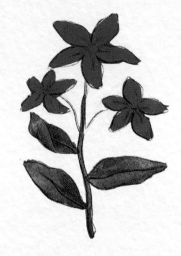

DESCRIPTION: It hath brownish shining round stalks, rising two by two, and sometimes three feet high, [with] two fair large leaves standing, of a dark blueish green colour on the upper side, and of a yellowish green underneath, turning reddish toward Autumn. At the top of the stalks stand large yellow flowers, and heads with seed.

PLACE: It grows in many [damp] woods, groves, and woody grounds, as parks and forests, and by hedge-sides. [Cultivated and escaped in the British Isles; from west and southwest Europe, the Caucasus, and northwest Africa; naturalized in scattered locations from California to British Columbia. John Parkinson in *Theatrum Botanicum* (1640) writes, "Some call it Parke leaves, because it is so familiar to parkes and woods, that it almost groweth no where else."]

GOVERNMENT AND VIRTUES: It is an herb of Saturn, and a most noble anti-venereal. Tustan purges choleric humours, as St. Peter's-wort, is said to do, for therein it works the same effects, both to help the sciatica and gout, and to heal burning by fire; it stays all the bleedings of wounds, if either the green herb be bruised, or the powder of the dry be applied thereto. It hath been accounted, and certainly it is, a sovereign herb to heal either wound or sore, either outwardly or inwardly, and therefore always used in drinks, lotions, balms, oils, ointments, or any other sorts of green wounds, ulcers, or old sores, in all which the continual experience of former ages hath confirmed the use thereof to be admirably good, though it be not so much in use now, as when physicians and surgeons were so wise as to use herbs more than now they do.

MODERN USES: Tustan is seldom used today, though Culpeper describes topical uses for this plant generally associated with common St.-John's-wort (*Hypericum perforatum*). A water extract of the plant's berry-like fruits has been shown to have experimental antioxidant and antidepressant effects. The fruits have shown potential to improve skin regeneration.

....

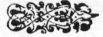

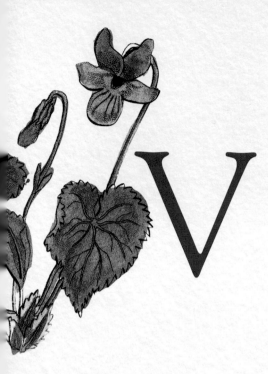

V

VALERIAN
(VALERIANA OFFICINALIS)
Garden Valerian

DESCRIPTION: From the head of these roots spring up many green leaves; and those upon a stalk with many small whitish flowers, sometimes with a pale purplish colour. The root smells stronger than either leaf or flower.

PLACE: It is generally in gardens. [Native to fields and forest edges throughout most of Europe; an herb garden plant naturalized in the British Isles. Introduced to North America and naturalized in the Northeast.]

GOVERNMENT AND VIRTUES: This is under the influence of Mercury. The decoction thereof taken, doth the like also, and takes away pains of the sides, provokes women's courses, and is used in antidotes. The root of Valerian boiled with licorice, raisins, and aniseed, is singularly good for those that are short-winded, and for those that are troubled with the cough, and helps to open the passages, and to expectorate phlegm easily. It is given to those that are bitten or stung by any venomous creature, being boiled in wine. It is of a special virtue against the plague, the decoction thereof being drank, and the root being used to smell too. It helps to expel the wind in the belly. The green herb with the root taken fresh, being bruised and applied to the head, takes away the pains and prickings there, stays rheum [watery discharge] and thin distillation, and being boiled in white wine, and a drop thereof put into the eyes, takes away the dimness of the sight, or any pin or web therein. It is of excellent property to heal any inward sores or wounds, and also for outward hurts or wounds, and drawing away splinters or thorns out of the flesh.

MODERN USES: Valerian may not be a cure for the plague, but just might help those suffering from insomnia. It is one of most widely used herbs for the treatment of insomnia, excitability, and nervous exhaustion. The fresh or dried root is used in commercial preparations standardized to valarenic acid content. Several controlled clinical studies on the safety and efficacy of valerian extract have shown generally positive but mixed results. Studies suggest that rather than using valerian occasionally for acute sleeplessless, consistent use for four weeks improves sleep disturbance patterns and daily mood, without the next-day hangover effect that many prescription sleep aids have. **CAUTION:** May cause stomach upset. Avoid during pregnancy and lactation.

....

VERVAIN
(*VERBENA OFFICINALIS*)

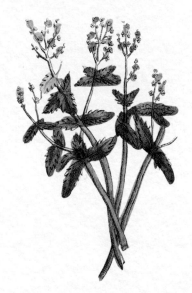

DESCRIPTION: The common Vervain hath somewhat long broad leaves next the ground deeply gashed about the edges. The stalk is square, rising about two feet high [with spikes of small blue to white flowers].

PLACE: It grows [near hedges] and way-sides, and other waste grounds. [Native to most of Europe, Asia, Africa, Australia; naturalized in North America and South America.]

GOVERNMENT AND VIRTUES: This is an herb of Venus, and excellent for the womb to strengthen and remedy all the cold griefs of it, as Plantain doth the hot. Vervain is hot and dry, opening obstructions, cleansing and healing. It helps the yellow jaundice, the dropsy and the gout; it kills and expels worms in the belly, and causes a good colour in the face and body, strengthens as well as corrects the diseases of the stomach, liver, and spleen; helps the cough, wheezing, and shortness of breath, and all the defects of the kidneys and bladder, expelling the gravel and stone. It is held to be good against the biting of serpents, and other venomous beasts, against the plague, and both tertian and quartan agues [malaria]. It consolidates and heals also all wounds, both inward and outward, stays bleedings, and used with some honey, heals all old ulcers and fistulas in the legs or other parts of the body; as also those ulcers that happen in the mouth; or used with hog's grease, it helps the swellings and pains of the secret parts in man or woman, also for the piles or hemorrhoids; applied with some oil of roses and vinegar unto the forehead and temples, it eases the inveterate pains and ache of the head, and is good for those that are frantic. The leaves bruised, or the juice of them mixed with some vinegar, doth wonderfully cleanse the skin, and takes away morphew [skin blemishes], freckles, fistulas, and other such like inflammations and deformities of the skin in any parts of the body. The distilled water of the herb when it is in full strength, dropped into the eyes, cleanses them from films, clouds, or mists, that darken the sight, and wonderfully strengthens the optic nerves. The said water is very powerful in all the diseases aforesaid, either inward or outward, whether they be old corroding sores, or green wounds. The dried root, and peeled, is known to be excellently good against all scrophulous and scorbutic habits of body, by being tied to the pit of the stomach, by a piece of white ribband round the neck.

MODERN USES: Vervain is used as a traditional medicine in European, Middle Eastern, and Chinese herbal traditions. Preparations of the aboveground parts are used for the treatment of diarrhea and enteritis; considered to be diuretic, antioxidant, anti-inflammatory, anticonvulsive, antidepressant, antimicrobial, neuroprotective (in Alzheimer's disease), and pain-relieving; It help to stimulate milk production and increase blood circulation.

Used externally to treat wounds. Traditionally used to treat anxiety, insomnia, asthma, coughs, gingivitis, and many other conditions. One seventeenth-century author expressed, "Strange that a plant which inherits no remarkable sensible quality should possess so many virtues!"

....

VIOLETS

(VIOLA ODORATA AND OTHER VIOLA SPP.)

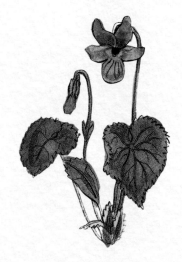

Both the tame and the wild are so well known, that they need no description. [Occurs throughout Europe and northwest Africa; naturalized in North America. There are more than four hundred *Viola* species in temperate climates.]

GOVERNMENT AND VIRTUES: They are a fine pleasing plant of Venus, of a mild nature, no way harmful. All the Violets are cold and moist while they are fresh and green, and are used to cool any heat, or distemperature of the body, either inwardly or outwardly, as inflammations in the eyes, in the matrix or fundament, in imposthumes [abscesses] also, and hot swellings, to drink the decoction of the leaves and flowers made with water in wine, or to apply them poultice-wise to the grieved places: it likewise eases pains in the head, caused through want of sleep; or any other pains arising of heat, being applied in the same manner, or with oil of roses. A dram weight of the dried leaves or flower of Violets, but the leaves more strongly, doth purge the body of choleric humours, and assuages the heat, being taken in a draught of wine, or any other drink; the powder of the purple leaves of the flowers, only picked and dried and drank in water, is said to help the quinsy, and the falling-sickness in children, especially in the beginning of the disease. The flowers of the white Violets ripen and dissolve swellings. The herb or flowers, while they are fresh, or the flowers when they are dry, are effectual in the pleurisy, and all diseases of the lungs, to lenify the sharpness in hot rheums, and the hoarseness of the throat, the heat also and sharpness of urine, and all the pains of the back or kidneys, and bladder. It is good also for the liver and the jaundice, and all hot agues, to cool the heat, and quench the thirst; but the syrup of Violets is of most use, and of better effect, being taken in some convenient liquor: and if a little of the juice or syrup of lemons be put to it, or a few drops of the oil of vitriol, it is made thereby the more powerful to cool the heat, and quench the thirst, and gives to the drink a claret wine colour, and a fine tart relish, pleasing to the taste. Violets taken, or made up with honey, do more cleanse and cool, and with sugar contrary-wise. The dried flower of Violets are accounted amongst the cordial drinks, powders, and other medicines, especially where cooling cordials are necessary. The green leaves are used with other herbs to make plasters and poultices to inflammations and swellings, and to ease all pains whatsoever, arising of heat, and for the piles also, being fried with yolks of eggs, and applied thereto.

MODERN USES: Violet extracts have been used in neuropsychiatric disorders and been found to have flavonoids with antidepressant activity. Used as an antihypertensive and treatment for headache, insomnia, and neurological conditions. Violet preparations include decoctions, sweet syrups, nasal sprays, and topical creams for the treatment of coughs, fever, colds, and various skin conditions. Pharmacological activities including anti-inflammatory, antioxidant, analgesic antibacterial, and diuretic activity, among other effects.

....

VIPER'S BUGLOSS

(ECHIUM VULGARE)

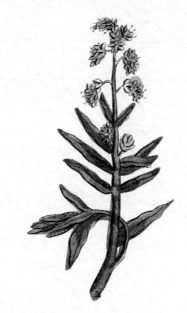

DESCRIPTION: This hath many long rough leaves, from among which rises up hard round stalks, very rough, set with prickles or hairs. The flowers stand at the top of the stalk [are] of a purplish violet colour, but more reddish while they are in the bud.

PLACE: Grows wild almost everywhere. [Found throughout most of Europe; a widespread weed in North America.]

GOVERNMENT AND VIRTUES: It is a most gallant herb of the Sun; it is a pity it is no more in use than it is. It is an especial remedy against the biting of the Viper, and all other venomous beasts, or serpents; as also against poison, or poisonous herbs. Dioscorides and others say, that whosoever shall take of the herb or root before they be bitten, shall not be hurt by the poison of any serpent. The root or seed is thought to be most effectual to comfort the heart, and expel sadness, or causeless melancholy; it tempers the blood, and allays hot fits of agues [malaria]. The same also being taken, eases the pains in the loins, back, and kidneys. The distilled water of the herb when it is in flower, or its chief strength, is excellent to be applied either inwardly or outwardly, for all the griefs aforesaid. There is a syrup made hereof very effectual for the comforting the heart, and expelling sadness and melancholy.

MODERN USES: Viper's bugloss is seldom used today, because of the known toxicity of the pyrrolizidine alkaloids in the plant. These compounds cause veno-occlusive disease of the liver, including fatalities in livestock. The pollen and honey collected by bees from the plant contain the toxic alkaloids, so analytic methods to help avoid toxicity from bee products have been developed. **CAUTION:** May cause contact dermatitis or irritation from spiny hairs.

....

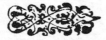

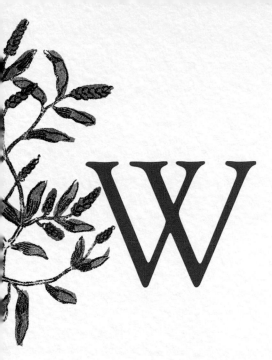

W

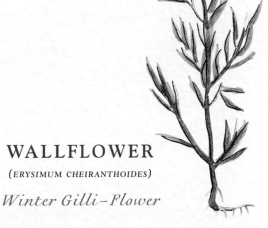

WALLFLOWER
(ERYSIMUM CHEIRANTHOIDES)

Winter Gilli–Flower

The garden kind are so well known that they need no description.

DESCRIPTION: The common single Wallflowers, which grow wild abroad, have small, long, narrow, dark green leaves, woody stalks, which bear at the tops diverse single yellow four-petaled flowers [with] a very sweet scent [often flowering in winter].

PLACE: It grows upon old stone walls. [Found throughout Europe and Asia; a weed in North America.]

GOVERNMENT AND VIRTUES: The Moon rules them. Galen, in his seventh book of simple medicines, saith, That the yellow Wallflowers work more powerfully than any of the other kinds, and are therefore of more use. It cleanses the blood, and fretteth the liver and kidneys from obstructions, provokes women's courses; helps the hardness and pain of the mother, and of spleen also; stays inflammations and swellings, comforts and strengthens any weak part, or out of joint; helps to cleanse the eyes from mistiness or films upon them, and to cleanse the filthy ulcers in the mouth, or any other part, and is a singular remedy for the gout, and all aches and pains in the joints and sinews. A conserve made of the flowers, is used for a remedy both for the apoplexy and palsy.

MODERN USES: Wallflower is seldom used today, except by practitioners in China for cardiac diseases, edema, and dyspepsia. Contains various potentially toxic cardiac glycosides. **CAUTION:** Only used by licensed practitioners in highly controlled dosages due to heart-affecting glycosides.

....

WALNUT
(JUGLANS REGIA)

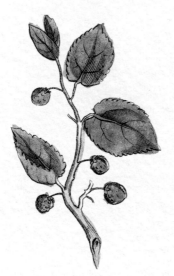

It is so well known, that it needs no description.

PLACE: [Introduced from southeast Europe and western Asia; commonly planted and naturalized in wild places throughout Europe and China.]

GOVERNMENT AND VIRTUES: This is also a plant of the Sun. Let the fruit of it be gathered accordingly, which you shall find to be of most virtues while they are green, before they have shells. The bark of the Tree doth bind and dry very much, and the leaves are much of the same temperature; but the leaves when they are older, are heating and drying in the second degree, and harder of digestion than when they are fresh, which, by reason of their sweetness, are more pleasing, and better digesting in the stomach. Taken with sweet wine, they move the belly downwards, but being old, they grieve the stomach; and in hot bodies cause the choler [bile] to abound and the headache, and are an enemy to those that have the cough. [They] are less hurtful to those that have a colder stomach, and are said to kill the broad worms in the belly or stomach. If they be taken with onions, salt, and honey, they help the biting of a mad dog, or the venom or infectious poison of any beast, etc. Caias Pompeius found in the treasury of Mithridates, king of Pontus, when he was overthrown, a scroll of his own hand writing, containing a medicine against any poison or infection; which is this; Take two dry walnuts, and as many good figs, and twenty leaves of rue, bruised and beaten together with two or three corns of salt and twenty juniper berries, which take every morning fasting, preserves from danger of poison, and infection that day it is taken. The juice of the green husks boiled with honey is an excellent gargle for sore mouths, or the heat and inflammations in the throat and stomach. The kernels, when they grow old, are more oily, and therefore not fit to be eaten, but are then used to heal the wounds of the sinews, gangrenes, and carbuncles. The said kernels being burned, are very astringent, and will stay lasks [diarrhea] and women's courses, being taken in red wine, and stay the falling of the hair, and make it fair, being anointed with oil and wine. The green husks will do the like, being used in the same manner. The kernels beaten with rue and wine, being applied, help the quinsy; and bruised with some honey, and applied to the ears, ease the pains and inflammation of them. A piece of the green husks put into a hollow tooth, eases the pain. The oil that is pressed out of the kernels, is very profitable, taken inwardly like oil of almonds, to help the cholic, and to expel wind very effectually; an ounce or two thereof may be taken at any time. The young green nuts taken before they be half ripe, and preserved with sugar, are of good use for those that have weak stomachs, or defluctions thereon. The distilled water of the green husks, before they be half ripe, is of excellent use to cool the heat of agues [malaria], being drank an ounce or two at a time: as also to resist the infection of the plague, if some of the same be also applied to the sores thereof. The same also cools the heat of green wounds and old ulcers, and heals them, being bathed therewith. The distilled water of the green husks being ripe, when they are shelled from the nuts, and drank with a little vinegar, is good for the place, so as before the taking thereof a vein be opened. The said water is very good against the quinsy, being gargled and bathed therewith, and wonderfully helps deafness, the noise, and other pains in the ears. The distilled water of the young green leaves in the end of May, performs a singular cure on foul running ulcers and sores, to be bathed, with wet cloths or sponges applied to them every morning.

MODERN USES: Green and dried walnut husks are considered strong antifungals. Traditionally, the leaves of the European walnut are used for the treatment of skin inflammation, chronic eczema, and excessive perspiration, especially of the hands and feet. Walnut leaf decoction is applied as a topical dressing to treat scalp itching, dandruff, and superficial burns. Walnuts themselves are a well-known food with high manganese content.

CAUTION: Walnut hulls can cause staining of the skin and contact dermatitis. Some individuals may be allergic to walnuts.

....

WATER CHESTNUTS

(TRAPA NATANS)

Water–Caltrops

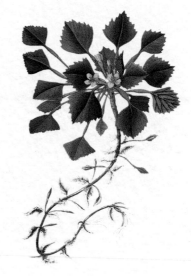

DESCRIPTION: As for the greater sort of Water Chestnuts it is not found here [in England], or very rarely. [Widely grown and cultivated in tropical and subtropical Asia and Africa, as well as temperate regions of southern Europe. Introduced in North America in the late nineteenth century; naturalized in some parts of New England.]

GOVERNMENT AND VIRTUES: They are under the dominion of the Moon, and being made into a poultice, are excellently good for hot inflammations, swellings, cankers, sore mouths and throats, being washed with the decoction; it cleanses and strengthens the neck and throat, and helps those swellings which, when people have, they say the almonds of the ears are fallen down. It is excellently good for the rankness of the gums, a safe and present remedy for the king's evil. They are excellent for the stone and gravel, especially the nuts, being dried. They also resist poison, and biting of venomous beasts.

MODERN USES: Better associated with Asian cuisines, the fleshy fruit of water chestnut, an aquatic annual, has been used as food in Europe since Neolithic times. In Ayurvedic medicine, water chestnut is used as a diuretic, nutrient, astringent, and cooling food and medicine. Science confirms mild analgesic, anti-inflammatory, anti-diabetic, and microbial activity.

....

WATERCRESS

(NASTURTIUM OFFICINALE;
SYN. RORIPPA NASTURTIUM-AQUATICUM)

Water Cresses

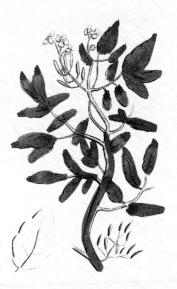

DESCRIPTION: The whole plant abides green in the winter, and tastes somewhat hot and sharp.

PLACE: [Watercress] grows, for the most part, in [shallow] standing waters, yet sometimes in small rivulets of running water, [flowering and going to seed by late spring. Native to most of Europe, North Africa, and central Asia; widely naturalized in North America and South America.]

GOVERNMENT AND VIRTUES: It is an herb under the dominion of the Moon. They are more powerful against the scurvy, and to cleanse the blood and humours, than Brooklime is, and serve in all the other uses in which Brooklime is available, as to break the stone, and provoke urine and woman's courses. The decoction thereof cleanses ulcers, by washing them. The leaves bruised, or the juice, is good, to be applied to the face or other parts troubled with freckles, pimples, spots, or the like, at night, and washed away in the morning. The juice mixed with vinegar, and the forepart of the head bathed therewith, is very good for those that are dull and drowsy, or have the lethargy.

Watercress pottage is a good remedy to cleanse the blood in the spring, and help headaches, and consume the gross humours winter has left behind; those that would live in health, may use it if they please; if they will not, I cannot help it. If any not fancy pottage, they may eat the herb as a salad.

MODERN USES: Watercress is an early spring green used fresh or, less frequently, dried. As a folk medicine it is used as a diuretic and spring tonic as well as in preparations to increase bile flow. The essential oil in watercress leaves contains organosulfur compounds, typical of the mustard family, which give a biting, piquant flavor. These compounds are also responsible for biological activity including antiviral, antifungal, and antibacterial effects. **CAUTION:** Watercress may uptake heavy metals or toxins from polluted waters.

....

WATER FIGWORT

(SCROPHULARIA AURICULATA)

Water Betony

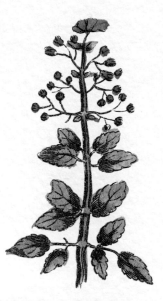

distilled water of the leaves is used for the same purpose; as also to bathe the face and hands spotted or blemished, or discoloured by sun burning.

I confess I do not much fancy distilled waters, I mean such waters as are distilled cold; some virtues of the herb they may haply have (it were a strange thing else;) but this I am confident of, that being distilled in a pewter still, as the vulgar and apish fashion is, both chemical oil and salt is left behind unless you burn them, and then all is spoiled, water and all, which was good for as little as can be, by such a distillation.

MODERN USES: Water betony is used externally as a poultice on cuts and wounds. Seldom used.

....

DESCRIPTION: [It] rises up with square, hard, greenish stalks, sometimes brown. The flowers are many, set at the tops of the stalks and branches, being round-bellied and open at the brims, the uppermost being like a hood, and the lowermost like a hip hanging down, of a dark red colour.

PLACE: It grows by the ditch side, brooks and other water-courses [in western Europe].

GOVERNMENT AND VIRTUES: Water Betony is an herb of Jupiter in Cancer, and is appropriated more to wounds and hurts in the breast than Wood Betony, which follows: It is an excellent remedy for sick hogs. It is of a cleansing quality. The leaves bruised and applied are effectual for all old and filthy ulcers; and especially if the juice of the leaves be boiled with a little honey, and dipped therein, and the sores dressed therewith; as also for bruises and hurts, whether inward or outward. The

WATER LILY

(NYMPHAEA ALBA)

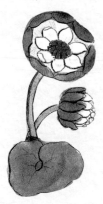

Of these there are two principally noted kinds, *viz.* the White (*Nymphaea alba*) and the Yellow (*Nuphar lutea*).

DESCRIPTION: The White Lily has very large and thick dark green leaves lying on the water, that arise from a great, thick, round, and long tuberous black root spongy or loose. The yellow kind is little different from the former, save only that it has fewer leaves on the flowers. The root of both is somewhat sweet in taste.

PLACE: [They are found growing in ponds and lakes throughout Europe, northeast Africa, and the Middle East. Naturalized in western temperate South America.]

GOVERNMENT AND VIRTUES: The herb is under the dominion of the Moon, and therefore cools and moistens. The leaves and flowers of the Water Lilies are cold and moist, but the roots and seeds are cold and dry; the leaves do cool all inflammations, both outward and inward heat of agues [malaria]; and so doth the flowers also, either by the syrup or conserve; the syrup helps much to procure rest, and to settle the brain of frantic persons, by cooling the hot distemperature of the head. The seed as well as the root is effectual to stay fluxes of blood or humours, either of wounds or of the belly; but the roots are most used, and more effectual to cool, bind, and restrain all fluxes in man or woman. The root is likewise very good for those whose urine is hot and sharp, to be boiled in wine and water, and the decoction drank. The distilled water of the flowers is very effectual for all the diseases aforesaid, both inwardly taken, and outwardly applied; and is much commended to take away freckles, spots, sunburn, and morphew [skin blemishes] from the face, or other parts of the body. The oil made of the flowers, as oil of Roses is made, is profitably used to cool hot tumours, and to ease the pains, and help the sores.

MODERN USES: In folk medicine, the large, spongy roots of dried water lily are used as an astringent and demulcent for dysentery. Water lily was described as an aphrodisiac in ancient times, but by the nineteenth century was thought of as an anaphrodisiac to reduce sexual desire. The fresh root is acrid. Experimentally, extracts have shown potential antiviral activity. Components of the leaves are antioxidant, liver protective, and have anxiolytic activity. Yellow water lily was used similarly. **CAUTION:** The fresh plant can be irritating. The root may concentrate heavy metals and pollutants from contaminated water.

....

WATER PEPPER

(PERSICARIA HYDROPIPER; SYN. POLYGONUM HYDROPIPER)

Arssmart

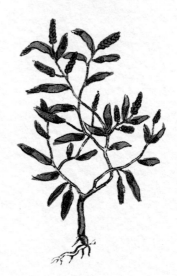

The hot Arssmart is called also Water-pepper, or Culrage.

DESCRIPTION: This has broad leaves set at the great red joint of the stalks; with semicircular blackish marks on them, usually either blueish or whitish.

PLACE: It grows in watery places, ditches, and the like, which for the most part are dry in summer. [Native to most of Europe and Asia; a naturalized weed throughout North America.]

GOVERNMENT AND VIRTUES: That which is hot and biting, is under the dominion of Mars, but Saturn, challenges the other, as appears by that leaden coloured spot he hath placed upon the leaf.

It is of a cooling and drying quality, and very effectual for putrefied ulcers in man or beast, to kill worms, and cleanse the putrefied places. The juice thereof dropped in, or otherwise applied, consumes all colds, swellings, and dissolveth the congealed blood of bruises by strokes, falls, etc. A piece of the root, or some of the seeds bruised, and held to an aching tooth, takes away the pain. The leaves bruised and laid to the joint that has a felon thereon, takes it away. The juice destroys worms in the ears, being dropped into them; if the hot Arssmart be strewed in a chamber, it will soon kill all the fleas. A good handful of the hot biting Arssmart put under a horse's saddle, will make him travel the better, although he were half tired before. The mild Arssmart is good against all imposthumes [abscesses] and inflammations at the beginning, and to heal green wounds.

MODERN USES: Water pepper is widely used as a folk medicine in China, Eastern Europe, India, and Japan as a diuretic and for the treatment of menstrual irregularities. Studies have found antioxidant, anti-inflammatory, antimicrobial, and pain-relieving activities. It is a promising research subject for pain-blocking activity and the inhibition of cellular obesity pathways. **CAUTION:** Associated with toxicity at high doses.

....

WHEAT
(*TRITICUM AESTIVUM*)

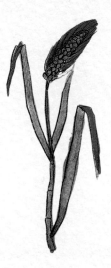

All the several kinds thereof are so well known unto almost all people, that it is all together needless to write a description thereof.

GOVERNMENT AND VIRTUES: This is under Venus. Dioscorides saith, that to eat the corn of green Wheat is hurtful to the stomach, and breeds worms. Pliny saith, That the corn of Wheat, roasted upon an iron pan, and eaten, are a present remedy for those that are chilled with cold. The oil pressed from wheat heals all tetters and ringworms, being used warm. Matthiolus commends the same to be put into hollow ulcers to heal them up, and it is good for chops in the hands and feet, and to make rugged skin smooth. The green corns of Wheat being chewed, and applied to the place bitten by a mad dog, heals it; slices of Wheat bread soaked in red rose water, and applied to the eyes that are hot, red, and inflamed, or blood-shotten, helps them. Hot bread applied for an hour, at times, for three days together, perfectly heals the kernels in the throat, commonly called the king's evil [unusual swelling of lymph nodes or scrofula].

The said meal boiled in vinegar, helps the shrinking of the sinews, saith Pliny; and mixed with vinegar, and boiled together, heals all freckles, spots and pimples on the face. Wheat flour, mixed with the yolk of an egg, honey, and turpentine, doth draw, cleanse and heal any boil, plague, sore, or foul ulcer. The bran of Wheat meal steeped in sharp vinegar, and bound in a linen cloth, and rubbed on those places that have the scurf, morphew [skin blemishes], scabs or leprosy, will take them away, the body being first well purged. The decoction of the bran of Wheat or barley is of good use to bathe those places that are bursten by a rupture; and the said bran boiled in good vinegar, and applied to swollen breasts, helps them, and stays all inflammations. It helps also the biting of vipers (which I take to be no other than our English adder) and all other venomous creatures. The leaves of Wheat meal applied with some salt, take away hardness of the skin, warts, and hard knots in the flesh. Wafers put in water, and drank, stays the lask [diarrhea] and bloody flux [dysentery], and are profitably used both inwardly and outwardly for the ruptures in children. Boiled in water unto a thick jelly, and taken, it stays spitting of blood; and boiled with mint and butter, it helps the hoarseness of the throat.

MODERN USES: Wheat is one of the first grains cultivated by humans thousands of years ago and is still responsible for up to 20 percent of calories consumed worldwide. Wheat germ oil, which is high in vitamin E, is used as a supplement to reduce inflammation and improve circulation to the extremities. Today, a major health concern with consuming wheat is the protein gluten, to which many individuals have allergic hypersensitive reactions. Wheatgrass—the young, green first-growth leaves—and wheatgrass juice are consumed as a health food. **CAUTION:** Avoid in cases of known intolerances or allergies to wheat, including, but not limited to, widely recognized gluten intolerances.

....

WILLOW

(SALIX ALBA AND OTHER SALIX SPP.)

The Willow Tree

BLACK WILLOW

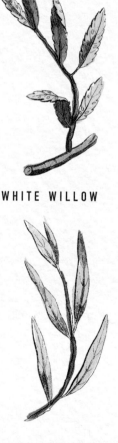

WHITE WILLOW

These are so well known that they need no description. I shall therefore only shew you the virtues thereof.

PLACE: [Willows usually grow in moist or wet soils along the edge of ponds or low areas in fields. Widespread in the Northern Hemisphere.]

GOVERNMENT AND VIRTUES: The Moon owns it. Both the leaves, bark, and the seed, are used to stanch bleeding of wounds, and at mouth and nose, spitting of blood, and other fluxes of blood in man or woman, and to stay vomiting, and provocation thereunto, if the decoction of them in wine be drank. The leaves bruised and boiled in wine, and drank, stays the heat of lust in man or woman, and quite extinguishes it, if it be long used. Water that is gathered from the Willow, when it flowers, the bark being slit, and a vessel fitting to receive it, is very good for redness and dimness of sight, or films that grow over the eyes, and stay the rheums [watery discharge] that fall into them; to provoke urine, being stopped, if it be drank; to clear the face and skin from spots and discolourings. Galen saith, the flowers have an admirable faculty in drying up humours, being a medicine without any sharpness or corrosion; you may boil them in white wine, and drink as much as you will, so you drink not yourself drunk. The bark works the same effect, if used in the same manner, and the tree hath always a bark upon it, though not always flowers. The burnt ashes of the bark being mixed with vinegar, takes away warts, corns, and superfluous flesh, being applied to the place. The decoction of the leaves or bark in wine, takes away scurf and dandruff by washing the place with it. It is a fine cool tree, the boughs of which are very convenient to be placed in the chamber of one sick of a fever.

MODERN USES: Willow has been used for at least two thousand years to treat inflammation, reduce fevers, thin the blood, and treat mild pain. Willow species contain salicylic acid; a derivative of that, acetylsalicylic acid, has pain-relieving, fever-reducing and anti-inflammatory compounds and is known today as aspirin. Willow bark itself is a traditional medicine used for minor pain from headaches, colds, joint pain, and fever associated with colds. CAUTION: Avoid use with prescription blood thinners. Some people have allergies to salicylates. Avoid use during pregnancy and lactation. Speak to your medical professional before using if on an aspiring regimen.

....

WINTERGREEN
(PYROLA ROTUNDIFOLIA)

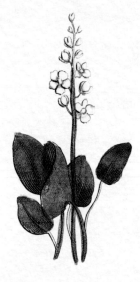

DESCRIPTION: This sends forth seven, eight, or nine leaves, every one standing upon a long foot stalk, bearing at the top many small white sweet-smelling flowers, laid open like a star.

PLACE: It grows seldom in fields, but frequent in the woods northwards. [Circumboreal in Europe, Asia, and North America.]

GOVERNMENT AND VIRTUES: Wintergreen is under the dominion of Saturn, and is a singularly good wound herb, and an especial remedy for healing green wounds speedily, the green leaves being bruised and applied, or the juice of them. A salve made of the green herb stamped, or the juice boiled with hog's lard, or with salad oil and wax, and some turpentine added to it, is a sovereign salve, and highly extolled by the Germans, who use it to heal all manner of wounds and sores. The herb boiled in wine and water, and given to drink to them that have any inward ulcers in their kidneys, or neck of the bladder, doth wonderfully help them. It stays all fluxes, as the lask [diarrhea], bloody fluxes [dysentery], women's courses, and bleeding of wounds, and takes away any inflammations rising upon pains of the heart; it is no less helpful for foul ulcers hard to be cured; as also for cankers or fistulas. The distilled water of the herb effectually performs the same things.

MODERN USES: Culpeper's wintergreen is most widely used as an Asian folk medicine, and scientists in China, Japan, and Korea have studied it for novel antibacterial, antioxidant, anti-inflammatory, and analgesic compounds. In traditional Chinese medicine, preparations of the herb have been used for neuralgia, gastrointestinal bleeding, high blood pressure, arthritis, and rheumatism. In northern China it is consumed as a beverage tea.
CAUTION: Not to be confused with the wintergreen-flavored North American herb known as wintergreen (*Gaultheria procumbens*), which contains toxic methyl salicylate.

·················

WOAD

(ISATIS TINCTORIA)

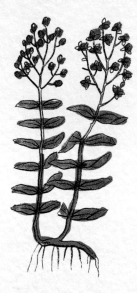

DESCRIPTION: It hath diverse large leaves, long, and somewhat blue. From leaves rises up a lusty stalk, three or four feet high; at the top it spreads diverse branches, [with] very pretty, little yellow flowers.

PLACE: [Cultivated as a dye plant throughout Europe, but declining due to less frequent cultivation. Found scattered throughout much of Europe, the Middle East, and much of central Asia and South Asia.]

GOVERNMENT AND VIRTUES: It is a cold and dry plant of Saturn. Some people affirm the plant to be destructive to bees, and fluxes them, which, if it be, I cannot help it. However, if any bees be diseased thereby, the cure is, to set urine by them, but set it in a vessel, that they cannot drown themselves, which may be remedied, if you put pieces of cork in it.

The herb is so drying and binding, that it is not fit to be given inwardly. An ointment made thereof stanches bleeding. A plaster made thereof, and applied to the region of the spleen which lies on the left side, takes away the hardness and pains thereof. The ointment is excellently good in such ulcers as abound with moisture, and takes away the corroding and fretting humours: It cools inflammations, quenches St. Anthony's fire, and stays defluxion of the blood to any part of the body.

MODERN USES: Woad leaf extracts are used in ointments (particularly in China) for inflammatory dermatitis, allergic skin reactions, and edema; it has antibacterial, antifungal, anti-inflammatory, immunostimulatory, and astringent activity. Also used to stop bleeding for wounds, ulcers, and hemorrhoids and to resolve skin growths. The root is more often used than the aboveground parts. Pharmacological activities are attributed to a combination of components in the plant, including alkaloids, polysaccharides and indigo-like dye components.

....

WOOD ANEMONE

(ANEMONE NEMOROSA; SYN. ANEMONOIDES NEMOROSA)

Anemone

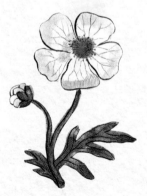

Called also Windflower, because they say the flowers never open but when the wind blows. Pliny is my author; if it be not so, blame him. The seed also (if it bears any) flies away with the wind.

PLACE: [Wood anemone is perennial that blooms in early spring. Native to open grasslands, hedgerows, and woods in most of Europe and Turkey. Numerous cultivars are grown in gardens.]

GOVERNMENT AND VIRTUES: It is under the dominion of Mars, being supposed to be a kind of Crowfoot. The leaves provoke the terms mightily, being boiled, and the decoction drank. The body being bathed with the decoction of them, cures the leprosy. And when all is done, let physicians prate what they please, all the pills in the dispensatory purge not the head like to hot things held in the mouth. Being made into an ointment, [it] is excellently good to cleanse malignant and corroding ulcers.

MODERN USES: Wood anemone is seldom if ever used today. When fresh, this and other anemones and buttercups contain the irritant protoanemonin, which may cause immediate irritancy and can lead to blistering and chemical burns, both internally and externally. Once dried or heated, the protoanemonin in the leaves becomes less toxic, but still irritating anemonin. The leaves are used to deter ants.

....

WOOD SAGE

(*TEUCRIUM SCORODONIA*)

*Sage-leaved Germander,
Wood Germander*

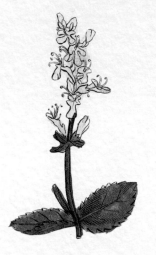

DESCRIPTION: Wood-sage rises up with square hoary stalks, two feet high, with two leaves set at every joint, and a little [crinkled] about the edges. The flowers [are] on a slender like spike, and are of a pale and whitish colour.

PLACE: It grows in woods, and by wood-sides. [Occurs throughout most of western Europe; naturalized in eastern Canada.]

GOVERNMENT AND VIRTUES: The herb is under Venus. The decoction of the Wood Sage provokes urine and women's courses: It also provokes sweat, digests humours, and discusses swellings and nodes in the flesh, and is therefore thought to be good against the French pox [syphilis]. The decoction of the green herb, made with wine, is a safe and sure remedy for those who by falls, bruises, or blows, suspect some vein to be inwardly broken, to disperse and void the congealed blood, and to consolidate the veins. The drink used inwardly, and the herb used outwardly, is good for such as

are inwardly or outwardly bursten, and is found to be a sure remedy for the palsy. The juice of the herb, or the powder thereof dried, is good for moist ulcers and sores in the legs, and other parts, to dry them, and cause them to heal more speedily. It is no less effectual also in green wounds, to be used upon any occasion.

MODERN USES: Wood sage is seldom used today except as a folk medicine. The extremely bitter leaves have a fragrance likened to hops and were once used in the English countryside as a flavoring for beer. Little research has been done, but it has confirmed antibacterial activity. It is a folk medicine for the treatment of mastitis in cows. Formerly used for colds, fever, inflammation, and menstrual disorders. **CAUTION:** Of unknown toxicity. Other species of *Teucrium* are known to cause severe kidney disease.

WOOD SORREL

(*OXALIS ACETOSELLA*)

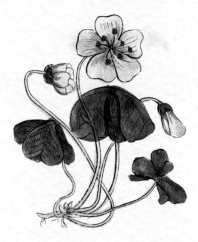

DESCRIPTION: This grows upon the ground, having a number of leaves coming from the root made of three leaves, like a trefoil, but broad at the ends, and cut in the middle, of a yellowish green colour, of a fine sour relish, and yielding a juice which will turn red when it is clarified, and makes a most dainty clear syrup. Among these leaves rise up a flower at the top, consisting of five small pointed [petals], star-fashion, of a white colour

PLACE: It grows in many places of our land, in [moist, shaded] woods [in most of Europe, east to Japan].

GOVERNMENT AND VIRTUES: Venus owns it. Wood Sorrel serves to all the purposes that the other Sorrels do, and is more effectual in hindering putrefaction of blood, and ulcers in the mouth and body, and to quench thirst, to strengthen a weak stomach, to procure an appetite, to stay vomiting, and very excellent in any contagious sickness or pestilential fevers. The syrup made of the juice, is effectual in all the cases aforesaid, and so is the distilled water of the herb. Sponges or linen cloths wet in the juice and applied outwardly to any hot swelling or inflammations, doth much cool and help them. The same juice taken and gargled in the mouth, and after it is spit forth, taken afresh, doth wonderfully help a foul stinking canker or ulcer therein. It is singularly good to heal wounds, or to stay the bleeding of thrusts or scabs in the body.

MODERN USES: Little used today, wood sorrel and other *Oxalis* species are of interest to wild food enthusiasts for the sour leaves, which are used sparingly for flavoring. In Poland, the leaves are nibbled as a children's snack and used as a green for flavoring soups. Considered antioxidant, wood sorrel contains oxalic acid and potassium oxalate, which gives it its sour taste. An ointment made from the herb is used topically to treat a recently acknowleged medical condition: "broken heart syndrome" (BHS). The ointment

is massaged into the abdomen for BHS-induced nervous digestive disturbances. Used topically for wound-healing and the treatment of cuts in various Asian cultures.

....

WORMWOOD

(*ARTEMISIA ABSINTHIUM*)

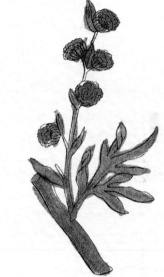

DESCRIPTION: Common Wormwood (*Artemisia absinthium*) I shall not describe, for every boy that can eat an egg knows it.

PLACE: [A widespread plant of wastelands and roadsides. Cultivated in herb gardens since ancient times. Found throughout Europe, Asia, northern Africa; widely naturalized in Australia, North America, and South America.]

GOVERNMENT AND VIRTUES: The seeds of the common Wormwood are prevalent, to expel worms in children, or people of ripe age; of both some are weak, some are strong. Let such as are strong take the common Wormwood, for the others will do but little good. It provokes urine, helps surfeits, or swellings in the belly; it causes appetite to meat, because Mars rules the attractive faculty in man: The sun never shone upon a better herb for the yellow jaundice than this. Why should men cry out so much upon Mars for an infortunate, (or Saturn either?). Did God make creatures to do the creation a mischief? This herb testifies, that Mars is willing to cure all diseases he causes; the truth is, Mars loves no cowards, nor Saturn fools, nor I neither. Besides all this, Wormwood provokes the terms. I would willingly teach astrologers, and make them physicians (if I knew how) for they are most fitting for the calling; if you will not believe me, ask Dr. Hippocrates, and Dr. Galen, a couple of gentlemen that our college of physicians keep to vapour with, not to follow. Whereby, my brethren, the astrologers may know by a penny how a shilling is coined. As for the college of physicians, they are too stately to college or too proud to continue. They say a mouse is under the dominion of the Moon, and that is the reason they feed in the night; the house of the Moon is Cancer; rats are of the same nature with mice, but they are a little bigger; Mars receives his fall in Cancer, *ergo*, Wormwood being an herb of Mars, is a present remedy for the biting of rats and mice. Mix a little Wormwood, an herb of Mars, with your ink, neither rats nor mice touch the paper written with it, and then Mars is a preserver.

Mushrooms (I cannot give them the title of Herba, Frutex, or Arbor) are under the dominion of Saturn, (and take one time with another, they do as much harm as good) if any have poisoned himself by eating them, Wormwood, an herb of Mars, cures him, because Mars is exalted in Capricorn, the house of Saturn, and this it doth by sympathy, as it did the other by antipathy. Wheals, pushes, black and blue spots, coming either by bruises or beatings. Wormwood,

an herb of Mars, (as bad you love him, and as you hate him) will not break your head, but he will give you a plaister. If he do but teach you to know yourselves, his courtesy is greater than his discourtesy. Mars eradicates all diseases in the throat by his herbs (for Wormwood is one).

The eyes are under the Luminaries; the right eye of a man, and the left eye of a woman the Sun claims dominion over: the left eye of a man, and the right eye of a woman, are privileges of the Moon. Wormwood, an herb of Mars cures both; what belongs to the Sun by sympathy, because he is exalted in his house; but what belongs to the Moon by antipathy, because he hath his fall in hers. Suppose a man be bitten or stung by a martial creature, imagine a wasp, a hornet, a scorpion, Wormwood, an herb of Mars, gives you a present cure.

I was once in the Tower and viewed the wardrobe, and there was a great many fine clothes: (I can give them no other title, for I was never either linen or woolen draper) yet as brave as they looked, my opinion was that the moths might consume them. Moths are under the dominion of Mars; this herb Wormwood being laid among clothes, will make a moth scorn to meddle with the clothes, as much as a lion scorns to meddle with a mouse, or an eagle with a fly.

A poor silly countryman hath got an ague, and cannot go about his business: he wishes he had it not, and so do I; but I will tell him a remedy, whereby he shall prevent it. Take the herb of Mars, Wormwood, and if infortunes will do good, what will fortunes do? Some think the lungs are under Jupiter; and if the lungs then the breath; and though sometimes a man gets a stinking breath. Give me thy leave by sympathy to cure this poor man with drinking a draught of Wormwood beer every morning. The Moon was weak the other day, and she gave a man two terrible mischiefs, a dull brain and a weak sight; Mars laid by his sword, and comes to her; Sister Moon, said he, this man hath angered thee, but I beseech thee take notice he is but a fool; prithee be patient, I will with my herb wormwood cure him of both infirmities by antipathy, for thou knows thou and I cannot agree; with that the Moon began to quarrel. Mars (not delighting much in women's tongues) went away, and did it whether she would or no.

He that reads this, and understands what he reads, hath a jewel of more worth than a diamond; he that understands it not, is as little fit to give physic. There lies a key in these words which will unlock, (if it be turned by a wise hand) the cabinet of physic. I have delivered it as plain as I [dare]; it is not only upon Wormwood as I wrote, but upon all plants, trees, and herbs; he that understands it not, is unfit (in my opinion) to give physic. This shall live when I am dead. And thus I leave it to the world, not caring a farthing whether they like it or dislike it. The grave equals all men, and therefore shall equal me with all princes; until which time the eternal Providence is over me. Then the ill tongue of a prating fellow, or one that hath more tongue than wit, or more proud than honest, shall never trouble me. *Wisdom is justified by her children.* And so much for Wormwood.

MODERN USES: Wormwood, as the name implies, was once regarded as a primary treatment for expelling worms. The extremely bitter leaves are traditionally nibbled as a digestive stimulant. They contain a potentially toxic compound, thujone, once thought to be responsible for the supposed psychoactive effects of absinthe, a liquor that is flavored with the flowers and leaves of the plant. Banned in most Western countries in the early twentieth century, by 2007, absinthe (with thujone re- moved) was again legally produced and sold around the world. **CAUTION:** Contains toxic thujone. Avoid use during pregnancy and lactation, and if taking anticonvulsants.

....

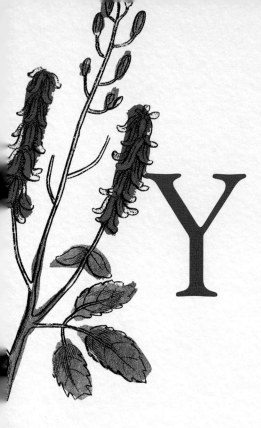

Y

YARROW
(ACHILLEA MILLEFOLIUM)

Nose–Bleed, Milfoil,
Thousand–Heal

DESCRIPTION: It has many leaves, finely cut, and divided into many small parts, [and white] flowers.

PLACE: It is frequent in all pastures [fields, roadsides, and wastelands throughout Europe, much of Asia, North America, South America, southern Africa, and Australia].

GOVERNMENT AND VIRTUES: It is under the influence of Venus. An ointment of them cures wounds, and is most fit for such as have inflammations; it stops the terms in women, being boiled in white wine, and the decoction drank; as also the bloody flux [dysentery]; the ointment of it is not only good for green wounds, but also for ulcers and fistulas, especially such as abound with moisture. It stays the shedding of hair, the head being bathed with the decoction of it; inwardly taken it helps the retentive faculty of the stomach: it helps the gonorrhea in men, and the whites in women, and helps such as cannot hold their water; and the leaves chewed in the mouth eases the tooth-ache, and these virtues being put together, shew the herb to be drying and binding. Achilles is supposed to be the first that left the virtues of this herb to posterity and certainly a very profitable herb it is in cramps, and therefore called Militaris.

MODERN USES: For centuries, yarrow has been used to staunch the bleeding of wounds and to resolve bruises, sprains, and swellins. Well-documented activities include anti-inflammatory, diuretic, mild depressant, antispasmodic, fever-reducing, styptic, and antioxidant effects. A tea is used to treat the common cold, thrombosis, hypertension, fevers, dysentery, and diarrhea. **CAUTION:** May cause allergic reactions in some individuals. Avoid use during pregnancy and lactation.

....

YELLOW FLAG

(IRIS PSEUDACORUS)

Flower–de–Luce, Yellow Water–Flag

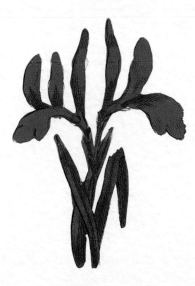

DESCRIPTION: [A showy yellow iris found in wet areas or the edge of ponds.]

PLACE: It usually grows in watery ditches, ponds, lakes, and moor sides, which are always overflowed with water. [Native to marshy areas of Europe; widely cultivated as an ornamental and naturalized elsewhere.]

GOVERNMENT AND VIRTUES: It is under the dominion of the Moon. The root of this Yellow Flag is very astringent, cooling, and drying; and thereby helps all lasks [diarrhea] and fluxes, whether of blood or humours, as bleeding at the mouth, nose, or other parts, bloody flux [dysentery], and the immoderate flux of women's courses. The distilled water of the whole herb, flowers and roots, is a good remedy for watering eyes, both to be dropped into them, and to have cloths or sponges wetted therein, and applied to the forehead. It also helps the spots and blemishes. The said water fomented on swellings and hot inflammations of women's breasts, upon cancers also, and those spreading ulcers called *Noli me tangere*, do much good: It helps also foul ulcers in the private parts of man or woman; but an ointment made of the flowers is better for those external applications.

MODERN USES: Yellow flag is seldom used today. The root was formerly used in a controlled dosage to treat diarrhea and dysentery. The root is considered cathartic. **CAUTION:** The leaves and root are considered toxic and may cause severe gastrointestinal distress or blistering of the skin if applied topically. The plant's tissues concentrate toxins from the water it grows in.

....

YELLOW LOOSESTRIFE

(LYSIMACHIA VULGARIS)

Willow-Herb

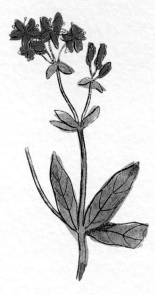

often used in gargles for sore mouths, as also for the secret parts. The smoke hereof being bruised, drives away flies and gnats, which in the night time molest people inhabiting near marshes.

MODERN USES: Yellow loosestrife has been used in the treatment of diarrhea and dysentery. In folk medicine it is considered an astringent, anti-inflammatory, and analgesic. Used externally to stop bleeding and clean wounds. Research suggests it has potential antioxidant, antibacterial, and experimental antitumor activity.

....

YELLOW SWEET CLOVER

(MELILOTUS OFFICINALIS)

Mellilot, King's Claver

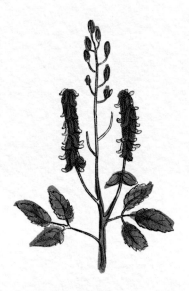

DESCRIPTION: Common yellow Loosestrife grows to be four or five feet high, or more [with] long and narrow leaves, somewhat like willow leaves, and at the tops of them also stand many yellow flowers. It has no scent or taste, and is only astringent.

PLACE: It grows in in moist meadows, and by water sides. [Found through Europe and northern Asia; naturalized in scattered locations in eastern North America.]

GOVERNMENT AND VIRTUES: This herb is good for all manner of bleeding at the mouth, nose, or wounds, and all fluxes of the belly, and the bloody-flux [dysentery], given either to drink or taken by clysters; it stays also the abundance of women's courses; it is a singular good wound-herb for green wounds, to stay the bleeding, and quickly close together the lips of the wound, if the herb be bruised, and the juice only applied. It is

DESCRIPTION: This hath many green stalks, two or three feet high, with small leaves, set three together. The flowers are yellow, and [pealike], but small, standing in long spikes.

PLACE: It grows plentifully in [fields, roadsides, and meadows throughout Europe. Widely naturalized elsewhere.]

GOVERNMENT AND VIRTUES: Melilot, boiled in wine, and applied, mollifies all hard tumours and inflammations that happen in the eyes, or other parts of the body. It helps the pains of the stomach, being applied fresh, or boiled with any of the forenamed things; and steeped in vinegar, or rose water, it mitigates the headache. The flowers of Melilot or Chamomile are much used to be put together in clysters to expel wind, and ease pains; and also in poultices for the same purpose, and to assuage swelling tumours in the spleen or other parts, and helps inflammations in any part of the body. The juice dropped into the eyes, is a singularly good medicine to take away the film or skin that clouds or dims the eye-sight. The head often washed with the distilled water of the herb and flower, or a lye made therewith, is effectual for those that suddenly lose their senses; as also to strengthen the memory, to comfort the head and brain, and to preserve them from pain, and the apoplexy.

MODERN USES: In European phytomedicine, yellow sweet clover is used externally for contusions and bruising. Internally, preparations are used for pain and heaviness in legs, calf cramping, itching, and swelling related to chronic venous insufficiency and capillary fragility. Also used for thrombophlebitis, hemorrhoids, and lymphatic congestion. The dried herb contains coumarins such as melilotin. In the 1940s, coumarins extracted from the plant were developed into rat poisons. In the 1950s, related compounds were developed by the Wisconsin Alumni Research Foundation (WARF) and led to development of the blood-thinning drug warfarin. **CAUTION:** May thin blood; avoid use before surgery or with certain medications. Consult your medical professional.

....

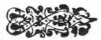

SOURCES

Allen, David E., and Gabrielle Hatfield. *Medicine Plants in Folk Tradition: An Ethnobotany of Britain & Ireland.* (Portland, OR: Timber Press, 2004).

Arber, Agnes Robertson. *Herbals, Their Origin and Evolution, a Chapter in the History of Botany.* (Cambridge, UK: Cambridge University Press, 1912).

Barnes, Joanne, Linda A. Anderson, and J. David Phillipson. *Herbal Medicines.* 3rd ed. (London: The Pharmaceutical Press, 2007).

Barton, Benjamin Herbert, and Thomas Castle. *The British Flora Medica, or, History of the Medicinal Plants of Great Britain.* 2 vols. (London: E. Cox, 1838).

Blumenthal, Mark, Alicia Goldberg, and Josef A. Brinckmann. *Herbal Medicine: Expanded Commission E Monographs.* (Austin, TX: American Botanical Council, 2000).

Blumenthal, Mark, Tara Hall, and Robert S. Rister, eds. *German Commission E Monographs, Therapeutic Monographs on Medicinal Plants for Human Uses by Commission E - A Special Expert Committee of the German Federal Health Agency.* (Austin, TX: American Botanical Council, 1996).

Bone, Kerry, and Simon Mills. *Principles and Practice of Phytotherapy: Modern Herbal Medicine,* 2nd ed. (St. Louis: Elsevier, Churchill Livingstone, 2013).

Bradley, Peter R., ed. *British Herbal Compendium: A Handbook of Scientific Information on Widely Used Plant Drugs,* vol. 1. (Bournemouth, UK: British Herbal Medicine Association, 1992).

———, ed. *British Herbal Compendium: A Handbook of Scientific Information on Widely Used Plant Drugs,* vol. 2. (Bournemouth, UK: British Herbal Medicine Association, 2006).

British Herbal Medical Association. *British Herbal Pharmacopoeia.* (Bournemouth, UK: British Herbal Medicine Association, 1971).

———. *British Herbal Pharmacopoeia.* (Bournemouth, UK: British Herbal Medicine Association, 1983).

———. *British Herbal Pharmacopoeia.* (Bournemouth, UK: British Herbal Medicine Association, 1990).

———. *British Herbal Pharmacopoeia.* (Bournemouth, UK: British Herbal Medicine Association, 1996).

———. *A Guide to Traditional Herbal Medicines: A Sourcebook of Accepted Traditional Uses of Medicinal Plants Within Europe.* (Bournemouth, UK: British Herbal Medicine Association, 2003).

Britten, James, and Robert Holland. *A Dictionary of English Plant-Names.* (London: Trübner & Co., 1886).

Coles, William. *Adam in Eden, or, Natures Paradise: The History of Plants, Fruits, Herbs and Flowers.* (London: Nathaniel Brookes, 1657).

Coles, William. *The Art of Simpling.* (London: Nathaniel Brookes, 1657).

Cowen, David L. "The Boston Editions of Nicholas Culpeper." *Journal of the History of Medicine and Allied Sciences* 11, no. 2 (1956), 156–65.

Cullen, J., J. C. M. Alexander, A. Brady, C. D. Brickell, P. S. Green, V. H. Heywood, P.-M. Jörgensen, et al., eds. *The European Garden Flora, Dicotyledons: Dilleniaceae to Leguminosae,* vol. IV. (Cambridge, UK: Cambridge University Press, 1995).

Cullen, J., J. C. M. Alexander, C. D. Brickell, J. R. Edmundson, P. S. Green, V. H. Heywood, P.-M. Jörgensen, et al., eds. *The European Garden Flora: Dicotyledons: Limnanthaceae to Oleaceae,* vol. V. (Cambridge, UK: Cambridge University Press, 1997).

———, eds. *The European Garden Flora: Dicotyledons: Loganiaceae to Compositae,* vol. VI. (Cambridge, UK: Cambridge University Press, 2000).

Culpeper, Nicholas. *A Physical Directory of a Translation of the London Dispensatory Made by the Colledge of Physicians in London: Being That Book by Which All Apothicaries Are Strictly Commanded to Make All Their Physick with Many Hundred Additions Which the Reader May Find in Every Page Marked with This Letter A. Also There Is Added the Use of All the Simples Beginning at the First Page and Ending at the 78 Page.* (London: Peter Cole, 1649).

———. *The English Physitian: Or an Astrologo-Physical Discourse of the Vulgar Herbs of This Nation. Being a Compleat Method of Physick. Whereby a Man May Preserve His Body in Health; or Cure Himself, Being Sick, for Three Pence Charge, with Such Things Only* as Grow in England, They Being Most Fit for English Bodies. (London: Peter Cole, 1652).

———. The English Physitian Enlarged: With Three Hundred, Sixty, and Nine Medicines Made of English Herbs That Were Not in Any Impression until This . . . Being an Astrologo-Physical Discourse of the Vulgar Herbs of This Nation: Containing a Compleat Method of Physick, Whereby Man May Preserve His Body in Health, or Cure Himself, Being Sick, for Three Pence Charge, with Such Things Only as Grow in England, They Being Most Fit for English Bodies, 2nd ed. (London: Peter Cole, 1653).

———. Culpeper's Last Legacy. (London: N. Brooke, 1655).

———. The English Physician. Containing, Admirable and Approved Remedies, for Several of the Most Usual Disease. Fitted to the Meanest Capacity by N. Culpepper [sic.] Doctor of Physick . . . (Boston: Nicholas Boone, 1708).

———. Pharmacopoeia Londinensis of the Long Dispensatory Further Adorned by the Studies and Collections of the Fellows Now Living of the Said College. (Boston: Nicholas Boone, 1720).

———. Culpeper's Complete Herbal: To Which Is Now Added, Upwards of One Hundred Additional Herbs, with a Display of Their Medicinal and Occult Qualities Physically Applied to the Cure of All Disorders Incident to Mankind to Which Are Now First Annexed His English Physician Enlarged. (London: R. Evans, 1814).

———. The Complete Herbal: To Which Is Now Added, Upwards of One Hundred Additional Herbs . . . To Which Are Now First Annexed, the English Physician Enlarged, and Key to Physic . . . Forming a Complete Family Dispensatory and Natural System of Physic . . . To Which Is Also Added . . . Receipts, Selected from the Author's Last Legacy to His Wife. (London: Thomas Kelly, 1847).

———. The Complete Herbal: To Which Is Now Added, Upwards of One Hundred Additional Herbs . . . To Which Are Now First Annexed, the English Physician Enlarged, and Key to Physic . . . Forming a Complete Family Dispensatory and Natural System of Physic . . . To Which Is Also Added . . . Receipts, Selected from the Author's Last Legacy to His Wife. (London: Thomas Kelly, 1850).

———. The British Herbal and Family Physician: For the Cure of Diseases Incident to the Human Frame. (London: William Nicholson & Sons, 1870).

Culpeper, Nicholas. The English Physician, Michael Flannery, ed. (1708; reprint ed., with new introduction, Tuscaloosa: University of Alabama Press, 2007).

Culpeper, Nicholas, Joshua Hamilton, and William Saunders. Culpeper's English Family Physician: or Medical Herbal Enlarged, with Several Hundred Additional Plants Principally from Sir John Hill Medicinally and Astrologically arranged, after the manner of Culpeper: and, a New Dispensatory from the ms. of the Late Dr. Saunders. 3 vols., (London: W. Locke, 1792).

Culpeper, Nicholas. The English Physician Enlarged. (London: J. Scatcherd, 1801).

Culpeper, Nicholas, and Ebenezer Sibly. Culpeper's English Physician and Complete Herbal: to which are Now First Added Upwards of One Hundred Additional Herbs, with a Display of their Medicinal and Occult Properties Physically Applied to the Cure of All Disorders Incident to Mankind, to Which Are Annexed Rules for Compounding Medicine according to the True System of Nature, forming a Complete Family Dispensatory and Natural System of Physic. (London: Green and Co., 1789).

Curtis, William. Flora Londinensis, or, Plates and Descriptions of Such Plants as Grow Wild in the Environs of London: With Their Places of Growth, and Times of Flowering, Their Several Names According to Linnæus and Other Authors: With a Particular Description of Each Plant in Latin and English: To Which Are Added, Their Several Uses in Medicine, Agriculture, Rural Economy and Other Arts. 6 vols. (London: William Curtis and B. White, 1777).

De Candolle, Alphonse. 1890. Origin of Cultivated Plants. (New York: D. Appleton and Company, 1890).

De Vos, P. "European Materia Medica in Historical Texts: Longevity of a Tradition and Implications for Future Use." Journal of Ethnopharmacology, vol. 132, no. 1. (Oct 28 2010): 28–47.

Dodoens, Rembert, Henry Lyte. *A New Herball, or, Historie of Plants: Wherein Is Contained the Whole Discourse and Perfect Description of All Sorts of Herbes and Plants: Their Divers and Sundrie Kindes: Their Names, Natures, Operations, & Vertues: And That Not Onely of Those Which Are Heere Growing in This Our Countrie of England, but of All Others Also of Forraine Realms Commonly Used in Physicke.* (London: Ninian Newton, 1586).

Duke, James A. *The Green Pharmacy: The Ultimate Compendium of Natural Remedies from the World's Foremost Authority on Healing Herbs.* (Emmaus, PA: Rodale Press, 1997).

Duke, James A., Bogenschutz-Godwin, Judi duCellier, and Peggy-Ann K. Duke. *CRC Handbook of Medicinal Herbs.* 2nd ed. (Boca Raton, FL: CRC Press, Inc., 2002).

Estes, J. Worth. *Dictionary of Protopharmacology: Therapeutic Practices, 1700–1850.* (Canton, MA: Watson Publishing International, 1990).

Fernie, William Thomas. *Meals Medicinal with "Herbal Simples" (of Edible Parts): Curative Foods from the Cook in Place of Drugs from the Chemist.* (Bristol, UK: John Wright, 1905).

Foster, Steven. *Herbal Bounty! The Gentle Art of Herb Culture.* (Layton, UT: Gibbs M. Smith, Inc., 1983).

———. *Herbal Renaissance: Growing, Using and Understanding Herbs in the Modern World.* (Salt Lake City, UT: Gibbs Smith, 1993).

———. *Herbs for Your Health.* (Loveland, CO: Interweave Press, 1996).

———. *101 Medicinal Herbs: An Illustrated Guide to History, Uses, Recommended Dosages & Cautions.* (Loveland, CO: Interweave Press, 1998).

Foster, Steven, and Yue Chongxi. *Herbal Emissaries: Bringing Chinese Herbs to the West.* (Rochester, VT: Healing Arts Press, 1992).

Foster, Steven, and James A. Duke. *Peterson Field Guide to Medicinal Plants and Herbs Eastern and Central North America.* 3rd ed. (Boston and New York: Houghton Mifflin Harcourt, 2014).

Foster, Steven , and Varro E. Tyler. *Tyler's Honest Herbal.* 4th ed. (New York: Haworth Press, 1999).

Gardner, Zoë and Michael McGuffin, eds. *American Herbal Product Association's Botanical Safety Handbook,* 2nd ed. (Boca Raton, FL: CRC Press).

Gerarde, John. *The Herball, or, Generall Historie of Plantes.* (London: John Norton, 1597).

———. *The Herball or Generall Historie of Plantes. Gathered by John Gerarde of London Master in Chirurgerie Very Much Enlarged and Amended by Thomas Johnson Citizen and Apothecarye of London.* (London: Adam Islip, Joice Norton and Richard Whitakers, 1633).

Grieve, Maude. *A Modern Herbal,* 2 vols. (London: Jonathan Cape, 1931).

Griggs, Barbara. *Green Pharmacy: A History of Herbal Medicine.* (New York: Viking Press, 1981).

Henrey, Blanche. *British Botanical and Horticultural Literature before 1800. The Sixteenth and Seventeenth Centuries History and Bibliography,* 3 vols. (London: Oxford University Press, 1975).

Hill, John. *The Useful Family Herbal, or, an Account of All Those English Plants, Which Are Remarkable for Their Virtues: and of the Drugs, which are Produced by Vegetables of Other Countries: with Their Descriptions, and Their Uses, as Proved by Experience,* 2nd ed. (London: W. Johnston and W. Owen, 1755).

———. *The British Herbal: An History of Plants and Trees, Natives Britain, Cultivated for Use, or Raised for Beauty.* (London: T. Osborne and J. Shipton, 1756).

Horwood, A. R. *A New British Flora: British Wild Flowers in Their Natural Haunts,* 6 vols. (London: Gresham Publishing Company, Ltd., 1919).

Jackson, Benjamin Daydon. *A Catalogue of Plants Cultivated in the Garden of John Gerard, in the Years 1596–1599, Edited with Notes, References to Gerard's Herball, the Addition of Modern Names, and a Life of the Author.* (London: Privately printed, 1876).

Johnston, Stanley H., Jr. *The Cleveland Herbal, Botanical, and Horticultural Collections.* (Kent, OH: The Kent State University Press, 1992.)

LaWall, Charles H. *Four Thousand Years of Pharmacy.* (Philadelphia: J. B. Lippincott Company, 1927.)

Linnaeus, Carlos. *Species Plantarum*, 2 vols. (Holmiae: Impensis Laurentii Salvii, 1753).

Mabberley, D. J. *Mabberley's Plant-Book: A Portable Dictionary of Plants, Their Classification and Uses*, 4th ed. (Cambridge, UK: Cambridge University Press, 2017).

McCarl, M. R. "Publishing the Works of Nicholas Culpeper, Astrological Herbalist and Translator of Latin Medical Works in Seventeenth-Century London." *Canadian Bulletin of Medical History* 13 (1996), 225–76.

McGuffin, M., J. T. Kartesz, A. Y. Leung, and A. O. Tucker. *Herbs of Commerce*, 2nd ed. (Silver Spring, Maryland: American Herbal Products Association, 2000).

Mills, Simon, and Kerry Bone. *The Essential Guide to Herbal Safety*. (St. Louis: Elsevier, Churchill Livingstone, 2005).

Molnar, J., G. J. Szebeni, B. Csupor-Loffler, Z. Hajdu, T. Szekeres, P. Saiko, I. Ocsovszki, *et al.* "Investigation of the Antiproliferative Properties of Natural Sesquiterpenes from Artemisia Asiatica and Onopordum Acanthium on Hl-60 Cells in Vitro." *Internal Journal of Molecular Science*, 17, no. 2 (Feb. 17, 2016), 83.

Newman, Edward, and T. N. Brushfield. *History of British Ferns, and Allied Plants*. (London: J. Van Voorst, 1844).

Parkinson, John. *Theatrum Botanicum: The Theater of Plants or an Herball of a Large Extent*. (London: Printed by Tho. Cotes, 1640).

Parkinson, John. *Paradisi in Sole Paradisus Terrestris, or, a Garden of All Sorts of Pleasant Flowers*. (London: Humfrey Lownes and Robert Young, 1629).

Pechey, John. *The Compleat Herbal of Physical Plants: Containing All Such English and Foreign Herbs, Shrubs and Trees, as Are Used in Physick and Surgery*. (London: R. and T. Bonwicke, 1707).

Phillips, Henry. *History of Cultivated Vegetables; Comprising Their Botanical, Medicinal, Edible, and Chemical Qualities; Natural History; and Relation to Art, Science, and Commerce*, 2 vols. (London: H. Colburn, 1822).

Poynter, F. N. L. "Nicholas Culpeper and His Books." *Journal of the History of Medicine and Allied Sciences* 17, no. 1 (1962), 152–67.

Preston, C. D., D. A. Perman, and T. D. Dines. *New Atlas of the British & Irish Flora*. (New York and London: Oxford University Press, 2002).

Rydén, Mats. *The English Plant Names in the Grete Herbal (1526): A Contribution to the Historical Study of English Plant-Name Usage*. Acta Universitatis Stockholmiensis: Stockholm Studies in English LXI. (Stockholm: Almqvist & Wiksell International, 1984).

Salmon, William. *Botanologia, the English Herbal, or, History of Plants*. (London: I. Dawks, H. Rhodes, and J. Taylor, 1710).

Scarborough, John. *Medical Terminologies: Classical Origins*. (Norman, OK: University of Oklahoma Press, 1992).

Schulz, Volker, Rudolf Hänsel, and Varro E. Tyler. *Rational Phytotherpy: A Physician's Guide to Herbal Medicine*. Translated by Terry C. Telger, 2nd English ed. of 4th German ed. (Berlin: Springer, 2000).

Sheldrake, Timothy. *Botanicum Medicinale: An Herbal of Medicinal Plants on the College of Physicians List*. (London: J. Millan, 1768).

Stace, Clive. *New Flora of the British Isles*. 3rd ed. (Cambridge, UK: Cambridge University Press, 2009).

Thornton, Robert John. *A Family Herbal*. (London: B. and R. Crosby and Co., 1814).

Tobyn, Graeme. "Nicholas Culpeper's Herbal Therapeutics." *Journal of the American Herbalists Guild*, (Spring/Summer, 2002), 19–27.

———. *Culpeper's Medicine: A Practice of Western Holistic Medicine*. (London: Jessica Kingsley Publishers, 2013).

Tobyn, Graeme, Alison Denham, and Margaret Whitelegg. *The Western Herbal Tradition: 2000 Years of Medicinal Plant Knowledge*. (London: Churchill Livingston Elsevier, 2011).

Turner, William. *A New Herball* (London: Steven Myerdman, 1551).

Tutin, T. G., V. H. Heywood, N. A. Burges, D. M. Moore, D. H. Valentine, S. M. Walters, and D. A. Webb, eds. *Flora Europaea* Vols. 1–5. (Cambridge, UK: Cambridge University Press, 1964-1980).

van Wyk, Ben-Erik. *Food Plants of the World: An Illustrated Guide*. (Portland, OR: Timber Press, 2005).

———. *Culinary Herbs & Spices of the World*. (Chicago and London: University of Chicago Press, Kew Publishing, Royal Botanic Gardens, Kew, 2013).

van Wyk, Ben-Erik, and Michael Wink. *Medicinal Plants of the World: An Illustrated Guide to Important Medicinal Plants and Their Uses*. (Portland, OR: Timber Press, 2004).

Walters, S. M., J. C. M. Alexander, A. Brady, C. D. Brickell, J. Cullen, P. S. Green, V. H. Heywood, et al., eds. *The European Garden Flora, Dicotyledons: Casuarinaceae to Aristolochiaceae*, vol. III. (Cambridge, UK: Cambridge University Press, 1989).

Walters, S. M., A. Brady, C. D. Brickell, J. Cullen, P. S. Green, J. Lewis, V. A. Matthews, et al., eds. *The European Garden Flora, Monocotyledons*, vol. II. (Cambridge, UK: Cambridge University Press, 1984).

———, eds. *The European Garden Flora, Pteridophyta, Gymnospermae, Angiospermae–Monocotyledons*, vol. I. (Cambridge, UK: Cambridge University Press, 1986).

Weiss, Rudolf Fritz, and Volker Fintelmann. *Herbal Medicine*. 2nd English ed. of the 9th German ed. (New York: Thieme, 2000).

White, Linda B., and Steven Foster. *The Herbal Drugstore*. (Emmaus, PA: Rodale Press, 2000).

World Health Organization. *WHO Monographs on Selected Medicinal Plants*, vol. 1. (Geneva: World Health Organization, 1999).

———. *WHO Monographs on Selected Medicinal Plants*, vol. 2. (Geneva: World Health Organization, 2002).

———. *WHO Monographs on Selected Medicinal Plants*, vol. 3. (Geneva: World Health Organization, (2007).

———. *WHO Monographs on Selected Medicinal Plants*, vol. 4. (Geneva: World Health Organization, (2009).

Witchtl, Max. *Herbal Drugs and Phytopharmaceutical: A Handbook for Practice on a Scientific Basis*. Edited and translated by Josef A Brinckmann and Michael P. Lindenmaier, translators. 3rd ed. (Stuttgart and Boca Raton, FL: Medpharm Scientific Publishers and CRC Press, 2004).

Woolley, Benjamin. *Heal Thyself: Nicholas Culpeper and the Seventeenth-Century Struggle to Bring Medicine to the People*. (New York: HarperCollins, 2004).

INDEX

curing disease using knowledge of herbs and, xi

governing body parts, xi

herb associations, xi. *See also specific herbs*

opposites curing disease, xi

Plantain. *See* Buck's-horn plantain (*Plantago coronopus*)

Plantain (*Plantago lanceolata* and *Plantago major*), 183–84

Plums (*Prunus domestica*), 185

Polypody of the oak (*Polypodium vulgare*), 185–86

Poplar tree (*Populus* spp.), 186–87

Poppies (*Papaver somniferum, Papaver hybridum, and Papaver rhoeas*), 188–89

Premenstrual syndrome (PMS). *See* Menstrual issues

Privet (*Ligustrum vulgare*), 189–90

Prostrate knotweed. *See* Knotgrass

Psoriasis, 26, 38, 92, 97, 115, 196

Purgatives, 6, 110, 115, 116, 178, 190, 228

Purslane (*Portulaca oleracea*), 190–91

Quince tree (*Cydonia oblonga*), 192–93

Ragwort (*Senecio jacobaea, Jacobaea vulgaris*), 194–95

Rattle grass (*Rhinanthus minor*), 195

Rephontic. *See* Rhubarb

Respiratory infections. *See* Colds; Upper respiratory tract

Restharrow (*Ononis spinosa*), 196–97

Rheumatism. *See* Arthritis and rheumatism

Rheumatoid arthritis, 104, 215

Rhubarb (*Rheum rhaponticum*), 197–98. *See also* Monk's rhubarb

Rocket, arugula (*Eruca vesicaria*; syn. *Eruca sativa*), 198–99

Rosa salis. *See* Sundew

Rose (*Rosa damascena, Rosa gallica, Rosa canina*), 199–201

Rosemary (*Rosmarinus officinalis*; syn. *Salvia rosmarinus*), 201–2

Round-leaved dock (*Rumex alpinus*), 202–3

Royal fern (*Osmunda regalis*), 203–4

Rue (*Ruta graveolens*), 204–5

Rupturewort (*Herniaria glabra*), 205–6

Rustyback, scale fern (*Ceterach officinarum*; syn. *Asplenium ceterach*), 206–7

Rye (*Secale cereale*), 207

Saffron (*Crocus sativus*), 208–9

Sage (*Salvia officinalis*), 209–10

Sage-leaved germander. *See* Wood sage

Samphire (*Crithmum maritimum*), 211–12

Sanicle (*Sanicula europaea*; syn. *Sanicula officinalis*), 212

Santolina (*Santolina chamaecyparissus*), 213

Saracen's confound, or saracen's woundwort (*Senecio ovatus*; syn. *Senecio sarracenicus*),

213–14

Sauce-alone. *See* Garlic mustard

Savine (*Juniperus sabina*), 214–15

Savory, winter and summer (*Satureja montana* and *Satureja hortensis*), 215

Scabies, 97, 216

Scabious, field (*Knautia arvensis, Centaurea scabiosa, Scabiosa atropurpurea,* and other species), 216

Scarlet pimpernel (*Lysimachia arvensis*; syn. *Anagallis arvensis*), 217

Sciatica, 107, 145, 201, 219

Sciatica (original text references only), 9, 13, 19, 30, 37, 50, 59, 71, 73, 78, 81, 89, 90, 93, 108, 110, 115, 116, 118, 120, 123, 132, 134, 146, 161, 164, 167, 182, 187, 195, 211, 221, 235, 239, 241

Scurvygrass (*Cochlearia officinalis*), 217–18

Sea-holly. *See* Eryngo

Sedatives, 50, 52, 55, 107, 115, 122, 139, 141, 145, 160, 161, 178, 189, 211

Self-heal (*Prunella vulgaris*), 218–19

Sengreen. *See* Houseleek

Septfoil. *See* Tormentil

Serpent's tongue. *See* Adder's tongue (*Ophioglossum vulgatum*)

Service tree (*Cormus domestica*; syn. *Sorbus domestica*), 219

Shepherd's purse (*Capsella bursa-pastoris*), 220

Silverweed (*Agertina anserina*; syn. *Potentilla anserina*), 220–21

Skin blemishes, 91, 237. *See also* Acne/pimples

Skin blemishes (original text references only), 7, 34, 41, 69, 75, 80, 82, 99, 112, 121, 147, 165, 167, 179, 199, 205, 216, 221, 244, 251, 252, 254, 263

Skin disorders, 61. *See also* Eczema; Psoriasis

Sleeping sickness, 7

Sloe-bush (*Prunus spinosa*), 221–22

Smallage. *See* Celery

Soapwort (*Saponaria officinalis*), 222–23

Solomon's seal (*Polygonatum multiflorum, Polygonatum biflorum*), 223–24

Sorrel (*Rumex acetosa*), 224–25

Southernwood (*Artemisia abrotanum*), 225

Sow fennel. *See* Hog's fennel

Sow thistles (*Sonchus asper, Sonchus oleraceus*), 226

Spearmint. *See* Mint

Spignel (*Meum athamanticum*), 226–27

Spleen (original text references only)

cleansing and strengthening, 5, 6, 9, 11, 18, 22, 49–50, 55, 57, 71, 84, 87, 95, 96, 105, 108, 109, 111, 139, 146, 156, 175, 179, 197, 218, 231

general benefit, 52, 76, 78, 128, 130, 140, 148, 173, 201, 206, 225, 238, 243

mollifying hardness of, 37, 50, 73, 87, 111, 112, (120–22), 147, 149, 186, 232, 233, 235, 247, 256–57

swelling of, 78, 87, 147, 229

tumors in, 265

Spleenwort. *See* Rustyback, scale fern

Spotted dead nettle (red archangel) (*Lamium maculatum*), 72–73

Sprains, 44, 63, 92, 205, 210, 236, 243

St. John's Wort (*Hypericum perforatum*), 210–11

Star thistle (*Centaurea calcitrapa*), 227–28

Stimulant, general, 139

Stimulant rubefacient, 202

Stonecrop (*Sedum acre*), 228

Strains, herb for, 63. *See also* Sprains

Strawberries (*Fragaria vesca*), 228–29

Succory. *See* Chicory

Sunburn, 187

Sunburn (original text references only), 67, 69, 80, 121, 179, 221, 251, 252

Sundew (*Drosera rotundifolia*), 229–30

Sweet cicely (*Myrrhis odorata*), 230–31

Sweet marjoram (*Origanum majorana*), 231

Sympathy, curing diseases using, xi

Tamarisk (*Tamarix gallica, Tamarix africana*), 232–33

Tansy (*Tanacetum vulgare*; syn. *Chrysanthemum vulgare*), 233–34

Tansy Ragwort. *See* Ragwort

Tapeworms. *See* Worm expellants

Teasel (*Dipsacus fullonum, Dipsacus sativus*), 234

Teeth, whitening/washing, 238. *See also* Toothaches

Teeth, whitening/washing (original text references only), 106, 140, 154, 162, 237

Thistle. *See* Cotton-thistle

Thoroughwax or thorough leaf. *See* Kale

Throat. *See also* Expectorants

gargle, 29, 121, 127, 215, 222, 239

inflamed/infected/sore throat, 4, 37, 40, 44, 45, 59, 63, 69, 81, 83, 108, 116, 121, 123, 127, 135, 142, 147, 149, 170, 190, 210, 215, 222, 239

mucous discharges, 67

Throat-wort. *See* Figwort

Thrombophlebitis, yellow sweet clover for, 265

Thrombosis, 263

Thyme (*Thymus vulgaris*), 235

Thyme, wild (*Thymus serpyllum*), 235–36

Toadflax (*Linaria vulgaris*), 236–37

Tobacco (*Nicotiana rustica*), 237–38

Toothaches, 120, 173

Toothaches (original text references only), 22, 23, 48, 57, 59, 78, 118, 127, 129, 139, (162–64), 179, 180, 191, 197, 201, 203, 221, 232, 237, 253, 262

easing pain of cavities, 9, 91, 120, 184, 189, 249. *See also* Toothaches

Tormentil (*Potentilla erecta*; syn. *Tomatillo erecta*), 238–39

Treacle mustard. *See* Field pennycress

Turnsole, or heliotropium (*Heliotropium europaeum*; syn. *Heliotropium majus*), 239–40

PICTURE CREDITS

Culpeper, Nicholas. *Culpeper's Complete Herbal . . .*, expanded edition. (London: Thomas Kelly, 1824): Cover—plants on front, back, flaps, and spine top; leaf dingbat throughout; i, ii, v, vi, xii, 1, 2, 3, 4, 5, 6, 7, 8, 10 right, 12, 13, 15 left, 16, 17 right, 19 right, 20, 22, 26, 27, 33, 34, 35, 36, 37, 39, 40, 45 left, 48, 49, 54, 55, 57 left, 61, 66, 67, 68, 69, 70, 71, 72, 73, 74, 75, 77, 78, 79, 81, 83, 84, 86, 88, 89, 90 left, 91, 92, 93, 94, 95, 96, 98, 100, 101, 102, 103, 105, 106, 107, 109, 112, 113, 114, 116, 119, 120, 123, 124, 125, 128, 133, 134, 135, 137, 138, 139, 140, 141, 142, 143, 144, 145, 146, 147 left, 148, 151, 152, 153, 154, 155 right, 157, 159, 160, 161, 162, 163, 166 left, 167, 169, 170, 171, 172 right, 173, 175, 176, 178, 179, 180, 181, 182, 183, 185, 186, 188,

189, 192, 193, 194, 195, 198, 202, 205, 207, 208 right, 210, 211, 212, 213 right, 215, 216, 217, 218, 219, 220 left, 221, 222, 223, 224, 226 right, 227, 228 right, 229, 231, 232 left, 233, 234, 235, 236, 237, 238, 239, 240, 242 left, 243, 244, 245, 247, 248, 250, 251, 252, 253, 254, 255, 256, 257, 258, 259, 260 left, 263, 264

Courtesy Internet Archive: Cover back bottom left, viii, 24

iStock: bauhaus1000: 15 right, 45 right, 58, 164; Cannasue: 147 right; eyewave: spine bottom, 10 left; ilbusca: 262 right; ivan-96: 29; mashuk: 62, 80; PLAINVIEW: 166 right; Ruskpp: 32, 226 left; THEPALMER: 177

Shutterstock: annarepp: 46

Thinkstock/GettyImages: Dorling Kindersley: 230

Wellcome Collection: 99

Courtesy of *Wikimedia* Commons: 1 (gutter), 11, 17 left, 19 left, 21, 23, 25, 28, 30, 31, 38, 41, 42, 43, 44, 47, 50, 51, 52, 53, 56, 57 right, 59, 60, 63, 64, 65, 76, 82, 85, 87, 90 right, 104, 108, 111, 115, 117, 118, 121, 122, 126, 127, 129, 131, 150, 155 left, 156, 158, 172 left, 190, 197, 199, 201, 203, 204, 206, 208 left, 209, 213 left, 214, 220 right, 225, 228 left, 232 right, 242 right, 249